PHARMACEUTICAL APPLICATIONS

PHARMACEUTICAL APPLICATIONS

By
Dr. S.K. Prasad
School of Studies of Zoology & Biotechnology
Vikram University
Ujjain (India)

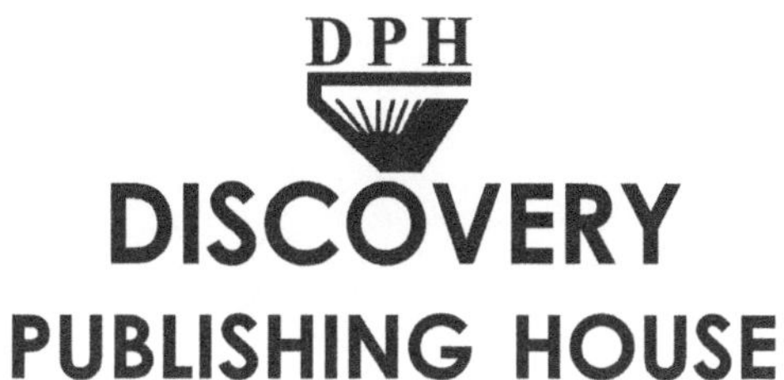

Published by:

DISCOVERY PUBLISHING HOUSE
4383/4B, Ansari Road, Darya Ganj
New Delhi-110 002 (India)
Phone : +91-11-23279245; 23253475; 43596065
E-mail : discoverybooksindia@gmail.com
discoverypublishinghouse@gmail.com
namitwasan9@gmail.com
web : www.discoverypublishinggroup.com

First Edition: **2011**
Reprinted: **2025**

ISBN: 978-81-8356-737-4

Pharmaceutical Applications

Printed at:
Infinity Imaging Systems
Delhi

Preface

The present title "Pharmaceutical Applications" has been written for those in the pharmaceutical research and those responsible for the education and training in pharmaceutical science and technology of graduate and undergraduate students. Medicine is an ever changing science. As new research and clinical experience broaden our knowledge, changes in treatment and drug therapy are required. This branch of life science has progressed enormously in recent years and the significant advances in therapeutics and an understanding of the need to optimize during delivery in the body have brought about an increased awareness of the valuable role played by the dosage forms. This statement is as true as it was back in ninteenth century and perhaps more so, given the increasing emphasis being placed on discovery, development, and use of large molecular entities as therapeutic and diagnostic agents. Development of these abilities requires an integration of knowledge, skills, attitudes, and values that can be acquired only through structured learning process including independent study, hands on practice and the availability of advanced literature. This tittle has designed to meet such needs of learners in the health professions.

In the last two decades, the pharmaceutical industry has experimented and successfully adopted several integrated and multidisciplinary approaches in the research areas of dring compound screening, toxicological evaluation, and pharmaceutical product development. The book is written in a concise style that facilitates an in-depth level of understanding of the essential concepts. The objectives of the present title are three folds: (i) to serve as a useful tool to help guide scientists in research and development by out-lining the theory and successful practice of in vitro - in vivo correlation, (ii) to help formulators apply the tool in designing and developing prototypes that enable selection of clinical formulations, and (iii) to help formulate strategy(ies) for product life-cycle management.

To make the work more comprehensive and informative, the author has consulted many authoritative books, research journals, abstracts, monographs etc., so there can be no claim to originality except in the manner of treatment.

The author expresses his thanks to his friends and colleagues whose continue inspirations have initiated him to bring out this book.

The author expresses his gratitude to Mr. Wasan and staff of M/s Discovery Publishing House Pvt. Ltd. for their whole hearted co-operation in the publication of this book.

Author

Contents

1

INTRODUCTION

Adsorption at solid surfaces is involved in nearly every aspect of pharmaceutical development, from formulation design, process development, and manufacturing to storage of finished dosage forms. Achieving content uniformity, especially for low-dose drugs, exhibits a challenge faced in the manufacturing of solid dosage formulations. One of the solutions is by adsorbing small drug particles onto the surface of large excipients. The adsorption of binder solution onto solid surfaces is the basis for granulation, which can improve excipient properties such as flowability, compactibility, and bulk density. In compaction, moisture adsorption generally facilitates particle deformation and increases the area of contact between particles during compression. However, when compressible and non-compressible excipients are mixed together, the adsorption of non-compressible excipients onto the surface of compressible excipients will reduce mixed powder compressibility. During storage, water molecules adsorbed on solid surface have significant impacts on pharmaceutical development such as compaction and tensile strength of tablets. Therefore hygroscopicity needs to be taken into consideration for selecting excipients in formulation design.

Solid dispersion is frequently used to improve the dissolution rate of poorly water-soluble compounds. By adsorbing drug molecules onto the surface of adsorbents with large surface areas, the total surface area of the drug is increased, and the drug may even be transformed from crystalline form to amorphous form. By adsorbing a surfactant onto the crystal surface of poorly water-soluble drugs, dissolution rate can also be enhanced, even though the mechanism is yet not fully understood. In many approaches used to increase dissolution rate, because drugs exist in higher-energy state than their crystal state, dissolved or amorphous drugs can be crystallized and may cause a decrease in dissolution rate. To maintain a high dissolution rate, polymers have been widely used to inhibit crystallization by adsorbing onto crystal surfaces.

Besides process development and dissolution rate enhancement, the phenomenon of adsorption at solid surfaces is also useful in many other aspects of pharmaceutics. By adsorbing moisture onto its large surface area, colloidal silica has been frequently used as a desiccant for stabilizing moisture-sensitive drugs such as aspirin. Some special formulation designs, such as dry powder inhalation (DPI) and sublingual nitroglycerin tablets, have been designed based on the adsorption of drugs onto a carrier surface. Additionally, the adsorption of liquid and gas on solid surfaces is utilized to measure the surface area of solid materials.

HISTORICAL VIEW

The basic approach regarding how adsorption at solid surfaces affects different aspects of pharmaceutical development, especially for solid dosage forms, is briefly reviewed. The three broad fields addressed are: general pharmaceutical processing, dissolution rate enhancement for poorly water-soluble compounds, and some other applications using adsorption at solid surfaces. Case studies are introduced to aid in understanding the applications and/or principles involved.

Adsorption could generally be classified as physical adsorption and chemical adsorption. Forces involved in adsorption include van der Waals force, hydrogen bonding or electrostatic force in physical adsorption, and covalent chemical bonds in chemical adsorption. Adsorption could occur between solid and solid, solid and liquid, or solid and gas. In pharmaceutical development, these adsorptions could take place during different processing stages, and affect the properties of the final products. There are cons and pros of these adsorptions, which will be discussed in this article.

Adsorption in General Pharmaceutical Processing

Because of the interactions existing between different materials as well as between like materials, the performance of excipients in a formulation could be different from the performance of the excipients themselves. The most frequently used procedures in pharmaceutical processing for solid dosage formulations are mixing, granulation, and compaction, as well as storage of finished dosage forms. The effects of adsorption on these procedures have been studied, observed, and utilized widely in the pharmaceutical industry.

Adsorption in Mixing

Adsorption of drugs onto the solid surfaces of excipients plays an important role in the preparation of pharmaceutical mixtures and can affect many aspects of the final formulations, especially the content uniformity of low-dose drugs. During mixing, there are many factors that can affect the content uniformity of mixtures, and adsorption generally plays a role when the average particle size is ≤ 400 μm. In drug manufacturing, it is a challenge to achieve content uniformity when mixing a small amount of one material with a much larger amount of another material. To achieve content uniformity for potent drugs in solid dosage forms, it is beneficial to produce mixes with good homogeneity if drugs can be dispersed very finely. If there are no interactions between mixed particles, ordered mixing and random mixing should achieve the same results. However, due to interactions between particles, such as aggregation between small particles and adsorption of small particles onto large carrier particles, ordered mixing and random mixing may have significantly different outcomes.

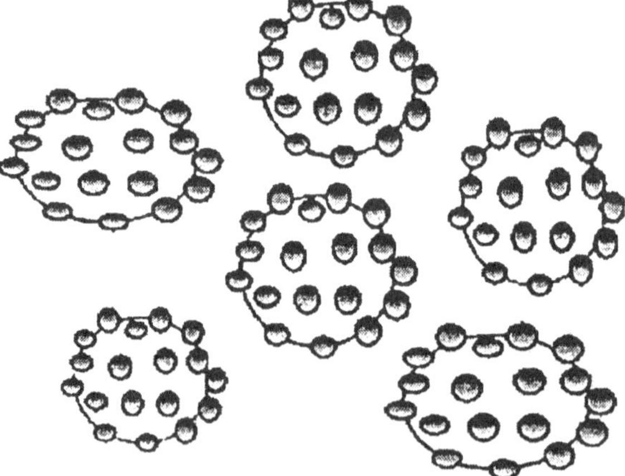

Fig. 1.1. Adsorption of small particles onto the surfaces of larger carrier particles.

Adsorbing drugs onto carrier particles by ordered mixing can be very beneficial in several ways, such as facilitating the preparation of master batches, avoiding segregation in stable systems, promoting excellent homogeneity in mixtures, and improving content uniformity of tablets especially at low dosage. For excipient particles, larger size and better flowability are beneficial for achieving content uniformity. Those excipients that can adsorb drugs more strongly exhibit a faster disintegration of agglomerates, and achieve higher homogeneity in both random and ordered mixing. Tablets of 120 mg containing 0.1 mg of digitoxin have been manufactured with very good content uniformity by adsorbing small particles onto larger carrier particles in ordered mixing. In the design, digitoxin, dissolved in a mixture of methylene chloride, and methanol, is first deposited onto milled critical micellar concentration (CMC). After mixing, the solvent is removed, and this dry blend is mixed with crystalline lactose. Other excipients are added later without affecting the content uniformity.

The most important factors in the adsorption process are moisture content and particle size distribution. Moisture content and the state of adsorbed water affect the adsorption of fine antibiotic powders onto the surface of sorbitol by plasticizing sorbitol, forming an adherent monoparticle layer that affects the capillary forces and hydrogen bonding interactions between sorbitol and the drugs, as well as masking the interparticle forces. It was observed that high moisture content has caused higher adsorption onto sorbitol for those fine antibiotic powders with low interfacial energy, internal location of adsorbed water, and the ability to form hydrogen bonding with sorbitol. When stored under high humidity, moisture adsorbed onto the surfaces of drugs and carriers could form a liquid bridge whose capillary interaction may significantly increase adhesion in the mixture.

However, high moisture does not always increase the adsorption of drugs onto the solid surface of excipients. For example, as to antibiotics with high interfacial energy and external location of adsorbed water, low moisture content is beneficial for achieving higher adsorption onto sorbitol. Overall, the mechanism by which moisture content affects the adsorption of drugs onto the solid surfaces of other excipients is very complex and can be affected by many factors.

Other factors such as the surface structure of particles, reduction of interparticle distance (e.g., by means of intensive mixing processes), as well as particle size also affect surface adsorption. It was observed that irregular particles of sorbitol with a structured surface could adsorb more vitamins than regular particles. By adjusting the ratio of three vitamins in the starting mixture, the proportions of vitamins B1, B2, and B6 in the adsorbed state can be changed. Because of the high fraction of vitamins not adsorbed onto sorbitol surface, the ordered mixing was arranged, at first, by mixing each vitamin with sorbitol separately, then by combining the individual mixtures to make the final mixture.

Milling can affect the adsorption of actives on the carrier surface by altering the surface properties of excipients. It was noticed that milled actives frequently failed blend uniformity criteria, but unmilled active batches consistently met the blend uniformity criteria. By adding lubricant magnesium stearate, the blending content uniformity of the milled batches can be significantly improved. A small amount of amorphous materials could affect the blending characteristics of a direct compression formulation.

Overall, factors that might affect the adsorption of actives on the carrier surface include surface properties, moisture content, the type and particle size/shape of carriers and actives, as well as the mixing ratio of actives and carriers. Pharmaceutical processes (i.e., milling and granulation) could affect the adsorption process by altering carrier and active properties (i.e., surface properties, size, and shape), hence the characteristics of blending and the quality of the final dosage form.

Adsorption in Granulation

In solid dosage forms, granulation is frequently used to improve excipient properties such as flowability, compactibility, bulk density, granule strength, dissolution rates, and so on. The granulation process generally includes binder atomization, fluidization, adsorbing and spreading on powder surfaces, particle agglomeration, and so on. In addition, binder adsorbed onto the particle surface can also provide solid bridges between particles. Of course, due to the complexity of the granulation process, many factors can affect the process and the final properties of the granules. However, the adsorption of the binder solution on solid surfaces, especially at the point of contact between particles or granules, is the key to the granulation process. The adsorption process can be affected by the surface tension and the viscosity of a binder, and more energy may be consumed during granulation. The surface tension and the viscosity of a binder play important roles in granulation because these properties influence the liquid bridges between the particles, as well as the distribution of the binder during the wet massing stage. For similar polymer binders, even at an equivalent viscosity, different molecular weights can affect binder surface tension and thus influence the granulation process and related granule properties. It is worthwhile to note that source and batch variation of both drugs and excipients can have profound effects on the final product performance.

A suitable amount of binder adsorbed onto the granular surface at the points of contact, as well as their physical properties such as viscosity and flowability, are very important for granule growth. Four mechanisms of granule growth and the mechanism that plays the main rôle is determined by the degree of binder dispersion in the powder. Many factors, such as binder atomization, addition rate, state of fluidization, and shear forces in the mixer, can affect the degree of binder dispersion. In the "*nucleation*" mechanism, particles stick together with the help of the liquid binder adsorbed on the powder surface; in the "*coalescence*" mechanism, through deformation and bonding, two large agglomerates combine to form one granule with the help of a surface-adsorbed binder; and in the "layering" mechanism, fine particles stick to either a large granule or a binder droplet. In a mixer, shear forces will cause particles to collide and bond together if some binder is present at the point of contact. Of course, two colliding particles may not always bond together, but may rebound and fail to achieve granule growth. Once granules have been formed and reach a certain size, they have to survive the shear forces in the mixer, which are determined by the relationship between shear forces of the outer shearing mass and the inner strength of the granules.

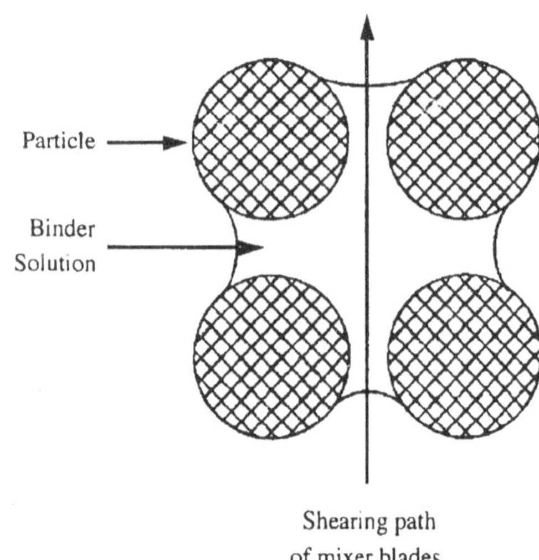

Fig. 1.2. Shearing path of mixer blades through wet mass at capillary state.

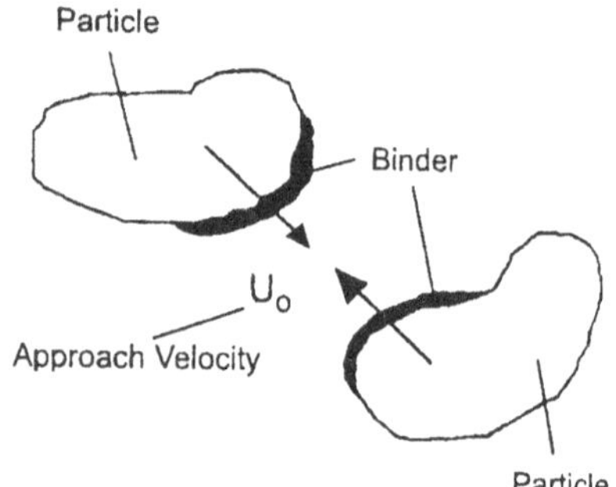

Fig. 1.3. Coalescence of two binder-covered particles.

Besides the traditional wet granulation, surface adsorbents, especially porous materials, are very helpful for maintaining liquid in a granulation. For example, calcium silicate, a fine porous powder, has been successfully used to adsorb an oily medicine, tocopheryl nicotinate. Due to the high capillarity of the pores inside calcium silicate, the adsorbent has an excellent liquid-holding ability. In the formulation preparation, after drug dissolved in ethanol was adsorbed on calcium silicate, hydroxypropylcellulose (HPC) was added to the mixture and granulated to improve flowability.

Adsorption in Compaction

In the manufacturing of tablets, compaction is a very important step, and many factors are involved in affecting the properties of excipients and final products, such as surface structure and wettability of excipients. For formulations, the larger is the surface area of compressible excipients, the greater is the compressibility.

When compressible and non-compressible excipients are mixed together, the adsorption of the non-compressible excipients onto the surface of the compressible excipients will reduce mixed powder compressibility. Lerk et al. and te Wierik et al. studied a new generation of starch products, which have a high surface area as excipients in pharmaceutical tablets, and confirmed that there is a positive relationship between the specific surface area and the binding capacity (i.e., compactibility). The surface area that takes part in the interparticle attraction is small, and only a minor fraction of the geometrical surface area may be available for tablet bonding. The addition of some materials, such as binder and lubricant, may decrease particle fragmentation during compression and affect the "true" bonding surface area. In tablet manufacturing, lubricants such as magnesium stearate act by adsorbing onto the surface of granules and forming a film, thus decreasing the crushing force and ejection force during compression. It was noticed that the distribution of adsorbed magnesium stearate was nonuniform on the surface of excipients, and much more lubricant existed on edges and defective parts of the sodium chloride crystals in their study, thus increasing the effective area for compaction.

Besides the surface area of the excipients, moisture adsorbed to the excipients is one important factor in compaction. Nyqvist reported that by affecting the surface structure of excipients, a small amount of water in furosemide could significantly affect the compaction properties of the direct compressible formulation. When water content was increased from 0.06% to 0.24%, the elastic recovery was increased and network was decreased at compaction. Besides, by adjusting the water content of furosemide, it was possible to avoid tablet capping as well. Because adsorption of water in furosemide did not change the internal structure of the crystals, water may be adsorbed onto the crystal surface with weak forces detectable with thermal analysis. The area of contact formed between particles was increased during compression due to the particle deformation facilitated by the higher moisture content. Two types of interparticulate bonds, adsorption bonds and diffusional bonds, have been involved in the increased bond strength between particles. It has been observed that increased moisture content in amorphous lactose particles could increase tablet tensile strength and reduce tablet porosity by direct compression. Overall, moisture content can influence bonding forces by affecting both the contact area between particles and the relative fractions of adsorption and diffusion bonds in the tablet.

Adsorption in Storage

The physical and chemical stabilities of finished dosage forms stored at high humidity have always been concerns in the pharmaceutical industry and have been extensively studied. The adsorption of water molecules onto the solid surface can affect tablet strength. For tablets stored under humid conditions, the tensile strength of tablets increases initially when relative humidity (RH) increases; however, as RH further increases, the tensile strength of tablets starts to decrease. During storage, the sublimation of drugs such as bromhexine HCl (BHCl) can be prevented by selecting suitable excipients based on their surface adsorption capacity.

Hygroscopicity of excipients

Based on hygroscopicity (i.e., the tendency of materials to absorb water under different conditions of humidity), solids have been classified into four categories, as follows:

1. *Non-hygroscopic*: No increase in water content at RH below 90%.
2. *Slightly hygroscopic*: No moisture increases at RH below 80% with less than 40% moisture increase at RH above 80% after 1 week.
3. *Moderately hygroscopic*: Less than 5% water content increase at RH below 60%, with less than 50% water content increase at RH above 80% after 1 week.
4. *Very hygroscopic*: Substantial water content increases at RH as low as 40–50%.

Different drugs and excipients have different hygroscopic properties, and the amount of moisture absorbed by drugs and excipients can affect not only their own properties but also the properties of the finished dosage forms, such as flowability, compression properties, and hardness of granules and tablets. The hygroscopicity of different excipients has been studied, and research on moisture adsorption may provide useful information in selecting excipients such as disintegrants, binders, and fillers in formulation design, as well as in choosing suitable manufacturing and storage conditions.

Effects of moisture on tablet strength

Increasing RH during storage will increase tensile strength and decrease the surface area of tablets initially. Water can adsorb onto solid surfaces at three locations: monolayer-adsorbed moisture, normally condensed moisture, and adsorbed moisture. Adsorbed water molecules affect tablet tensile strength by influencing interparticle separation and interparticle forces, especially van der Waals interactions, as well as the ratio of the binding to diffusion forces for water molecules on the solid surface. The initially adsorbed water molecules on the solid surface may form a monomolecular layer, increase the van der Waals interactions between particles, smooth out surface microirregularities, and reduce interparticle separation, thus increasing tensile strength. As more water molecules adsorb onto the particle surface, they are subjected to both surface binding and diffusion forces, and the diffusion forces induce water to penetrate into the particles. The penetrated water may soften the particle surface, increase contact area between particles under high pressure due to plastic deformation, and form more solid bonds. All those effects may explain the observed initial increase in tensile strength when RH increases.

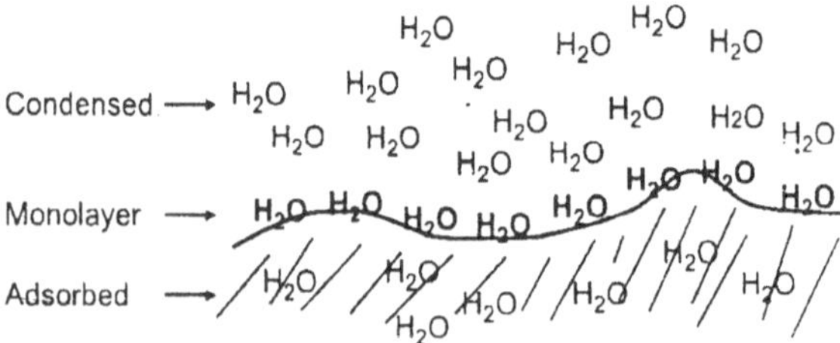

Fig. 1.4. Three locations of adsorbed water molecules in solid materials: monolayer adsorbed moisture, condensed moisture, and moisture adsorbed inside solid.

However, as RH further increases, tablet strength decreases for most tested tablets, and it was suggested that condensed water on the solid surface at high RH weakens intermolecular attraction forces between particles in the tablets and the further softened particles and solid bonds cause the tensile strength to decrease. In addition, at high RH, water may form multilayers on the solid surface, which can act as a lubricant and reduce the frictional forces between particles, thus decreasing tensile strength as well. Ultimately, the effects of adsorbed moisture on particle surfaces are very complex, affected by many factors, especially the properties of the tablet excipients.

Preventing drug sublimation during storage

During storage, BHCl can sublime away from solid dosage formulations and reduce the dosage potency. It was observed that BHCl prefers to adsorb to the surface of magnesium aluminum silicate (MAS) rather than to the package material polyethylene film. The adsorption to MAS was accelerated at high temperature and reduced pressure, and the BHCl adsorbed onto the surface of MAS was amorphous rather than crystalline. BHCl could also adsorb onto many other solid excipients, such as kaolin, Avicel PH101, and Avicel PH102, and many factors affect the adsorption. When pH increased, adsorption by microcrystalline cellulose (MCC) increased moderately. As particle size increased, adsorption decreased. Within the range of 20–46°C, temperature did not affect the adsorption of BHCl on MCC. Thermodynamic analysis showed that both entropy and enthalpy changes favored the adsorption on MCC. Overall, selecting suitable excipients to keep BHCl from sublimating during storage proved a very useful application of adsorption at solid surfaces.

Effects of Adsorption on Dissolution

Solid Dispersion

Solid dispersions are frequently used to improve the bioavailability of poorly soluble compounds for enhancing the dissolution profiles of these compounds. Boraie, El-Fattah, and Hassan have successfully used the approach of adsorbing poorly water-soluble compounds onto the surface of adsorbents to improve dissolution rate. The main idea is to increase the surface area of the compound in contact with the dissolution medium, thus increasing dissolution rate. Aerosil, MCC, montmorillonite, and modified starch were tested as adsorbents. An obvious improvement of dissolution rate is observed—

100% of the drug was released from tablets containing 50% Avicel, whereas only 32% was released from pure drug tablets. The weak physical bonding between the drug and the adsorbent was proposed to explain the rapid release of the drug from the adsorbent surface.

Due to their large surface area for adsorption, porous materials are useful excipients for solid dispersions. For example, 2-naphthoic acid (2-NPA) solid dispersion with porous crystalline cellulose (PCC) has been successfully prepared by heat treatment of 2- NPA and PCC mixture. PCC is derived from MCC, but with a larger surface area. Different from 2-NPA mixed with PCC, 2-NPA mixed with MCC still maintained a crystalline form under the same mixing and heating conditions. Various experimental data such as X-ray powder diffraction, Fourier transform infrared (FT-IR) spectroscopy, and solid-state fluorescence measurements suggest that 2-NPA is adsorbed onto the surface of PCC and becomes molecularly dispersed into the system.

Using a combination of solid dispersion and surface adsorption, the dissolution of a poorly water-soluble drug, BAY 12-9566, has been enhanced significantly. Gelucire 50/13 was used as the solid dispersion carrier, and the melt of the drug and Gelucire 50/13 was adsorbed onto the surface of Neusilin US2 (magnesium aluminosilicate), the surface adsorbent, using hot melt granulation. The dissolution of BAY 12-9566 increased as Gelucire 50/13 and Neusilin US2 loading increased, but decreased as drug loading increased. The solid dispersion granules were successfully compressed into tablets. Different from the usually observed decrease in dissolution on storage at 40°C/75% RH, the dissolution rate increased at 2 and 4 weeks.

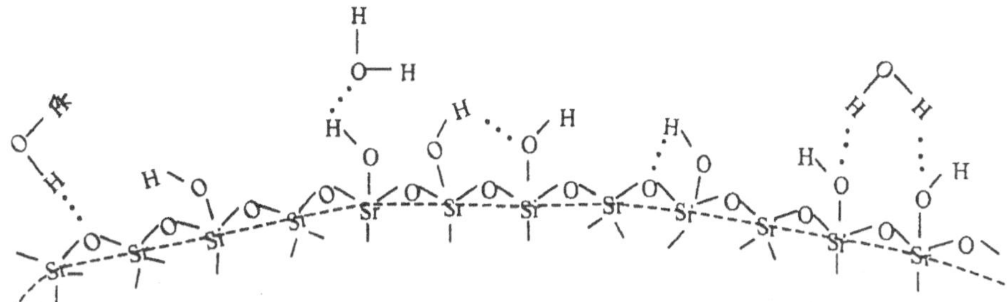

Fig. 1.5. Some possible hydrogen bonding arrangements on the surfaces of silica gel particles.

The transformation of drugs in solid dispersion from amorphous form to crystalline form is one critical obstacle to making solid dispersion a practical approach in pharmaceutical industry. Utilization of surface adsorbents can be used as one approach to solve the problem. Gupta et al. used seven different poorly water-soluble compounds and observed that the dissolution rates for some compounds in solid dispersions increased when stored at 40°C/75% RH. In their study, crystalline drugs were prepared as ternary solid dispersion granules using hot melt granulation, two solid dispersion carriers, poly(ethylene glycol) (PEG) 8000 and Gelucire 50/13, as well as Neusilin US2 as surface adsorbent.

Drug adsorption onto Neusilin US2 through hydrogen bonding interactions was proposed to explain the drug transformation from crystalline form to amorphous form, and to cause the increase in drug dissolution during storage. However, during storage especially under high humidity, crystallization will decrease the dissolution rate of drugs. Whether or not a drug is highly soluble in the dispersion carrier is a very important factor in determining which of the two competing mechanisms, tendency to crystallize or to stay in amorphous state, plays the dominant role in solid dispersions during storage. When a drug is highly soluble (>10% wt/wt) in the dispersion carrier, the molecularly dispersed drug can diffuse significantly onto the surface of Neusilin and form more hydrogen bonds with Neusilin in the formulations. For a drug with low solubility in the dispersion carrier, the drug in a molecularly dispersed state cannot readily diffuse onto the surface of Neusilin and form more hydrogen bonds with the

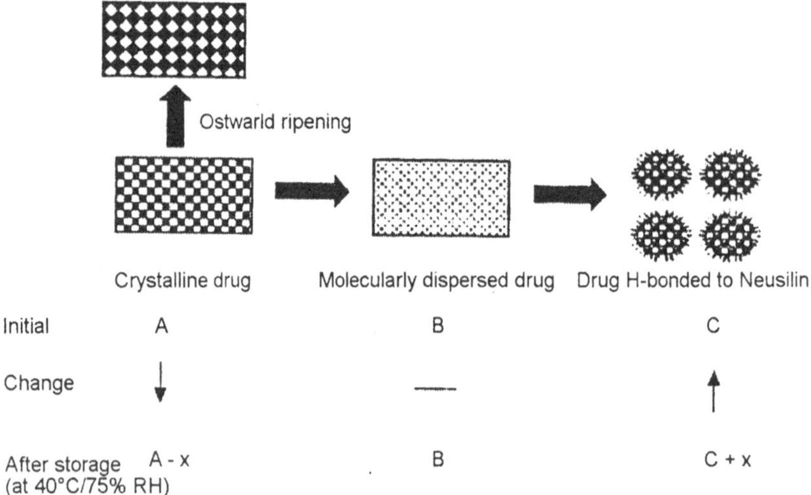

Fig. 1.6. Proposed mechanism for further increase in dissolution after storage.

adsorbent. For drugs with low solubility, even though they may have formed hydrogen bonds with Neusilin and will not revert to the crystalline state, crystallization will become the dominant mechanism and cause the dissolution rate to decrease during storage.

As to the mechanism of drug adsorption onto the surface of adsorbents, besides hydrogen bonding interactions, Pignatello, Ferro, and Puglisi noticed that there exist electrostatic interactions between ammonium groups in a polymer backbone and the carboxyl group in selected drugs. The polymers examined were Eudragit S100 (RS) and RL100 (RL), and the drugs were three non-steroidal anti-inflammatory drugs: diflunisal (DIF), flurbiprofen (FLU), and piroxicam (PIR). In the presence of Tris–HCl buffer (pH 7.4), due to the competition between the chloride ions and drug anions for the polymer-binding sites, drug adsorption on polymer particles was reduced. Overall, these interactions are stronger for drugs with a carboxylic moiety and lower pK_a values, and the interactions can be utilized to design a suitable drug release profile from a solid dispersion.

Effects of Surfactant on Dissolution

It has been observed that by adsorbing surfactants onto the crystal surfaces of poorly water-soluble drugs, dissolution rate can be enhanced. Chen et al. showed that the dissolution rate of CI-1041, a poorly water- soluble compound, in 0.1 N HCl may be affected by the surfactant Tween 80. The effects of surfactant are complicated, and many factors are involved. Above the CMC of Tween 80, the adsorption of the surfactant onto the crystal surface may inhibit crystal nucleation on the surface, and causes the dissolution rate to increase. By adsorbing a very small amount of poloxamer onto the hydrophobic drug particle surface, the dissolution profile can be significantly improved compared with untreated drugs.

Utilizing the adsorption of surfactants at solid surfaces, the release profile of a drug can be controlled. For example, the release profile of oxprenolol can be controlled by adsorbing different amounts of the wetting agent sodium laurylsulphate (SLS) onto microporous polypropylene powder. In the process, matrix tablets containing oxprenolol HCl, polypropylene powder, and other excipients were made first, then were dry-coated with a drug–polymer mixture by a single compression. The coat contained polypropylene powder pretreated with a suitable amount of SLS and a small amount of oxprenolol HCl. With the adsorbed SLS, both wetting problems of hydrophobic polypropylene powder and food effects on release profile were successfully solved.

The reason why the adsorption of some polymers onto a drug particle surface can improve the dissolution rate, but some cannot, is not fully understood. Some surfactant molecules may adsorb onto solid surfaces by utilizing the strong hydrophobic interactions between hydrophobic moieties of drugs and surfactants and orient the polar headgroups to the aqueous phase, thus increasing the overall wettability of the drug surface. Some polymers may specifically interact with drug molecules at the drug crystal surface, and either increase or decrease the dissolution rate of drugs. Acetaminophen has been dissolved in aqueous solutions of different polymers. In the absence of polymers, on the (010) face, the etching patterns follow the *a*-axis and *c*-axis exactly. However, polymers such as polyvinyl-alcohol (PVA), PEG, and polyvinylpyrrolidone (PVP) can adsorb onto crystal surface, and alter the etching patterns of acetaminophen on the (010) face, thus affecting dissolution rate.

Crystallization Inhibition

In the formulation designs used to improve dissolution rate, drugs adsorbed onto the surface of adsorbents exist completely or partially in the amorphous state. The drug in solution becomes supersaturated relative to the solubility of the crystalline drug. Because the free energy of both amorphous drug and supersaturated drug in solution is higher than the free energy of the crystalline drug, crystallization may occur for both amorphous drugs and supersaturated drugs in solution.

Polymers that can interact with drug molecules especially adsorbed onto crystal surfaces have been widely used to inhibit drug crystallization to maintain supersaturated states for drug delivery systems. Raghavan et al. observed that methylcellulose (MC) and HPMC could significantly inhibit the crystallization of supersaturated hydrocortisone acetate (HA). The mechanism of nucleation retardation was believed to be due to the hydrogen bonding interactions between HA and the polymers. As to the inhibition of crystal growth and crystal morphology change by polymers, it is believed to be due to the hydrodynamic boundary layer surrounding the crystal, and the adsorption of polymer molecules onto the crystal surface. Hasegawa et al. found that carboxy-methylethylcellulose (CMEC) could inhibit the crystallization of drugs from supersaturated solutions. The inhibitory effect of CMEC might be due to the adsorption of CMEC at the solid–water interface in which a hydrophobic drug crystal surface is formed, and hinders the deposition of drug molecules on the crystal surface. There were significant differences for the dissolution profiles of nifedipine, spironolactone, and griseofulvin solid dispersions in the presence or absence of CMEC in the dissolution medium. Because CMEC is an anionic polymer whose hydrophobicity increases with decreasing pH, the inhibitory effect of CMEC on crystallization increases as pH decreases. The observation of the pH effect also supports the hypothesis that CMEC inhibits drug crystallization by adsorbing onto the hydrophobic surface of poorly water-soluble drugs.

Due to the difference of the polymer adsorption onto different faces of different crystal forms, polymer adsorption onto the crystal face has played an important role in crystal polymorphic transformation. Garti and Zour have studied the effects of surfactants on the polymorphic transformation of glutamic acid. Glutamic acid has two crystal forms, α and β, with the β-form being more stable than the α-form. Those surfactants that preferentially adsorb onto the surface of the α-growing crystals retard the transformation of the α-form to the β-form. A Langmuir analysis indicates that the kinetic coefficient of crystal polymorphic transformation is related to the volume of the surfactant adsorbed at the crystal surface.

Trace amounts of impurity that adsorbed onto the surface of a growing crystal can cause a marked difference in dissolution rate. Grant, Chow, and Chan reported that in the presence of even trace amounts of n-alkanoic acid, the adipic acid crystal grown from an aqueous solution will have changes in crystal energy and dissolution rate. It was suggested that additive *n*-alkanoic acid could adsorb onto the surfaces of growing crystals even when incorporated into adipic acid crystals. The additive-induced difference in intrinsic dissolution rate (IDR) cannot be ignored.

Other Applications Using Adsorption at Solid Surfaces

Desiccant for Stabilizing Moisture-Sensitive Drug

Colloidal silica has been successfully used by Gore and Banker to improve the chemical stability of aspirin, whose hydrolytic tendency is well-known. Colloidal silicas have a large surface area and a highly polar silanol surface, which imparts a high moisture adsorption capacity. Water adsorbs onto the surface of colloidal silicas by forming hydrogen bonds with silanol. Colloidal silicas are commonly used as desiccants in the pharmaceutical industry, especially for hygroscopic or hydrolabile drugs. Even though the desiccant effect of colloidal silica is not the only factor that helps to stabilize aspirin in the studied formulation, its strong moisture adsorption capacity has played a very important role.

Dry Powder Inhalation

The surface adsorption approach has been used to make a DPI device. First, a fatty acid or fatty alcohol derivative or a poloxamer is dissolved or dispersed in a solvent in which drugs and carriers are insoluble. The preferred solvent is *n*-hexane or cyclohexane. Second, the fatty acid solution or suspension is adsorbed onto the surface of soluble micronized drugs and/or acceptable carriers such as lactose mono- hydrate, anhydrous glucose, polylactides, or PVA. The surface modification of drugs via adsorption has several advantages in making DPI formulations, such as the reduction of electrostatic charge during processing and handling, reduction of adhesion on contact surfaces, improvement of powder flowability in pneumatic transport, and improvement of drug content uniformity. This approach has made the scaling up of DPI formulations easier, and has significantly improved the inhalation properties of powders.

Sublingual Nitroglycerin Tablets

Waaler et al. have successfully applied the adsorption approach to make sublingual nitroglycerin tablets by direct compression with better content uniformity, lower weight variation, and much higher stability than tablets made from a molding approach. In the molding approach, nitroglycerin will migrate to the surface of a tablet during the drying process. During manufacturing as well as storage, there may be potency loss due to the volatility of nitroglycerin. Tablets can also be made by wet granulation, where drying may also induce unblending. In the direct compression approach, nitroglycerin dissolved in alcohol was first added to MCC, and triturated slowly for about 5 min to assure content uniformity. The powder is left at room temperature for 12 hr with occasional stirring. Then alcohol is evaporated and nitroglycerin becomes adsorbed onto MCC. Afterward, MCC/nitroglycerin is mixed with other excipients to achieve suitable properties for the finished tablets, including solubility and disintegration rate.

Surface Area Measurement

Besides liquid adsorption on solid surfaces, gas adsorption on solid surfaces is also very useful in measuring surface area in the pharmaceutical industry. Based on the Brunauer–Emmet–Teller (BET) equation, Vertommen, Rombaut, and Kinget used krypton adsorption to measure the specific surface area of pellets made from wet granulation, extrusion, and spheronization. Westermarck et al. noticed that nitrogen adsorption was more sensitive to changes in the surface area of mannitol tablets caused by compression. In measuring pore size, nitrogen adsorption can measure smaller pores (diameter range 3–200 nm) than high-pressure mercury porosimetry, with a range of 7 nm–14 μm. It is the large number of small pores with diameters <200 nm that contribute to the increased compactibility of granules and, ultimately, greater tablet strength.

The surface morphology of five commonly used excipients has been studied using both particle size distribution and nitrogen adsorption methods. The five tableting excipients were unmilled dicalcium phosphate dihydrate (Di-Tab), MCC (Avicel PH102), corn starch, croscarmellose sodium (Ac-di-sol), and sodium starch glycolate. A surface irregularity index (SII) was established to indicate surface roughness due to porosity, and its value was consistent with the direct microscopic observation of a powder sample. The nitrogen adsorption–desorption isotherms showed certain hystereses, especially for Avicel PH102, Di-Tab, and Ac-di-sol, and the remaining nitrogen adsorbed on the surface during desorption process was believed to be due to pores on the powder surface.

Adsorption at solid surfaces has been addressed in relation to many aspects of pharmaceutical development. Besides process development and dissolution rate enhancement, the phenomenon of adsorption at solid surfaces is also useful in many other aspects of the pharmaceutical industry, such as making special formulations such as DPI, surface area measurement, and so on. In pharmaceutical processing, adsorbing drugs onto the solid surface of other excipients can help to achieve content uniformity, especially for low-dose drugs, during the mixing process. The adsorption of binder solution onto solid surfaces is important in granulation for improving excipient flowability, compactibility, and so on. The adsorption of moisture onto excipients not only facilitates compression, but also affects both the physical and chemical properties of finished solid dosage forms during storage. Desiccants can help to control environmental humidity by adsorbing moisture via their large hydrophilic surface and to stabilize moisture-sensitive drugs.

Adsorption at solid surfaces has also been applied in different approaches to improve the dissolution rate of poorly soluble compounds. In solid dispersions, by adsorbing drug molecules onto the surface of adsorbents with a large surface area, the dissolution rate can be significantly increased due to the increase in surface area and/or the decreased crystallinity of drugs. Adsorbing surfactant onto solid surfaces of poorly soluble drugs can enhance the dissolution rate by mechanisms that are not fully understood. The adsorbed surfactant may affect dissolution rate through mechanisms such as improving the wettability of drug surfaces, having specific interactions with drug molecules on the crystal surface, or increasing equilibrium drug solubility in aqueous solution. By adsorbing onto crystal surfaces, polymers have been widely used to inhibit the crystallization of dissolved drugs or unstable amorphous drugs during dissolution, to maintain good dissolution rate during dissolution, and to improve the bioavailability of poorly soluble compounds. Exactly how polymers adsorb onto, and interact with, solid surfaces and why some polymers are more effective as crystallization inhibitors than others are topics of ongoing investigation.

Isolators for Pharmaceutical Application

The use of isolators in research and manufacturing in the health care and life science industries continues to develop rapidly. An overview shows many new applications being conceived, designed, constructed, and set into operation to satisfy many different processing needs. These applications frequently fall outside the accepted concepts and practice found in human scale rooms. It is only in the last 2 or 3 years that the technology has been recognized within cGMP guidelines and regulations. This article attempts to describe the practical experience gained from consultancy and design of isolators from the early 1970s up to and including state of the art applications developed today. For clarity, an isolator can be defined as: "A device creating a small enclosed controlled or clean classified environment in which a process or activity can be placed with a high degree of assurance that effective segregation will be maintained between the enclosed environment, its surroundings, and any personnel involved with the process or manipulation. Isolators can be closed or open designs, and may be maintained at positive or negative pressure to their surroundings."

The following list summarises some essential features that help to expand on the definition as it is applied in the life science and pharmaceutical industry context:

1. An isolator is an enclosed controlled environment of minimum volume.
2. Isolators segregate people from processes.

3. Isolators can contain processes hazardous to the surroundings, processes that are at risk from the surroundings, or in some cases activities where both types of risk coexist.
4. Isolator walls or envelopes may be rigid or flexible; typical primary materials are stainless steel and glass, and polyvinyl chloride (PVC) flexible sheet welded to form an enclosure.
5. Isolators are internally pressurized with air or inert gas to help achieve the required segregation between inside and outside. Pressurization can be positive or negative.
6. Air filtration through High Efficiency Particulate Air (HEPA) or Ultra Low Particulate Air (ULPA) filters is used to control the quality of air entering, leaving, and recirculating. For some applications in which very small inert gas quantities are used, nitrogen, for example, can be delivered through sterilizing-grade membrane filters.
7. Isolators are frequently connected intimately to items of process equipment to provide an effective locally controlled environment.

The principal industry drivers generating the interest in isolators in the last few years have been focused on improvements in process integrity. This includes operator protection from potent and hazardous materials and, in the case of sterile products manufacturing, to reduce the potential of contaminated non-sterile units from being produced by a specific process. There are some circumstances in which reductions in occupied space and operational cost savings have been essential objectives.

Technical Guidelines and Standards

Although guidelines, such as the UK Pharmaceutical Isolator Guideline, and standards for microbiological safety cabinets and those for flexible-film isolators, satisfy part of the need for effective standards, further support is needed. During 2001, the ISO Technical Committee 209 should publish EN/ISO (DIS) 14644-7. This standard will be entitled "*Enhanced Clean Devices.*" Although it is not pharmaceutical industry specific, it will contain much excellent basic good practice guidance. 2001 should also see publication of PDA's Monograph "Design and Validation of Isolator Systems for the Manufacturing and Testing of Health Care products." Useful sources of reference can also be obtained from the nuclear industry. ISO 10648 "*Containment enclosures*" contains some valuable sections.

For isolators, the barrier between the critical controlled environment and its surroundings is created by a single element, rather than the multilayer protection approach used in cleanroom technology. It is essential, therefore, to realize that the engineering solution, integrity, and reliability of the final operational isolator will have a direct impact not only on the enclosed process, but also on the quality required of the surrounding environment. This is particularly so when an isolator is used to contain a vulnerable aseptic process. This is usually be the most critical task for isolators, and the one that is most difficult to prove.

The design and construction of isolators should be carried out in an appropriate quality-assured way because the devices are frequently complex and require a high level of documentation to comply with both safety and good quality requirements. ISO 9000 compliant or similar quality assurance systems provide an appropriate management environment in which to design and build systems destined for quality or safety critical applications.

Health Care Industry Regulatory Demands and Expectations

Many operational applications are now in place, particularly in Europe. They can be found in manufacturing, R&D, and QC sectors. Experience continues to develop, and the users are at the forefront of the knowledge. Regulatory guidance can now be found in the European Union Guide to Good Manufacturing Practice (EU GMP) and will shortly appear in "Pharmaceutical Inspection Co-operation Scheme" (PICS) inspection guidelines. It is the responsibility of the isolator user, together with the designer or supplier, to effectively demonstrate an appropriate level of system integrity and performance.

Regulators primarily hope to see that the use of isolators has been targeted at improvements in sterility or other attributes of quality assurance, as well as operator health and safety, and environmental protection. Such regulators may be less impressed by issues relating to reduction of unit manufacturing cost or amount of capital employed.

At present, the pharmaceutical industry regulatory requirements refer to isolators specifically in the context of the manufacture of sterile products. There is no reference to their role in broader areas of cross-contamination and operator safety control. Within Europe, the current EU GMP clearly states that isolators might produce improvements in sterility assurance of sterile products, and that aseptic processing manufacturing isolators should be placed in at least a Grade D surrounding environment. The Food and Drug Administration (FDA) requirements are less well defined, but it is likely that in equivalent circumstances, they would like to see an isolator located in a class 100,000 or M6.5 environment "In Operation."

As far as the configuration and performance of isolators is concerned, the pharmaceutical regulators have not made specific demands in their documentation. However, some of the main issues that have been identified by U.S. and European investigators or inspectors include:

1. Concern that the use of isolators engenders a false sense of security, and that cGMP standards might be abandoned.
2. Concern over the effects of vibration caused by the process and the critical environment being physically connected.
3. Integrity of glove and half-suit systems.
4. Effective leak testing regimes that should be established.
5. Effectiveness of the physical cleaning of isolators applied in conjunction with gaseous or aerosol disinfection systems.
6. Evidence of good ergonomic design.
7. A well-defined and implemented personnel intervention policy, including intervention recording.
8. Tailored process simulation programs for aseptic processing.
9. Inappropriate sterility assurance level claims.

Applications

Isolator systems can be used for quality-critical, safety-critical, or combined applications. The examples given here are not exhaustive but focus on some of the most important applications, and clearly illustrate the broad range of devices that are created to satisfy particular needs.

Sterility Testing

For many years, isolators have provided a valuable tool for providing very clean conditions in the microbiological laboratory for testing the sterility of the end product. Both flexible-film and rigid-wall devices have been successfully utilized. These isolators are used to carry out manipulations with a growth-promotion medium. Any failures in the security of the isolator are likely to manifest themselves as growth in the culture medium. Such growths would be deemed false positives, and would result in a requirement to investigate the source of contamination. The security and effectiveness of isolators, operating in conjunction with sanitization techniques and transfer systems such as interlocking transfer ports, have been demonstrated to provide a more secure system than the traditional cleanrooms for this type of analytical work.

Sterility testing requires a strict control of microbial contamination challenge from outside the controlled environment, but not of the particulate contamination liberated by the process itself. Hence, a positive-pressure isolator in a controlled environment, using non-unidirectional airflow, is satisfactory.

Flexible-film devices using half-suit manipulation techniques are frequently used in these applications. These isolators are usually configured as "closed" isolators because they don't have continuous-process discharges from the contained volume.

Subdivision and Dispensing of Potent Compounds

As pharmaceutical products contain increasingly potent active constituents and as health, safety, and environmental protection issues increase in importance, isolators have been developed in many shapes and forms to permit the safe weighing and subdivision of highly active compounds. The most sophisticated applications, such as the subdivision of bulk sterile active compounds, require that the isolator maintain aseptic processing conditions internally at the same time as satisfying the safety requirements. An isolator device designed to allow a keg of potent raw material to be introduced into an isolator environment, and be securely subdivided into lots suitable for a subsequent formulation batch process. The device includes systems for mechanical handling of the kegs, and for washing their exterior to decontaminate them after completion of the manipulation.

Powder Processing Systems

A natural extension from the simple handling of potent compounds is to use barrier technology to provide highly secure mechanisms for processing and more complex manipulation of powders. Isolators of this type and configuration have the objectives of operator and environmental protection as well as the provision of a secure clean and aseptic environment around the process. It provides a clean classified environment for handling bulk powder, a containment of the potent compound, and a nitrogen environment to allow the safe use of flammable solvents. It is a rigid positive-pressure device located in a EU GMP Grade D cleanroom. The cleanliness of the internal nitrogen environment is maintained using non- unidirectional airflow. Manipulations are achieved using a combination of glove and half-suit systems.

Small-Scale Manipulations

Many isolator applications at the clinical trial scale of manufacturing are based on the same scale of technology used for sterility testing. The aseptic dispensing of pharmaceutical products in hospital pharmacies is also carried out on this scale. Such manufacturing is not carried out on a continuous basis, but in relatively small batches that can be transferred from the isolator with the help of one of the more secure transfer systems. In this type of application, one isolator is being used to dispense a variety of products or several isolators are used for separate tasks. The isolators are configured to provide an aseptic environment interfacing with a depyrogenating oven for handling and holding dry-heat-sterilized components. Additional individual isolators are provided in which separate formulation and/or filling operations can be undertaken. Materials are moved from one isolator to another using closed containers that dock with alpha/beta docking ports mounted in the sidewall and floor of the isolators. Internal cleanliness is maintained through positive pressurization and the supply of double HEPA-filtered unidirectional airflow to the critical process zones within the isolators.

Large-Scale Aseptic Production

Isolators are now used in industrial scale aseptic processing for both formulation and filling.The internal control of the environment is achieved by a combination of non-unidirectional and unidirectional airflow within positively pressurized cells. The individual cells are separated by "airlock" flap valves. The product flow through to aseptic filling operations is largely automatic, with gloves provided for specific manual interventions. The complete line is placed in a room in which the environment is controlled but unclassified in terms of cleanroom standards. Hydrogen peroxide vapor is used for the surface sterilization of the isolator network, and for the continuous surface disinfection of containers of product components that enter the system.

Technical Considerations for the Design, Manufacture, and Testing of Isolators

The susceptibility of the process to contamination is critical in terms of risk assessment. In aseptic processing, for example, open processes are at far greater risk than closed processes. Furthermore, systems requiring complex aseptic assembly prior to use are more difficult to manage in a small isolator environment than if cleaning and sterilization-in-place techniques were employed. It is essential, therefore, to evaluate all the process steps, including equipment transfers, assembly manipulations, and the processing activity itself. Effective documentation of such analysis is good practice in a validated operational scenario.

Barrier-integrity characteristics

Complex isolators are unlikely to be leak free. It is obvious that the better the barrier integrity is, the less will be the opportunity for contamination to be transferred across the isolator wall. The integrity is influenced by the basic materials of construction, design effectiveness, damage caused by cleaning, resistance to process chemicals, and robustness. The first fundamental option to consider is a rigid or a soft-wall construction. The former normally utilizes a combination of stainless steel and glass or Perspex windows; the latter uses a welded transparent PVC envelope connected to a stainless steel floor tray or machine bedplate. After choosing either a rigid or soft-wall solution, it is most important to ensure that an effective mechanism is selected to measure the leakage-air tightness of the isolator. Such tests should form part of the construction acceptance testing of a device, and should become part of routine operational leak testing. A pressure-hold test is the simplest method of determining that the complete assembly satisfies a set of acceptance criteria. Provided that the isolator, including its internal and external air systems, is configured in an appropriate way, simple isolating valves can be used to isolate the isolator, thus allowing convenient leakage-rate tests to be carried out. Such tests could ultimately be carried out on a batch basis if required. The most commonly used test methods are:

1. Evaluation of pressure decay rate.
2. Leakage-rate measurement at constant pressure.
3. Tracer gas leak-rate detection.
4. Tracer particle transfer measurement (sometimes called a leak-induction test).

Manipulation technique

The manipulation technique influences the overall integrity of an isolator system, as in virtually all cases, the manipulation device presents a potential breach to the barrier of the isolator. Additionally, where the manipulation involves placing part of the human body within a specialised system component, such as gloves or a half-suit, a greater potential exists for process or product contamination than would occur with tong manipulators, remote manipulators, or robotics devices. Utilizing a simple pressure-hold or leakage test on a glove port and glove before and after a process work session can achieve a high level of glove integrity assurance. Such a technique is virtually impossible with half-suit applications due to their size and construction. Strategic inspections and pressure tests for integrity at less frequent intervals are required for such devices. Alternative manipulation methods using tongs and remote manipulators (mainly for handling radioactive substances) can be of advantage in isolators, but currently are rarely found in pharmaceutical applications. However, it should be noted that tong manipulators, for example, have their own special problems and use a gaiter system to ensure air pressure integrity around the rotation and sliding gimbals. This gaiter is failure are just as important.

Manipulations should always be minimised. An event report should be made, and a preprepared action plan must be implemented should damage occur to a glove. The selection of glove and gauntlet materials is most important. Half-suit and sleeve/glove systems use a technique where the glove can be detached from the sleeve by way of a specialized fitting in the wrist region. Some of these devices have the capability of allowing glove change while the system is in use. Gauntlet or one-piece systems are generally more durable, but do not have the same change in use capability. A balance has to be maintained between durability and "feel." Typical available materials are:

1. Latex (natural rubber) allows great dexterity; if thick enough, these can be wear and abrasion resistant. It is chemically resistant to many mild chemicals, detergents, and disinfectants.
2. Neoprene (synthetic) has high flexibility and allows good dexterity. It has low tensile strength, and is chemically resistant to materials with the exception of oxidizing agents such as hydrogen peroxide.
3. Nitrile (synthetic copolymer) has poor flexibility, but is strong and highly chemical resistant.
4. PVC (synthetic polymer) is strong and chemically resistant to materials except ketones and aromatic hydrocarbons; it is inflexible and subject to tearing.
5. Urethanes have good abrasion, chemical resistance, and good tensile strength, but are not suitable for high temperatures.
6. Laminated polymers exhibit high strength and selective resistance to chemicals; they are subject to failure when used with sharp objects.

A variation of the pressure-hold test can be used to test the integrity of manipulation gloves in situ. This provides a convenient way of determining the integrity of the glove without entering the controlled environment or unnecessarily changing an expensive commodity. An alternative, provided by a particular vendor, involves inert gas purging of a glove volume, followed by measurement of the build-up of oxygen that diffuses through glove pinhole leaks.

Transfer techniques

The transfer of materials into and out of an isolator represents the most likely and most common source of loss of internal environmental integrity. The more secure the transfer system, the less demanding is the surrounding environment. The simplest devices, such as single doors, present very little ability to separate the external from the internal environment. In fact, in these applications, the only facet of the device's performance that provides any protection is outward airflow when the door or cover is open. Security can be improved by a double-door pass-through hatch. The performance and effectiveness of such a device can be improved by introducing mechanical or electromechanical interlocking of the opposing doors. Furthermore, adding positive ventilation of the airlock space to dilute and remove contamination that may enter when the external door is open adds security to this form of transfer. The most secure techniques include a direct process connection to the isolator, interlocked docking port systems (often called alpha/ beta systems), and airflow protected tunnels for continuous component discharge. Although no specific tests or standards exist to define the performance of such devices, tests can be adopted from other applications. Containment tests such as those used for open-fronted microbiological safety cabinets can be effectively used to determine a protection factor for airflow-protected product-discharge tunnels. In the case of alpha/beta interlocked docking port systems, certain manufacturers have developed and applied particulate and microbiological challenge tests to determine the effectiveness or a protection factor of these devices. This quantifies the segregation achieved by such a device in operation. Such tests may become the basis of type or performance testing and subsequent selection of specialized transfer devices.

Internal pressurization

Internal pressure within an isolator clearly has a major influence on the ability of the isolator to exclude the external environment. The level of the pressurization should also be considered in relation to its ability to withstand the piston effect of rapid glove movement, and whether or not the internal isolator air system should achieve a specific outflow of air in the event of partial or total glove loss. The integrity and performance of pressurisation equally apply to negative- pressure systems. However, negative-pressure systems, used for clean and aseptic processing, are more likely to require a higher class of surrounding environment than that required for equivalent positive pressure systems. The glove piston effect is relative volume related (i.e., the volume displaced by the glove compared to the volume of the isolator). As a rule of thumb, devices with a pressure of 15–25 Pa compared to the surrounding atmosphere, are likely to be less secure (due to the piston effect) than devices with a pressure of 50–80 Pa compared to the surrounding area. When lost glove airflow protection is required, air velocities of 0.5–0.7 m/s should be considered. If extremely high velocities above these figures occur, reentrainment of external contamination due to high turbulence is a distinct possibility. In testing the effectiveness of the pressurisation, it is necessary to challenge not only the steady state conditions but also the transient conditions. It is therefore expected that a series of tests be carried out to investigate start and stop modes of the isolator control system, the influence of glove or other device manipulation, and of course, the interaction of the process itself. The most demanding processes in aseptic pharmaceutical applications are usually continuous depyrogenation tunnels, where the air leakage into the tunnel due to isolator overpressure, varies with time, and may well vary with different machine settings for various sizes. In this type of application, it is absolutely critical that the qualification of the isolator environment is carried out in conjunction with all states of operation. Similarly, it is essential that the depyrogenation process in the tunnel is fully qualified with all states of the isolator.

Airflow configuration

As with cleanroom applications, isolators can use unidirectional or non-unidirectional airflow regimes, or in larger systems a combination of both. Isolators are very different from cleanrooms in that generally a physical barrier separates critical from non-critical zones rather than the use of managed airflow. It is possible therefore in isolators to obtain the necessary levels of environmental cleanliness with very low air velocities. Unidirectional airflow systems designed to achieve class 100/M3.5/ISO 5 cleanliness can be achieved with velocities as low as 0.10m/s. When the velocity is set at such low levels, it is necessary to carefully evaluate the influence of heat sources and process disturbance. Having defined the airflow characteristics required for the isolator, it is necessary to determine both the airflow rate using flow anemometers and the uniformity of the airflow in the case of unidirectional airflow systems. The latter is best achieved using flow visualization smoke-tracing techniques. This is particularly important if an isolator environment itself contains a mixture of unidirectional and turbulent and/or conventional flow zones. Filtered-air exchange rate in non-unidirectional flow systems should be based on the rate required to dilute internally generated contamination. The contamination decay rate of an enclosed volume can be used as a measure of effectiveness of the air-movement system in an isolator. This can be helpful for assessing the degassing rate at the conclusion of a gaseous sanitisation or sterilizing procedure. The decay rate can be measured using artificial aerosol generation combined with measuring the decay profile broadly in accordance with the method set out in IES recommended practice 006.2. Alternative gas-decay methods can be adapted from tracer-gas methods used to prove the effectiveness of ventilation systems.

HEPA filtration

The provision and location of air filters and the filtration integrity in isolators are as important as in clean or containment room technology. The filter and its installation must be designed with the utmost care, and special consideration should be given to the effect of vibration transferred from the isolator mechanical systems or the process. Final filters should be placed as close as possible to the critical zone. However, this sometimes makes the task of fitting the filters difficult due to restricted space and access. Maintenance convenience can be improved by locating filters close to, but away from the critical zone, in carefully engineered housings. When this technique is used, the duct between the filter and the isolator should be constructed of non shedding materials. Natural or artificial aerosol challenge tests are the appropriate way to test in situ final HEPA or ULPA filters and existing cleanroom oriented standards, and requirements are directly relevant to isolator applications.

Airborne cleanliness classification

Classification of the working environment by measuring the particulate concentration is normally carried out in accordance with the requirements stated within the accepted airborne-particle classification standards. If the isolator working volume is extremely small, it may be necessary to increase the number of test locations from the single point determined by using the formula within the standards. Two, three, or more locations focused on the critical points of process or product exposure. When continuous or cyclic automatic particle monitoring is being considered, care should be taken to ensure that the volume of air taken as a sample does not adversely influence the isolator pressurization.

Open aperture integrity

Open aperture protection is an important feature of some isolators. In addition to designing and testing for isolator pressurisation, some isolators need to be engineered to maintain segregation in case of partial or total glove loss. This is particularly the case when biological or chemical hazards are present internally, and need to be contained for safety reasons. Furthermore, in many production-scale isolator networks, particularly those filling parenteral containers, it is an advantage to pass the filled closed containers out of the isolator continuously via an airflow protected tunnel. In such cases, there is a protecting air velocity, entering or leaving the isolator, to contain a hazard or minimize the opportunity of internal contamination, respectively. The effectiveness of this inrush or out-rush of air (protection factor) can be quantified by a biological or aerosol challenge test derived from adaptation of the method defined in British Standard 5726 or the U.S. Standard NSF 49. Both these standards relate to microbiological safety cabinets where the test is specified for the purposes of quantifying a containment factor. The containment test challenges the aperture with a test aerosol, and measures the quantity that escapes through the opening. The ratio of escape to generated quantity is used to calculate a containment factor. This test method can also be effectively deployed for testing and demonstrating the effectiveness of any other aperture inward or outward and is used to protect and segregate the internal from the external environment. In the classic case, there is a continuous discharge of filled containers across a dead plate, leaving an aseptic processing environment. Here it is important to determine that there is no turbulence causing induction of external contamination into the critical aseptic zone.

Cleaning and Sanitization of Isolators

Effective cleaning and biodecontamination of the internal surfaces of isolators and their intimate product contact parts is of greatest importance, particularly for aseptic processing. The effectiveness and repeatability of the sanitisation method also has an impact on the quality of the surrounding environment required. This is particularly the case if it is anticipated that batch and machine format changes are carried out with the isolator open. If this procedure is adopted, it is necessary first to minimize the introduction of room contamination into the open isolator, and then to apply an effective cleaning procedure. If some contamination has entered the device, it is essential to use a repeatable and effective sanitization or surface sterilization method. The requirement to clean and disinfect would be lessened if change over were achieved with a closed isolator. The least effective processes, such as surface swabbing and aerosol spraying with disinfectant, are unlikely to satisfy the requirements of a repeatable process of high efficacy. However, the use of highly controlled gaseous-phase processes, using materials such as formaldehyde, hydrogen peroxide, peracetic acid, and chlorine dioxide, can be very effective. These gaseous-phase processes are generally intolerant of soiling deposits on the surface. Therefore, the methods must be deployed in conjunction with effective physical cleaning.

Design Considerations for the Surrounding Environment

Finally, having taken all the above issues into account, and determined the type and nature of the isolator to be used and the quality of the surrounding environment, it is important to consider some of the broader issues relating to the design of the surrounding environment. It is essential to thoroughly consider all the attributes of the facility in which the isolator is placed, as this can have a major influence on the product. The facility in which the isolator is placed must provide a clear departmental separation from less critical adjacent activities. By layout and configuration, it must achieve the following:

1. Provide appropriate physical security for the operation.
2. Control and manage access of personnel and materials.
3. Ensure the required background environment is maintained.
4. Provide the utilities required by the isolator.

2

Microsphere Technology and Applications

The range of techniques for the preparation of microspheres offers a variety of opportunities to control aspects of drug administration. The term "control" includes phenomena such as protection and masking, reduced dissolution rate, facilitation of handling, and spatial targeting of the active ingredient. This approach facilitates accurate delivery of small quantities of potent drugs; reduced drug concentrations at sites other than the target organ or tissue; and protection of labile compounds before and after administration and prior to appearance at the site of action. The characteristics of microspheres containing drug should be correlated with the required therapeutic action and are dictated by the materials and methods employed in the manufacture of the delivery systems.

The behavior of drugs in vivo can be manipulated by coupling the drug to a carrier particle. The clearance kinetics, tissue distribution, metabolism, and cellular interactions of the drug are strongly influenced by the behavior of the carrier. Exploitation of these changes in pharmacodynamic behavior may lead to enhanced therapeutic effect. However, an intelligent approach to therapeutics employing drug-carrier technology requires a detailed understanding of the carrier interaction with critical cellular and organ systems and of the limitations of the system with respect to formulation procedures and stability. A variety of agents have been used as drug carriers, including immunoglobulins, serum proteins, liposomes, microspheres, nanoparticles, microcapsules, and even cells such as erythrocytes.

Antineoplastic drugs, narcotic antagonists, steroid hormones, luteinizing hormone releasing hormone analogs, elastase, and other macromolecules have been incorporated into microspheres. In addition, vaccines, living cells, and tissues have been encapsulated.

Definition and General Description

Microspheres can be defined as solid, approximately spherical particles ranging in size from 1 to 1000 μm. They are made of polymeric, waxy, or other protective materials, that is, biodegradable synthetic polymers and modified natural products such as starches, gums, proteins, fats, and waxes. The natural polymers include albumin and gelatin; the synthetic polymers include polylactic acid and polyglycolic acid.

The solvents used to dissolve the polymeric materials are chosen according to the polymer and drug solubilities and stabilities, process safety, and economic considerations. Substances can be incorporated within microspheres in the liquid or solid state during manufacture or subsequently by absorption. There are two types of microspheres: Microcapsules, where the entrapped substance is completely surrounded by a distinct capsule wall, and micromatrices, where the entrapped substance is dispersed throughout the microsphere matrix.

Microspheres are small and have large surface-to-volume ratios. At the lower end of their size range they have colloidal properties. The interfacial properties of microspheres are extremely important, often dictating their activity. In fact, the principle of microsphere manufacture depends on the creation of an interfacial area, involving a polymeric material that will form an interfacial boundary and a method of cross-linking to impart permanency. The methods of manufacturing described later are by no means comprehensive and the reader should bear in mind that if the aforementioned criteria are adhered to, the only limitation to the manufacture of microspheres is the researcher's imagination.

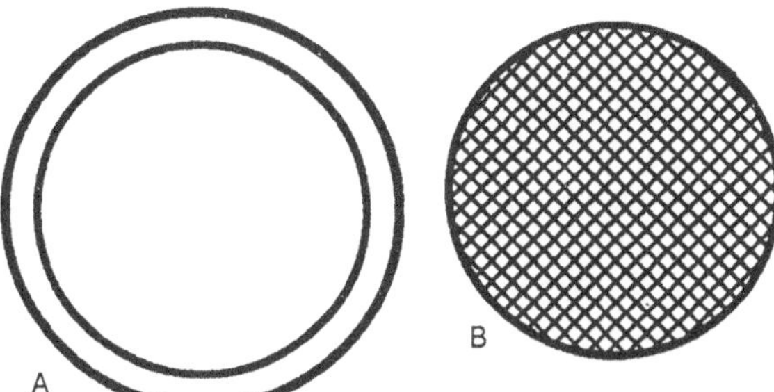

Fig. 2.1. Schematic diagram illustrating microspheres. A–Microcapsule consisting of an encapsulated core particle and B–micromatrix consisting of homogeneous dispersion of active ingredient in particle.

Historical and Contextual Perspective

The concept of packaging microscopic quantities of materials within microspheres dates back to the 1930s and the work of Bungenberg de Jong and coworkers on the entrapment of substances within coacervates. The first commercial application of encapsulation was by the National Cash Register Company for the manufacture of carbonless copying paper. The technology and applications have advanced over the last several decades. This technology is used by the agricultural, food, household products, medical, graphics, and cosmetics industries. The potential use of microspheres in the pharmaceutical industry has been considered since the 1960s for the following applications:

1. Taste and odor masking
2. Conversion of oils and other liquids to solids for ease of handling
3. Protection of drugs against the environment (moisture, light, heat, and/or oxidation) and vice versa (prevention of pain on injection)
4. Delay of volatilization
5. Separation of incompatible materials (other drugs or excipients such as buffers)
6. Improvement of flow of powders
7. Safe handling of toxic substances
8. Aid in dispersion of water-insoluble substances in aqueous media, and
9. Production of sustained-release, controlled-release, and targeted medications
10. Reduced dose dumping potential compared to large implantable devices

Microencapsulation has also been used medically for the encapsulation of live cells and vaccines. Biocompatibility can be improved by the encapsulation of artificial cells and biomolecules such as peptides, proteins, and hormones, which can prevent unwanted immunological reactions that would lead to inactivation or rejection. Microspheres are used for isolating materials until their activity is needed. The biotechnology industry employs microspheres to contain organisms and their recombinant products to aid in the isolation of these products.

Pharmaceutical Applications

A number of pharmaceutical microencapsulated products are currently on the market, such as aspirin, theophylline and its derivatives, vitamins, pancrelipase, antihypertensives, potassium chloride, progesterone, and contraceptive hormone combinations. Microencapsulated KCl is used to prevent gastrointestinal complications associated with potassium chloride. The dispersibility of the microcapsules and the controlled release of the ions minimize the possibility of local high salt concentrations, which could result in ulceration, hemorrhage, or perforation. Microspheres have also found potential applications as injection or inhalation products. The number of commercially available products does not reflect the amount of research that has been carried out in this area, nor the benefits that can be achieved using this technology. Economic considerations have been a key factor in determining the number of pharmaceutical micro- encapsulated products. Most encapsulation processes are expensive and require significant capital investment for equipment. An exception is pan or spray coating and spray drying, since the necessary equipment may already be available within the company. An additional expense is due to the fact that most microencapsulation processes are patent protected.

Other Applications

Applications of microencapsulation in other industries are numerous. The best known micro-encapsulated products are carbonless copying paper, photosensitive paper, microencapsulated fragrances, such as "scent-strips" (also known as "snap-n-burst"), and microencapsulated aromas ("scratch-n-sniff"). All of these products are usually prepared by gelatin–acacia complex coacervation. Scratch-n-sniff has been used in children's books and food and cosmetic aroma advertising. Micro- capsules are also extensively used as diagnostics, for example, temperature-sensitive microcapsules for thermographic detection of tumors.

In the biotechnology industry microencapsulated microbial cells are being used for the production of recombinant proteins and peptides. The retention of the product within the microcapsule can be beneficial in the collection and isolation of the product. Encapsulation of microbial cells can also increase the cell-loading capacity and the rate of production in bioreactors. Smaller microcapsules are better for these purposes; they have a larger surface area that is important for the exchange of gases across the microcapsule membrane. Microcapsules with semipermeable membranes are being used in cell culture. A feline breast tumor line, which was difficult to grow in conventional culture, has been successfully grown in microcapsules. Microencapsulated activated charcoal has been used for hemoperfusion. Paramedical uses of microcapsules include bandages with microencapsulated antiinfective substances. A unique application of microencapsulation technology is for feeding organisms. Sea bass larvae have been fed with all-protein microcapsules or with microcapsules containing lipids to supplement their diet.

Microsphere Manufacture

The most important physicochemical characteristics that may be controlled in microsphere manufacture are:

1. Particle size and distribution
2. Polymer molecular weight
3. Ratio of drug to polymer
4. Total mass of drug and polymer

Each of these can be related to the manufacture and rate of drug release from the systems. The following discussion presents methods of manufacture of coated or encapsulated systems, referred to as microcapsules, and matrix systems containing homogeneously distributed drug, referred to as micromatrices.

Wax Coating and Hot Melt

Wax may be used to coat the core particles, encapsulating drug by dissolution or dispersion in the molten wax. The waxy solution or suspension is dispersed by high speed mixing into a cold solution, such as cold liquid paraffin. The mixture is agitated for at least one hour. The external phase (liquid paraffin) is then decanted and the microcapsules are suspended in a non-miscible solvent, and allowed to air dry. Multiple emulsions may also be formed. For example, a heated aqueous drug solution can be dispersed in molten wax to form a water-in-oil emulsion, which is emulsified in a heated external aqueous phase to form a water-in-oil-in-water emulsion. The system is cooled and the microcapsules collected. For highly aqueous soluble drugs, a non- aqueous phase can be used to prevent loss of drug to the external phase. Another alternative is to rapidly reduce the temperature when the primary emulsion is placed in the external aqueous phase.

Wax coated microcapsules, while inexpensive and often used, release drug more rapidly than polymeric microcapsules. Carnauba wax and beeswax can be used as the coating materials and these can be mixed in order to achieve desired characteristics. Wax-coated microcapsules have been successfully tableted. Small aerosol particles, 1–5 μm in diameter, have been condensation coated from a vapor of a fatty acid or paraffin wax. These particles have been shown to exhibit reduced dissolution rates in vitro, corresponding to reduced absorption rates following deposition in the lungs of Beagle dogs. Polyanhydrides have been chosen for the preparation of microspheres because of their degradation by surface erosion into apparently non-toxic small molecules. The mixture of polymer and active ingredient is suspended in a miscible solvent, heated 5°C above the melting point of the polymer and stirred continuously. The emulsion is stabilized by cooling below the melting point until the droplets solidify.

Spray Coating and Pan Coating

Spray coating and pan coating employ heat-jacketed coating pans in which the solid drug core particles are rotated and into which the coating material is sprayed. The core particles are in the size range of micrometers up to a few millimeters. The coating material is usually sprayed at an angle from the side into the pan. The process is continued until an even coating is completed. This is the process typically used to coat tablets and capsules.

Coating a large number of small particles may provide a safer and more consistent release pattern than coated tablets. In addition, several batches of microspheres can be prepared with different coating thicknesses and mixed to achieve specific controlled release patterns.

The Wurster process, a variation of the basic pan coating method, is an adaptation of the fluid-bed granulator. The solid core particles are fluidized by air pressure and a spray of dissolved wall material is applied from the perforated bottom of the fluidization chamber parallel to the air stream and onto the solid core particles. Alternatively, the coating solution can be sprayed from the top or the sides into an upstream of fluidized particles. This adaptation allows the coating of small particle s The fluidized-bed technique produces a more uniform coating thickness than the pan-coating methodology. Problems can arise with inflammable organic solvents because of the high risk of explosion in the enclosed fluidizer chamber. Explosion proof units have been designed; however, over the past two decades aqueous coating solutions are being used more and more.

Examples of aqueous coating solutions include water- soluble low molecular weight cellulose ethers, emulsion polymerization latexes of polymethacrylates, and dispersions of water-insoluble polymers such as ethyl-cellulose in the form of pseudolatex. These solvent-free coating solutions provide a range of different coatings from fast disintegrating isolating layers to enteric and sustained-release coatings. Lehmann has reviewed different commercial methods, the conditions required for coating, and various coating formulas including illustrations of the types of equipment used.

Coacervation

Coacervation is the simple separation of a macromolecular solution into two immiscible liquid phases, a dense coacervate phase, which is relatively concentrated in macromolecules, and a dilute equilibrium phase. Coacervates may be described as liquid crystals and mesophases. In the presence of only one macromolecule, this process is referred to as simple coacervation. When two or more macromolecules of opposite charge are present, it is referred to as complex coacervation. Simple coacervation is induced by a change in conditions, which results in dehydration of the macromolecules. This may be achieved by the addition of a non-solvent, the addition of microions, or a temperature change, all of which promote polymer–polymer interactions over polymer–solvent interactions. Complex coacervation is driven by electrostatic interactive forces between two or more macromolecules.

Bungenberg de Jong, Kruyt, and Lens first showed that solid particles could also be entrapped in coacervate systems. On phase separation by simple or complex methods tiny coacervate droplets are formed, which sediment or coalesce to form a separate coacervate phase. The coacervate forms around any core material that may be present, such as drug particles. Agitation of the coacervate system can prevent coalescence and sedimentation of the droplets, which can be cross-linked to form stable microcapsules by addition of an agent, such as glutaraldehyde, or the application of heat. Drug micro-encapsulation by coacervation has been reviewed by Madan and by Nixon. The large number of variables involved in complex coacervation (pH, ionic strength, macromolecule concentration, macromolecule ratio, and macromolecular weight) affect microcapsule production, resulting in a large number of controllable parameters. These can be manipulated to produce microcapsules with specific properties. Complex coacervate microcapsules have been formulated as suspensions or gels, and have been compounded within suppositories and tablets. Although many successful coacervate microencapsulation systems have been prepared, coacervate microcapsules have a number of limitations. They can be produced only at specific pH values, they require stabilization by cross-linking agents or heat, and the retention of the encapsulant depends on the extent of cross-linking. The pH limitation can be overcome to some extent by the addition of water-soluble non-ionic polymers, such as polyethylene oxide or polyethylene glycol. The presence of a small amount of these polymers allows microencapsulation to occur over an expanded pH range. For example, the pH range for coacervation of gelatin and acacia can be extended from pH 2.6–5.5 to pH 2–9. In addition, these polymers induce simple coacervation, as has been shown for macromolecules such as gelatin, carboxymethylcellulose, and ethylene- maleic anhydride copolymer. The pH range for simple coacervation is also expanded in the presence of these water-soluble non-ionic polymers. For example, the pH range for simple coacervation of gelatin can be increased from only pH values close to the isoelectric point to the pH range of 5.5–9.5.

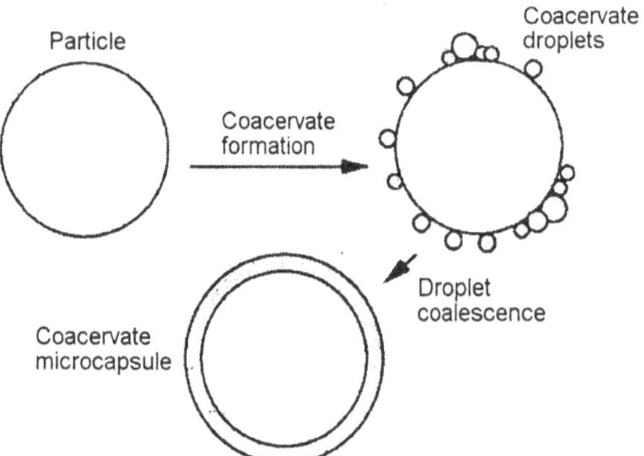

Fig. 2.2. Schematic diagram of the formation of a coacervate around a core material.

Cross-linking of coacervates is necessary to stabilize coacervate emulsion droplets and hence form microcapsules. Both chemical cross-linking agents and the application of heat may be harmful to the encapsulant materials, such as thermolabile and chemically labile drugs and live cells. A stable coacervate system, formed without the use of chemical cross-linking agents or the application of heat, has been developed by Burgess and Singh. This system is potentially useful for the delivery of protein and polypeptide drugs and other materials unable to withstand cross-linking procedures.

Calcium Alginate Microcapsules

Dropping or spraying a sodium alginate solution into a calcium chloride solution produces microcapsules. The divalent calcium ions cross-link the alginate, forming gelled droplets. These gel droplets can be permanently cross-linked by addition to a polylysine solution. Lim and Sun developed this method for the encapsulation of live cells. Variations on this method with different polymers have been developed. Chitosan is a preferred polymer, because it has a better biocompatibility than alginate. Traditionally alginate beads were formed by dropping the alginate solution into the calcium chloride with a fine-bore pipette. However, the droplets were relatively large, because the drops do not fall until they reach a critical mass. Smaller droplets can be formed by using a pump to force the alginate through the pipette, a vibration system to help remove the drops from the end of the pipette, and an air atomization method.

Spray Drying

Spray drying is a single-step, closed-system process applicable to a wide variety of materials, including heat-sensitive materials. This process is often used commercially since the necessary equipment is frequently available at the manufacturing site. As a closed system, it is ideal for good manufacturing practice and the production of sterile materials. The drug and the polymer coating materials are dissolved in a suitable solvent (aqueous or non-aqueous) or the drug may be present as a suspension in the polymer solution. Alternatively, it may be dissolved or suspended within an emulsion or coacervate system. For example, biodegradable polylactide microcapsules can be prepared by dissolving the drug and polymer in methylene chloride. Methylcellulose and sodium carboxymethylcellulose spray-dried microspheres are prepared by dissolving the polymers in aqueous systems. The microsphere size is controlled by the rate of spraying, the feed rate of the polymer drug solution, the nozzle size, the temperature in the drying and collecting chambers, and the size of these two chambers. The quality of spray-dried products is improved by the addition of plasticizers that promote polymer coalescence and film formation and enhance the formation of spherical and smooth-surfaced microcapsules.

Solvent evaporation

This is one of the earliest methods of microsphere manufacture. The polymer and drug must be soluble in an organic solvent, frequently methylene chloride. The solution containing the polymer and the drug may be dispersed in an aqueous phase to form droplets. Continuous mixing and elevated temperatures may be employed to evaporate the more volatile organic solvent and leave the solid polymer–drug particles suspended in an aqueous medium. The particles are finally filtered from the suspension.

Precipitation

Precipitation is a variation on the evaporation method. The emulsion consists of polar droplets dispersed in a non-polar medium. Solvent may be removed from the droplets by the use of a cosolvent. The resulting increase in the polymer drug concentration causes precipitation forming a suspension of microspheres.

Freeze Drying

This technique involves the freezing of the emulsion; the relative freezing points of the continuous and dispersed phases are important. The continuous-phase solvent is usually organic and is removed by sublimation at low temperature and pressure. Finally, the dispersed phase solvent of the droplets is removed by sublimation, leaving polymer-drug particles.

Chemical and Thermal Cross-Linking

Microspheres made from natural polymers are prepared by a cross-linking process; polymers include gelatin, albumin, starch, and dextran. A water–oil emulsion is prepared, where the water phase is a solution of the polymer that contains the drug to be incorporated. The oil phase is a suitable vegetable oil or oil-organic solvent mixture containing an oil-soluble emulsifier. Once the desired water–oil emulsion is formed, the water soluble polymer is solidified by some kind of cross-linking process. This may involve thermal treatment or the addition of a chemical cross-linking agent such as glutaraldehyde to form a stable chemical cross-link as in albumin. If chemical or heat cross-linking is used, the amount of chemical and the period and intensity of heating are critical in determining the release rates and swelling properties of the microspheres. If glutaraldehyde is the cross-linking agent, residual amounts can have toxic effects.

NANOPARTICLES

Nanoparticles, 10–1000 nm polymeric particles, are prepared from the same natural and synthetic biodegradable polymers as microspheres. Albumin nanoparticles are prepared by the cross-linking processes mentioned previously. For the preparation of particles from synthetic polymers, heterogeneous bulk polymerization techniques of suspension, emulsion, and micelle polymerization are often used.

Suspension polymerization of water-insoluble liquid monomer and drug may be achieved by agitating a dispersion of droplets, 10–1000 nm in diameter, in a continuous aqueous phase. The temperature must be carefully controlled. An initiator is frequently employed to increase the reaction rate in the droplets, and the aqueous phase may contain stabilizers to prevent coalescence and thickening agents to increase the viscosity. The polymer is formed by reaction of the functional groups of the monomer. This process has the advantage that the continuous phase absorbs the heat of the polymerization reaction and minimizes the temperature change within the droplets. However, aggregation of the particles may arise as the polymer molecules in suspended particles coalesce. Unfortunately, it is difficult to eliminate stabilizers and additives, used to prevent coalescence, from the final product.

Emulsion polymerization involves the dispersion of the monomer liquid in an aqueous phase to form droplets, 0.05–5 nm in diameter. An initiator and a surfactant, in a concentration higher than its critical micelle concentration, are present in the aqueous phase. Excess surfactant molecules form micelles whose hydrophobic interiors take up part of the available monomer, causing them to swell. Initiator radicals diffuse into these swollen micelles and begin the polymerization process. As the monomer is consumed, it is replaced by progressive diffusion of the remaining monomer from its location in the emulsified droplets to the interior of the micelles. The micelles continue to swell in size as polymerization proceeds. The enlarging surfaces compete for available surfactant, thus influencing the number of available micelles that can participate in the polymer formation. This method yields particles of very small size and predictable number at low temperatures. However, the particles usually have a high concentration of associated monomer, which may be toxic.

Micelle polymerization differs from emulsion polymerization in that all of the monomer and the drug is contained within micelles composed of surfactant. Diffusion of the monomer from the micelles is prevented by the non-solvent properties of the outer phase. Therefore, the increase in particle size is negligible as the polymerization proceeds.

CHARACTERIZATION

Materials

The polymer employed to prepare microspheres must be characterized in terms of molecular weight and purity, however this topic is beyond the scope of this article. Characterization of the materials may have implications for the formation of the micro- spheres. The viscosity and film-forming properties of the polymers used should be known. Viscosity can affect the tendency to form microspheres, their size, and even their shape. Burgess and coworkers have shown that albumin–acacia coacervates do not form microcapsules under certain conditions of pH and ionic strength, if the viscosity of the coacervate phase is too high. Burgess and Carless developed a method to predict the optimum conditions for complex coacervation based on the charge carried by the two polymers involved.

Microspheres

Size characterization may be conducted by various methods including light microscopy, resistance blockage techniques (Coulter analysis), light blockage techniques, light scattering, laser diffraction analysis, and for particles less than 1 *mm*, photon correlation spectroscopy. Electron microscopy, scanning electron microscopy, and scanning tunneling microscopy are used for surface characterization of microspheres. Fourier transform Raman spectroscopy or X-ray photoelectron spectroscopy may be used to determine if any of the material which should have been entrapped is present on the surface and if any other contaminants are present. Other surface characterization techniques include surface charge analysis using microelectrophoresis. Surface charge can provide information regarding microsphere aggregation. Surface charge is an important parameter with respect to the interaction of microspheres within the body.

Surface forces are important in the entrapment, wetting, and adhesion of core material by the coating material. The wettability of solids by different liquids is usually assessed by contact-angle measurement. When wetting of the core material is poor, it is difficult or impossible to form microcapsules. For example, Eudragit RS dissolved in THF-cyclohexane failed to encapsulate charcoal particles but was successful in encapsulating potassium dichromate. The surface hydrophobicity of oil droplets has been shown to affect their uptake into complex coacervate droplets. Oil uptake was directly related to the hydrophile–lipophile balance (HLB) value at the droplet interface. Additives, such as surfactants, which alter surface properties were shown to affect the uptake of core materials.

Biological Distribution

The disposition of microspheres upon entry to the body has been studied extensively. They are frequently labeled with a radionuclide to allow study by scintillation counting or scintigraphy. This work has largely focused on tissue distribution as a function of particle size, with the conclusion that particles below 7 μm tend to locate predominantly in the reticuloendothelial system of the liver, whereas particles 7–15 μm in size tend to be collected in the capillary system of the lung. The acute toxicity, tissue interaction, cell interaction, and protein interaction of various microspheres have been investigated. These studies demonstrated that the toxicity of microspheres is related to the number and size administered. Initial inflammatory responses to the administration of microspheres were consistent with observations that phagocytosis by neutrophils and macrophages may occur. The extent and nature of the cell and tissue affects of microspheres may be related to the surface characteristics of the polymer employed and to the particle size. For example, fibrinogen has been shown to associate with poly-DL-lactide microcapsules, affecting the surface-charge characteristics. This phenomenon is related to the hydrophobic nature of the surface. Indeed, hydrophilic coatings can reduce the uptake of microspheres by the liver and peritoneal macrophages.

Therapeutic Applications

Targeting

Drugs can be targeted to specific sites in the body using microspheres and other colloidal carrier systems. Targeting by colloid delivery systems is dealt with elsewhere in this encyclopedia. Targeting by micro- spheres may be passive, active, diversional, or physical. In passive targeting the microspheres follow their natural distribution in the body (which depends on particle size, shape, surface characteristics, particle deformation, and route of administration). In active targeting the natural distribution of the microspheres is altered (for example, by attachment of site-specific vectoring agents such as monoclonal antibodies and lectins). Diversional targeting means blocking the natural distribution of the microspheres, for example, partly or completely impairing the cells of the reticuloendothelial system, which would otherwise take up the microspheres. Physical targeting involves an external influence, such as a change in temperature or a magnetic field to direct the microspheres to the desired site. Degrees of targeting can be achieved by localization of the drug to a specific area in the body, to a particular organ in the body (for example, the lungs), to a particular group of cells within the body (for example, the Kupffer cells), and even to intracellular structures (such as the lysosomes or the cell nucleus). The problems associated with directing microspheres to specific areas in the body following parenteral administration.

'Oral targeting can be achieved using microspheres; those less than 10 μm in diameter have been shown to target the Peyer's patch. Microspheres less than 5 μm were shown to be transported through the lymphatics within macrophages and those larger than 5 μm remained in the Peyer's patch. Toxoid vaccine microcapsules were effectively delivered and released in the gut-associated lymphoid tissue following oral administration.

Controlled Release

The rate of drug release from microspheres dictates their therapeutic action. Release is governed by the molecular structure of the drug and polymer, the resistance of the polymer to degradation, and the surface area and porosity of the microspheres. Reservoir delivery systems extend the residence time of drug within the systemic circulation and were originally focused on zero-order dissolution kinetics. This mathematical expression describes a linear relationship between rate of appearance in plasma and time. Ideally, the plasma drug concentration is independent of time for most of the dissolution period and is optimally maintained in the therapeutic window.

In non-porous polymeric systems the rate of drug release is dictated by the device surface area which is linked directly to its shape. Drug release from polymeric systems with a variety of geometries has been described. Zero-order release kinetics may be more easily achieved with slab or rod geometries than spheres. The rate of release from spheres may result from polymer diffusion or erosion. Diffusion-mediated release has been studied extensively and described mathematically. The internal structure of microspheres may vary as a function of the microencapsulation process employed. Reservoir microcapsules have a core of drug coated with a polymer. The drug is distributed homogeneously throughout the polymeric matrix in monolithic microspheres.

Controlled drug release from microspheres occurs by diffusion of drug through a polymeric excipient, diffusion of entrapped drug as the polymer erodes, and release of drug through pores in the polymeric microspheres. If the drug is released by diffusion through the polymer without erosion, the release depends on the surface area of the microspheres and the path length of the drug in transit to the surrounding environment. For example, increasing the surface area, by reducing particle size, results in an increased release rate. The path length of motion for the drug in the matrix can be controlled by manipulating the microsphere loading. Microspheres with a high drug content release the active ingredient more rapidly than those with a low load. Physicochemical properties of the drug and excipient such as permeability of one in the other, identity of the polymer, degree of crystallinity, inclusion of plasticizers and fillers, and thickness of the polymer influence the drug release rate.

Release from reservoir microcapsules

The factors affecting drug release may be elucidated by a study of drug release from the simplest system, a reservoir microcapsule. Diffusion of drug through such a structure may involve transport not only through an isotropic medium, such as the drug in solution, but also through a polymeric membrane. Transport of drug through such a membrane involves dissolution of the drug in the polymer at the high-concentration side of the membrane interface and diffusion across the membrane in the direction of decreasing concentration. In addition, the concentration difference across the membrane, which is taken as the driving force for drug transport, tends to decrease as the solubility of the drug on the upstream side of the membrane decreases. Therefore, the dissolution rate of poorly soluble the thermodynamic activity of the core material is maintained constant within the device, and the coating is inert, homogeneous, and of uniform thickness. The steady-state release rate derived from Fick's law is

$$\frac{dM}{dt} = 4DKC\frac{r_0 \cdot r_i}{r_0 - r_i} \qquad \ldots(1)$$

where r_0 and r_i are the outside and inside radii, respectively, D is the diffusion coefficient of the drug molecule, K is the partition coefficient, and C is the concentration difference between either side of the coating. Assuming all parameters on the right side of Eq. (1) remain constant, consistent with no change in activity of the core material, C does not change. Integration of Eq. (1) over a finite period of the steady state would indicate that the drug release was zero-order. This is explained by the pathlength and surface area remaining constant since the membrane the drug has to traverse is of uniform thickness. If, however, the thermodynamic activity of the core material does not remain constant, then release is first-order.

It may be necessary to consider the effect of a boundary layer on the release rate. A boundary layer of appreciable drug concentration on the surface of the device would hinder drug release by diffusion. The effect of the layer is more marked with drugs of low solubility and with microparticles having irregular surfaces. From this simple example, it can be seen that various factors affect the release rate from reservoir microcapsules.

Release from monolithic micromatrices

In a monolithic microsphere the path length does not remain constant, since the drug in the center has a longer path to travel than the drug near the surface, and therefore the rate of release decreases exponentially with time. Nevertheless, monolithic microspheres can be made to release drug at an approximately constant rate. The core loading of these microspheres may be increased to create structures similar to those of reservoir micro-capsules. An optimum combination of particle sizes (a size distribution), may be prepared to achieve a constant rate of drug release. Preparing microspheres with an erodible polymer in such a way that maximum erosion occurs in conjunction with minimum diffusion may establish a constant release rate. Although the principles described here appear simple, they are difficult to utilize because of their dependence on a number of factors, each of which can complicate the process.

Live-Cell Encapsulation

Microcapsules have been investigated as potential artificial cells and as a means to immobilize live cells. Potential medical applications of artificial cells have been investigated such as artificial liver, artificial kidney, and red blood cell substitutes. The encapsulation of living cells has been investigated as a means to transplant tissues without immune rejection. The capsule membrane must be semipermeable in order to be impermeable to high molecular weight antibodies, which would cause rejection or destruction of the transplanted cells, but be permeable to lower molecular weight species such as oxygen, nutrients, and internally generated therapeutic agents (for example, hormones such as insulin). The encapsulation process must not be harmful to the cells and therefore must not involve harsh conditions, such as those caused by the use of organic solvents and heat during processing. The finished microcapsules must be sterile, stable, and biocompatible. The encapsulation of mammalian cells is more difficult than that of microbial cells since their membranes are more fragile, and these must be preserved during encapsulation. The temperature, pH, ionic strength, and toxicity of solvent and reagent must be carefully controlled. A common method of micro- encapsulating live cells is to entrap the cells in a protective gel and form a permanent membrane around the gel droplets. A calcium alginate gel method was developed by Lim and Sun, has been successfully applied to mammalian cells. A microencapsulation system combining the easy setting characteristics of alginate and the stability and biocompatibility of hydrogel polymers has been devised; it involves an alginate-HEMA graft copolymer.

Immobilized islets of Langerhans are able to respond to external glucose concentrations and release insulin into the systemic circulation. A number of animal studies have shown that alginate-polylysine encapsulated pancreatic islets were successful in correcting the diabetic state in rats for periods of two to three weeks. Immobilized cells are also used in biotechnology in the production of protein molecules. For example, entrapped hybridoma cells have been used for the production of monoclonal antibodies which are secreted into the microcapsules. This allows for easier collection of the antibodies compared to growing the hybridoma cells directly in the culture medium. The microcapsules are easily separated from the culture medium and broken to collect the antibodies. Isolation of the antibodies from the culture medium involves numerous purification steps, and product is lost during each of these steps to an extent which depends on the efficiency of the process. Live vaccines have been encapsulated. For example. Bacillus Calmette Guerin has been encapsulated in an alginate polylysine-alginate system.

Sterilization

Microspheres that are administered parenterally must be sterile. Sterilization is usually achieved by aseptic processing. The final product may not be able to undergo terminal sterilization, which may be detrimental to the delivery system, altering the release pattern or destroying the targeting properties. In addition, the entrapped drug or biological substance may not be able to withstand the heat of sterilization. Although the exterior of the microspheres can be investigated for sterility by conventional plating methodology, it is difficult to determine whether the interiors of the microspheres are free from contamination. The microspheres can be broken, although this introduces the possibility of false positive or false negative results. A method has been developed whereby the presence of viable organisms in the interior of microsphere systems can be determined without breaking the microcapsules using a detection method for organism metabolism. Sterilization is one of many aspects that must be addressed when considering microspheres for commercial purposes. The development of a product is achieved most effectively by parallel approaches to formulation and process design. Very little has been published with regard to industrial-scale manufacturing of microspheres for the delivery of pharmaceuticals.

3

HAZARDOUS CHEMICALS AND PHARMACEUTICALS

Over the last few years, legislation on the safety of chemical substances for humans and for the environment has been completed. Chemicals manufactured, imported and, in any way, handled by pharmaceutical and chemical companies are covered by a number of laws, which have been reinforced at all national levels. The United States and European requirements differ in some ways as to the application of safety parameters, but a good reciprocal acceptance on safety data exists. The safety of chemicals is evaluated through a number of physicochemical, toxicological, and ecotoxicological studies standardized by the international evaluation agencies. Risk Assessment (RA) of these chemicals is performed based on such experimental data, the use of the chemical, and possible exposure to humans and the environment. In Europe, there is a long-standing harmonized system (since 1981) that evaluates the final classification and labeling of a chemical and the so-called new or existing chemicals. In the United States, chemical safety is regulated by the Toxic Substance Control Act (TSCA) and the Code of Federal Regulation (CFR), and is managed by the Environmental Protection Agency (EPA). The Food and Drugs Administration (FDA) focuses on the registration of novel drugs in the American market. One basic step of the approach for handling a hazardous chemical is its classification and subsequent labeling.

The classification is reported in the Safety Data Sheet (SDS), which is a tool that informs workers and operators about the possible hazards and risks related to the substance. The handling of hazardous chemicals must also observe the occupational exposure limits as well as medical advice rules, which provide first aid in case of accidental spillage or exposure to the chemical. To handle a hazardous chemical correctly, we need to know a lot about it [e.g., legislation that covers its handling, methods for testing the hazards and consequent risks for humans, possible efficacy (in case of Active Principle Ingredient, or API), epidemiological data, and classification and labeling]. Pharmaceuticals are substances intended for human therapy, but because they are internally handled during the manufacturing phases (production, formulation, packaging, etc.), concerns for the safety of workers and the environment arise.

In this article, we will go through the safety concepts that can be applied to a chemical substance to give the readers a general overview of the matter. The safety of hazardous pharmaceuticals is a field that can be included in this approach, and many suggestions or proposals regarding pure chemicals will be discussed. The term "*chemicals*" is used interchangeably with pharmaceuticals because all pharmaceuticals are, in essence, chemicals.

Legislation and Requirements

We will refer to two main approaches to the safety of new chemicals: that applied in the United States and that applied in Europe.

United States

The so-called premanufacturing notification (PMN) is regulated by the EPA through the TSCA, which has been in force since January 1, 1977. The notification process and the assessment system for new chemicals became operative in July 1979. All substances imported into the United States (including pharma intermediates, which are considered chemicals from a regulatory point of view) have to be listed in the TSCA Inventory of Chemical Substances, unless they are imported in low quantities for research and development (R&D) purposes. Requests for limited notifications may be accepted for the following types of products: new chemicals imported or produced in quantities of 1000 kg/year or less, new chemicals used for the production or processing of instant photographic or peel-apart film articles, and some polymers.

The PMN approach also applies for known substances destined for a significant new use. If the substance is on the list and it is still destined for the use shown (no SNUR), the production/importation can take place. If the substance is not listed, the PMN process is followed. The PMN must be presented at least 90 days before the production of the new substance. New substances presented with a PNM are added to the list only after a 90-day review period and after the producer has submitted the so-called Notice of Commencement (NOC) within 30 days of the start of production. The notifier is asked for the following information: Chemical Abstracts Service (CAS) number, chemical name, structural and molecular formulas, trade name, spectral analysis, type and percentage of impurities, and use. Initially, no experimental data are requested; but if valid data are available, they must be included. Existing chemicals (those already listed) can be classified and consequently handled based on criteria given by the Occupational Safety and Health Agency (OSHA) and the National Institute for Occupational Safety and Health (NIOSH).

Europe

The European procedure involves the conduction of a testing program (toxicology, ecotoxicology and physicochemical properties) based on the tonnage of the substance (annual or total production) to be notified in the European Union (EU) market. A final dossier containing all the data on safety, production, storage, handling, and disposal must be prepared. The dossier must also include a proposal for the classification and labeling of the test substance, along with an RA for humans and the environment. The levels of notification requested in Annexes VIIC, VIIB, and VIIA of EEC Directive 92/32 are to be considered standard programs (minor changes may be introduced depending on the physicochemical features of the substance); for subsequent levels, all the European Authorities must discuss and agree on the testing program to be carried out. The ecotoxicological profile of the substance from the previous level is obviously taken into account.

The EU Directive 67/548 and its latest amendment (EEC 92/32) consider "new" those chemicals not listed in European Inventory of Existing Chemical Substances (EINECS) and not belonging to the following categories for which specific community laws are in place: pharmaceuticals such as API, pesticides, cosmetics, biocides, and food additives. Exemptions may be obtained for products under R&D or for process-oriented R&D (PORD) products. Particular attention is paid to the use of animals in testing; a product already notified cannot undergo a new testing program, but the two applicants are obliged to share toxicology data. Existing chemicals are covered by specific regulations that set up a priority list system. Preparations are classified and labeled by adopting a theoretical approach based on the hazard of each single component as detailed in the European Directive 45/1999.

Testing on Chemicals

The actual evaluation of the possible hazards of chemicals and the risk to humans handling such chemicals is based on data obtained from animal studies. This approach is constantly under discussion in terms of the ethical use of animals and some difficulties in adapting animal data to humans. Thanks to years of research, a huge amount of data on chemicals already exists, and the availability of data banks means that it is easy to access. Nevertheless, many chemicals are still unclassified for safety, and much research still needs to be done. Over the last 3 or 4 years, some industry associations have launched programs focused on testing chemicals to cover the lack of safety information, namely ICCA and HPV initiatives. Furthermore, some theoretical new tools such as the family approach and the quantitative structure- activity relationship (QSAR) are now available. These approaches are now under validation processes, which hopefully will lead to their use for regulatory purposes. The current testing package, which checks the hazards of a chemical, consists of the following studies:

1. Oral, dermal, and inhalation acute toxicity testing.
2. Dermal and ocular irritation studies.
3. Skin sensitization studies.
4. Mutagenicity studies (basically Ames and chromosomal aberration).
5. Repeated dose toxicity (subacute and chronic) studies.
6. Reproductive and carcinogenicity studies.
7. Ecotoxicology studies for the environmental impact.
8. Studies to identify endocrine-disrupting chemicals.
9. Physicochemical profile.

The research program has a tiered approach starting from the acute profile up to the most important studies such as chronic toxicology, carcinogenicity, and reproductive studies.

At the end of the process, we will be able to classify the chemical substance and to understand which handling safety procedures are the most suitable.

The aim of the experimental studies is to determine a number of toxicological parameters that will serve as a basis in classifying a substance. The most important are:

1. LD50, the lethal dose that kills 50% of the treated animals; this is determined by acute studies.
2. The potential to be irritating to skin and eyes, and the sensitization effects.
3. The No Observed Adverse Effect Level (NOAEL) and the No Observed Effect Level (NOEL) determined by repeated dose studies.
4. Some intrinsic physicochemical properties that can lead to risks for humans or the environment.

Normally, those chemicals classified as highly toxic, highly sensitizing, carcinogenic, or affecting the reproductive/fertility field are considered very dangerous and very risky for humans, and special containment and safety procedures are required for them. In some cases, they are banned from the market or from use in chemical industries.

Classification and Labeling

The classification of a chemical substance is focused on three main areas: physicochemical properties, toxicology, and ecotoxicology. The next step is to label the substance based on the classification obtained. The label must include all necessary information to inform the users about the hazards of the substance.

Safety Data Sheet

The SDS is a document for users, which contains all the information on the substance. In particular, it provides information that is useful for the handling of chemicals. It is normally composed of a number of paragraphs focused on specific information.

Table 3.1.

Possible classification	*Letter*
Explosive	E
Oxidizing	O
Highly flammable	F
Extremely flammable	F^+
Toxic	T
Very toxic	T^+
Corrosive	C
Harmful	Xn
Irritant	Xi
Dangerous to the environment	N

Handling

The handling of hazardous chemicals or pharmaceuticals is a consequence of all the above-mentioned activities. It is obviously affected by different parameters that enter into the final evaluation. The first is the intrinsic hazard of the chemical. This is evaluated, as discussed, through a number of appropriate tests. However, the knowledge of such elements is not sufficient to calculate the risk of the chemical for humans. A simple rule says that the final risk is related to the exposure of the chemical to humans. This leads us to believe that handling is something that can considerably decrease the rate of exposure and, consequently, the risk. Low toxic substances with high exposure can be more dangerous than highly toxic substances with a low (or no) exposure. This means that handling/manipulation procedures are the key factor to reducing possible effects on workers or, if not applied correctly, to amplifying adverse effects on humans that can lead to very severe heath problems, especially after long exposures.

When approaching the problem, the first parameter that needs to be carefully evaluated is the possible route of exposure. Inhalation route related to the presence of thin powders is the most dangerous way of affecting the human body. This can cause respiratory problems in the lungs, or sensitizing problems, or, in worst cases, cancer of the lungs. The second route of exposure is, without doubt, the dermal route, through which local effects (irritation, dermatitis, and redness) or systemic effects (toxicity or sensitization) can be determined. The third route is the oral route, which is less common but causes high toxicity in case of accidental ingestion of the chemical. This route is used less among skilled company workers but maybe used in the public at large due to accidental reasons.

Compounds classified as harmful or toxic in these routes of exposure must be handled with specific procedures and Personal Protection Equipment (PPE) in almost all phases of their manipulation during chemical processes. Compounds classified as highly toxic, highly sensitizing, carcinogenic, or affecting the reproductive system should be used in sealed areas or closed systems with no possible exposure to humans by any route. Medical advice from the company medical doctor is required if any symptom appears within a few minutes after exposure, or in cases of considerable acute exposure.

The medical doctor is responsible for adopting all the suitable therapies based on the symptoms observed and in relation to the information written on the label of the chemical. Based on physicochemical testing, a different approach to the manipulation of the chemical is needed: this is more related to storage conditions than to the handling itself. Particular care must be taken with explosives, flammables, and oxidizing substances in terms of labeling, packaging, storing, and handling. Table 6 shows the containment/handling procedures based on the intrinsic characteristics of the substance.

Special handling provisions are foreseen for those chemicals classified as dangerous to the environment. Do not allow the substance to enter the drainage system, surface water, ground water, and soil. Therefore, storage must be severely controlled. The release of the substance in the environment is severely banned and reference to local/national rules/laws must be followed. All residuals from empty containers and cleaning of reactors must be stored, well labeled, and disposed of by specialized waste disposal companies. Incineration is normally suggested as the best method of disposal. The amount of waste must be controlled and kept to a minimum. All substances classified as highly toxic, highly sensitizing, carcinogenic, or affecting the reproductive system must be used in a sealed area or in a closed system in the chemical plant to avoid any possible exposure to humans. If the chemical plant has some weak points where a possible leakage or exposure could occur, all the PPE must be available.

Occupational Exposure Levels

The so-called Occupational Exposure Level (OEL) is a key parameter for people responsible for the safety issues in pharmaceutical and chemical industries. The assessment and the application of the OEL are particularly important also for hazardous pharmaceuticals that are routinely handled within the pharmaceutical companies. There are different approaches to determine the OEL of a certain chemical and its relation to the handling/use of the substance. We are oriented to applying a tiered approach, which assesses all possible parameters that compose the hazard evaluation of a chemical substance.

Such a tiered approach is carried out in different phases:

Phase I: Identify NOEL–NOAEL in animal studies and also the possible effects in healthy human beings; kinetics/absorption data are also important.

Phase II: Find out all occupational toxicology data from available sources, treating the route of exposure as highly significant.

Phase III: Identify available epidemiological data (post-marketing surveillance and industrial hygiene).

Phase IV: Apply suitable and good safety factors.

Phase V: Calculate OEL using the following formula: (see equation above).

The final calculated value of the OEL will be considered during all procedures involving the chemical, in particular the possible human exposure consequent to its handling and use. As we realize from the information provided in this article, the handling of hazardous chemicals and pharmaceuticals is a process involving many different areas of expertise. A company that intends to adopt a serious policy concerning the safety of their compounds (raw materials, intermediates, or bulks/API) needs to set up a multidisciplinary team with experts in pharmacology (for efficacy and epidemiology data), industrial toxicology (for classification), medicine (in relation to health), and management (in relation to legal responsibility in case of accidents). The key area is clearly industrial toxicology because of its capacity to interpret toxicological data derived from various experimental activities and its use for safety. The presence of an industrial toxicologist is common in large organizations, but infrequent in small/medium companies where safety issues will become a problem in the near future. The last step that is becoming more and more requested by competent authorities in terms of chemical safety is the preparation of a final RA on the basis of the intrinsic hazard features of the studied chemical, its use, and its possible exposure to humans. The final RA evaluation will give us the index of possible risk for humans and the containment measures to be adopted when the risk is too high. The handling of substances classified as highly toxic, highly sensitizing, carcinogenic, or affecting the reproductive system should be kept to a minimum and, in some cases, banned if replacement is possible.

4

Use of Pharmacophores in Predictive ADME

The earliest proposed definition of the term '*pharmacophore*' was made by Ehrlich, who defined it as the molecular framework that carries (phoros) the essential features responsible for a drug's (pharmacon) biological activity. More-recent definitions of what a pharmacophore entails have been proposed by various researchers; many of these newer definitions can be found in the first published book on pharmacophores. Today, elucidation of the pharmacophore is considered as one of the most-important first step towards understanding ligand–target interaction, and hence pharmacophore-modeling methodology is widely used in drug discovery research as an aid in the early identification of new chemical entities.

The pharmacophore concept derives its coinage from an intuitive perception of which chemical functional entities are important in ligand–target recognition, especially where no information about the structure of the native or bound receptor or protein target is available to researchers. Until recently, the pharmacophore concept has been mostly applied to ligand-based approaches in drug discovery research. Today, increasing advancements in high-throughput crystallography, NMR imaging techniques, and protein-modeling tools have significantly increased the number of protein structures available to researchers, concomitantly elevating application of the pharmacophore concept to protein-guided drug discovery research.

As mentioned earlier, pharmacophore modeling has been mostly applied to the discovery of new lead candidates in the absence of target structural information. Much less use of this approach has been applied to candidate evaluation for clinical viability, i.e., use of pharmacophore models as predictive tools for understanding the ADME properties and potential toxicities of new lead candidates. The earliest pioneering studies of pharmacophore modeling of cytochrome P450 enzyme inhibition and/or substrate specificity were described by Wolff et al., Meyer et al., Islam et al., Koymans et al., Jones et al., and Mancy et al. The models derived in these earlier studies were qualitative with no predictive ability, yet provided significant insights into substrate specificity or ligand inhibition for cytochrome P450 mediated metabolism.

Predictive pharmacophore-based 3D-QSAR models of substrates and inhibitors of some cytochromes P450 have been reported by Mancy et al., Ekins et al., and de Groot et al. These studies applied pharmacophore-modeling methodology to investigate drug–drug interactions mediated by several cytochrome P450 metabolism enzymes, e.g., CYP2D6, CYP1A2, CYP3A4, and CYP2C9.

Predictive ADME Models Derived by Pharmacophore Modeling

CYP Enzymes

As a rule, metabolism increases the aqueous solubility of a drug such that it is easily excreted from the body. Such metabolism is mediated by a host of CYP enzymes, notably CYP2D6, CYP3A4, CYP1A2, and CYP2C9. Out of the ca. 20% of all relevant CYPs known to date, the 3A4 subsystem accounts for ca. 50% of CYP metabolism, 2D6 accounts for ca. 30%, while 1A2, 2C9, 2C10, 2C19, and 2E1 account for the remaining 20%. Since eukaryotic CYPs are membrane-bound proteins, crystal-structure information has been difficult to obtain. The first reported structure of a CYP enzyme was reported for CYP51 from *Mycobacterium tuberculosis* (MTCYP51) recently appeared in the literature. Recently, Williams et al. reported a crystal-structure determination of the human CYP2C9 enzyme with bound warfarin. Prior to these two reports, a number of homology models of CYP-dependent enzymes were generated to aid research efforts dedicated to the study of drug–drug interactions and drug metabolism involving the CYP enzyme subtypes.

There are vast amounts of in vitro and in vivo CYP data available in the public domains that are suitable for use in molecular-modeling studies. Data exists for 1A1, 1A2, 1B1, 2A6, 2B6, 2C9, 2C19, 2D6, and 3A4. With the large amount of data generated for substrate specificity or inhibition of these enzymes, studies involving in silico model development for predicting drug–drug interactions and drug metabolism have become very important. Applications of pharmacophore modeling techniques for evaluating ligand requirements for specificity and/or inhibition of the CYP enzymes have recently been summarized. The studies described below expand on this previous review and includes recent work, which employed the pharmacophore concept to elucidate difficult information on predicting potential drug–drug interactions and drug metabolism.

CYP2B6

The CYP2B6 enzyme represents <0.2% of total human hepatic CYPs, yet it plays a very prominent role in the metabolism of many xenobiotics. There is no crystal-structure information for this enzyme due to its membrane-bound nature, but the residues believed to be responsible for enzyme interaction were deduced from a homology model of a rat CYP2B1 aligned with P450-BM3. This homology model allowed researchers to deduce that substrate specificity for the CYP2B6 enzyme may involve π-stacking interactions among the side chains of Phe^{181} and/or Phe^{263}.

The earliest study of pharmacophore modeling of ligands with potential specificity or inhibition of the CYP2B6 enzyme was reported by Ekins et al. The study involved two different statistical methods using a pharmacophore-based 3D-QSAR modeling package available within the Catalyst software, and a partial-least-squares (PLS)-based approach termed MS-WHIM, or molecular surface weighted holistic invariant molecular modeling technique. For the pharmacophore-based study, 16 compounds were selected as training set for model generation. Conformations of each compound were sampled within 20 kcal/ mol energy threshold, with a maximum number set to 255. Biological activity data in the form of K_i, the kinetic rate constant for enzyme inhibition, was used as input data for the QSAR model generation. For substrate binding to the CYP2B6 enzyme, the pharmacophore hypothesis identified four geometric binding features-three hydrophobic features and one H-bond acceptor at distances of 5.3, 3.1, and 4.6 A. The

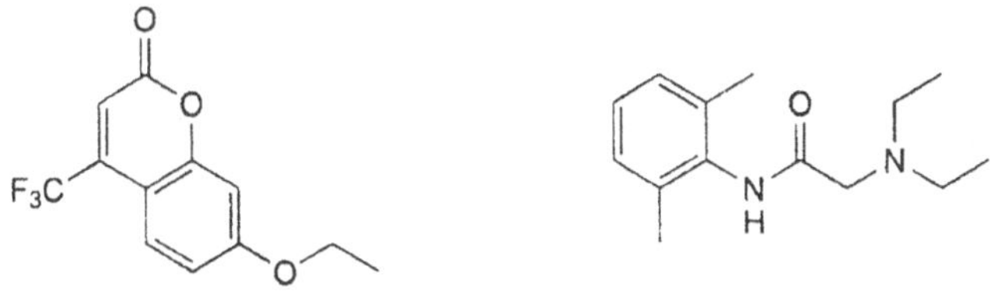

7-Ethoxy-4-(trifluoromethyl)coumarin Lidocaine

Fig. 4.1. Examples of CYP2B6 substrates used in the pharmacophore model generation study: 7-ethoxy-4-irifluoromethylcoumarin and lidocaine.

pharmacophore model was shown to correlate the variations in the biological activities of training-set compounds as a function of the geometric features in the model. The model was used to predict the activities of four test compounds, and the estimated activities were within 1 log unit with r = 0.85. In general, some agreement was found between the Catalyst pharmacophore model for substrate binding to CYP2B6, and the active-site characterization of a homology model of CYP2B6 reported by Lewis and Lake.

CYP2C9

Pharmacophore perception of substrate specificity and active-site characterization of the CYP2C9 enzyme is the second-most investigated of the CYP enzymes. The first study involving a pharmacophore-based elucidation of requirements for substrate specificity for a CYP metabolism enzyme was conducted by Jones et al. Using a manual pharmacophore mapping of the active site of a homology model of CYP2C9, these workers suggested that the active site is dominated by H-bond interaction features. A follow-up study involving alignment of eight substrates and one inhibitor implicated a H-bond donor heteroatom situated at a distance of ca. 7 Å from the catalytic site. Mancy et al. identified a similar inter-feature distance (ca. 7.8 Å) between an anionic site and a hydrophilic site for tight substrate binding to CYP2C9 based on manual superposition of 20 substrates of the enzyme. This study corroborated earlier findings reported by Jones et al. with regard to the geometric features required for substrate binding to CYP2C9, as well as the location constraints between these features.

An extension of this work to sulfaphenazoles confirmed findings that strong ligand–CYP2C9 binding involves hydrophobic interactions as well as a cationic functional group, which can be represented as a positive ionizable N-atom. The studies conducted by Jones et al. and Mancy et al. provided the first glimpse into geometric features responsible for substrate binding to the CYP2C9 enzyme. However, the models generated from these studies were qualitative with no predictive ability. The first predictive pharmacophore model for estimating binding affinities for the CYP2C9 enzyme was reported by Ekins et al., using the Catalyst/Hypogen program. The dataset was partitioned into three training sets to build models that would identify the requisite geometric functional groups responsible for the substrate specificity of the enzyme. Each training set was subjected to a pharmacophore-modeling run, and results were compared against each other. Each model differed from the other and contained different combinations of requisite binding features. All models implicate at least one hydrophobic group and one H-bond acceptor function as an important feature for binding to the enzyme, with the location of a H-bond donor at 3.4-5.7 Å from a neighboring H-bond acceptor.

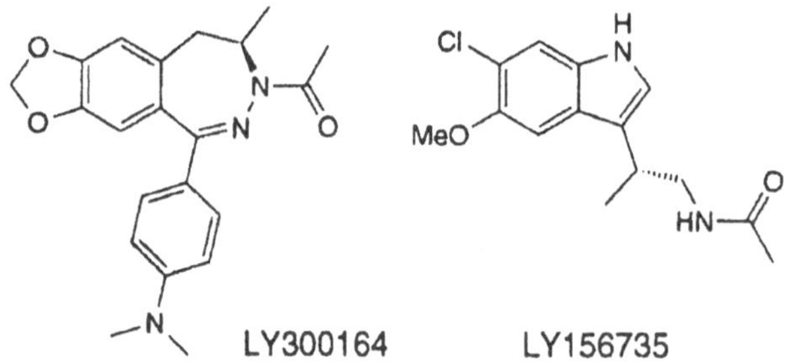

LY300164 LY156735

Fig. 4.2. Examples of compounds used in the pharmacophore modeling of inhibitors of CYP2C9.

The pharmacophore models for inhibition of the CYP2C9 enzyme derived using Catalyst/Hypogen was found to be in good agreement with a CoMFA analysis of a collection of 27 CYP2C9 compounds, which identified two cationic sites, an aromatic group, and a steric region as important to substrate recognition by the CYP2C9 enzyme. Additionally, Ekins et al. employed a PLS-optimized MS-WHIM technique against the same dataset, and the sets of QSAR models obtained from this approach were found to contain chemical descriptors, which were internally consistent with chemical functional groups identified in the Catalyst/ Hypogen pharmacophore model. As mentioned earlier, a new crystal structure of human CYP2C9 has been reported, and it is hoped that this will spur additional structure-based investigation of inhibitors and substrates for this enzyme.

CYP2D6

Earliest reports of small molecule based computational models for inhibition or substrate specificity for this enzyme were based on manual alignments of a variety of substrates or inhibitors of this enzyme. These models were found to be inconsistent in rationalizing substrate specificity requirements for this enzyme. Later studies conducted by Islam et al. using information from related crystal structure of CYP101 and by Koymans et al. provided a more-detailed picture of substrate specificity for this enzyme.

A pharmacophore model for inhibition of CYP2D6 was derived using a template of six strongly reversible inhibitors of the enzyme. The two most-important geometric features in the pharmacophore model were a positive ionizable N-center (protonated at physiological conditions), and an aromatic hydrophobic group. The presence of a H-bond interaction was also linked to enhanced inhibitory potency. This inhibitor-based model consisting of a tertiary N-center, an aromatic hydrophobic group, where enhanced inhibitory potency is observed with inclusion of H-bond interactions, and another aromatic hydrophobic site, which plays no role in inhibitory potency, compared favorably with the substrate specificity models reported by others. It is of note that the model for substrate specificity derived by these workers was used to successfully design a novel and selective CYP2D6 substrate and to investigate the hydroxylation of debrisoquine.

More recently, de Groot et. al. reported a combined pharmacophore/homology modeling study of the CYP2D6 enzyme. The study identified two pharmacophore models: one for O-dealkylation and oxidation reactions, and another for CYP2D6-catalyzed N-dealkylation reactions. The latter model correctly predicted the metabolism of a wide range of compounds.

Predictive 3D/4D-QSAR pharmacophore-based models for competitive inhibition of CYP2D6 were also reported by Ekins et al. The first model was generated from an in-house dataset of 20 inhibitors of bufuralol-1′-hydroxylation. The correlation coefficient (r) for estimated activities (K_i) of the training set compounds was 0.75. A second model was derived using 31 compounds from the literature. The observed correlation coefficient for estimated activities (K_i) was 0.91. Both models correctly estimated activities (K_i) of 9–10 of 15 test compounds. Fukushima et al. also employed the Catalyst/Hypogen program to generate predictive models for ligand inhibition of CYP2D6. In the study, four pharmacophore models were generated from training and test sets derived from either published data or in-house data. Predictive models were built with input of four chemical features defined for the Hypogen program–hydrophobe, H-bond donor, H-bond acceptor, and a basic amine.

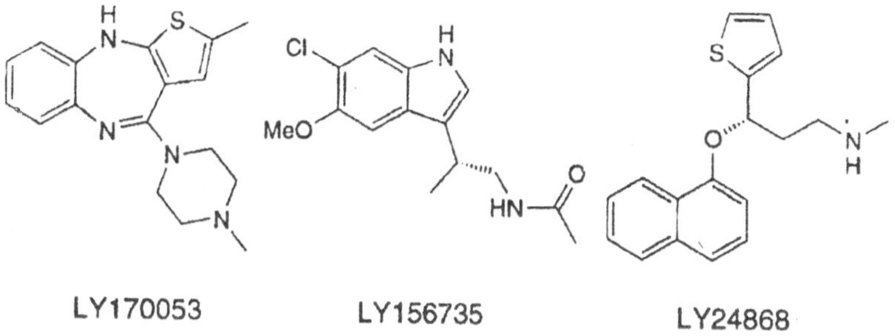

LY170053 LY156735 LY24868

Fig. 4.3. Examples of inhibitors of CYP2D6 used to generate the 3D pharmacophore model for enzyme inhibition.

The latter feature was used in place of a positive ionizable feature, since most CYP2D6 inhibitors are basic compounds, and it is not clear what the functional form of such feature is. Interestingly, all four pharmacophore models generated contained the basic amine function as a required feature for enzyme inhibition, along with one or more hydrophobic groups and a H-bond donor group. The four models correctly estimate activities of ca. 60% of a test set of 41 compounds. Poor estimated activities were obtained for (a) compounds with aromatic nitrogen groups, which can act as a heme chelator, (b) compounds containing basic functional groups other than amines, and (c) compounds with poor fits to any of the four pharmacophores generated in the study.

CYP3A4

This enzyme is important in the metabolism of many classes of drugs and can be described as the most-significant human CYP enzyme involved in drug metabolism. A homology model of the CYP3A4 enzyme derived from soluble bacterial CYP structures as templates found that the active site of this enzyme is likely dominated by hydrophilic groups, but includes H-bond donor/acceptor features. In addition, the homology model suggested a conformationally flexible active site, which is believed to account for the wide range of structurally diverse ligands that interact with this enzyme.

Three sets of pharmacophore-modeling experiments of ligand requirements for CYP3A4 inhibition were performed by Ekins et al. The first run consisted of inhibitors of CYP3A4-mediated midazolam-1′-hydroxylase. The pharmacophore model derived for this class of ligands contained four chemical functional requirements – three hydrophobic centers and a H-bond acceptor, located 5.2–8.8 Å apart. The model had a correlation coefficient of 0.91 between observed and estimated activities (K_i). The second pharmacophore experiment was conducted on ligands that competitively inhibit CYP3A4-mediated cyclosporin A metabolism. The model derived for this class of compounds contained five chemical functional requirements – three hydrophilic centers and two H-bond acceptor groups. As a predictive tool, the model had a correlation coefficient of 0.77, between observed and estimated activities (K_i). The third pharmacophore model experiment was conducted on data from inhibition (IC50) of CYP3A4-mediated quinine hydroxylation. The derived model contained four feature types – one hydrophobic center and three H-bond acceptors. The correlation coefficient between observed and estimated activities was 0.92.

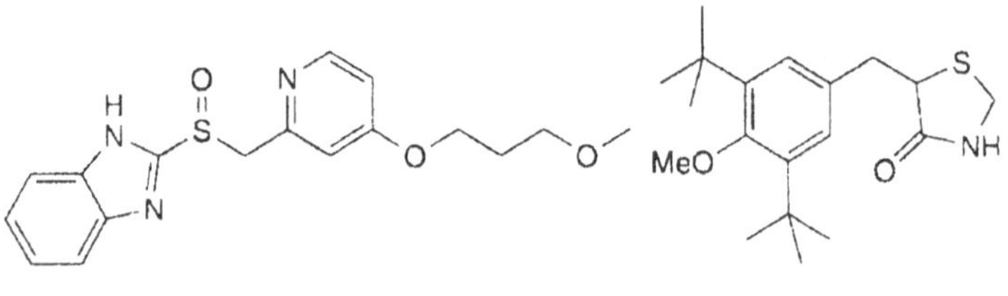

LY307640 LY213829

Fig. 4.4. Examples of competitive inhibitors of CYP3A4 used for generating a pharmacophore model for the enzyme.

Comparing the two pharmacophore models generated using K_i data showed strong similarities in location and type of chemical features. The merged model identified the critical requirements for CYP3A4 inhibition: two hydrophobic regions separated by H-bond acceptor groups. Another study to evaluate requirements for substrate specificity for CYP3A4 enzyme was conducted using a dataset of 38 known substrates of the enzyme. The pharmacophore model so derived contained four geometric features – two hydrophobic centers, one H-bond donor, and one H-bond acceptor group. Although the correlation coefficient of the difference between observed and estimated K_m was poor ($r = 0.67$), predicted activities for 12 test compounds were well within an order of magnitude of their observed activities. Both the inhibition model and the substrate-binding model had a level of commonality with presence of at least one H-bond-acceptor feature. This finding supports information derived from the homology model of CYP3A4 which implicated interaction with Asn^{74} in both substrate binding and ligand inhibition processes.

CYP51

The enzyme 1 4α-lanosterol demethylase (CYP51) is widely distributed in various biological species as the major sterol 14-demethylase. This enzyme catalyzes the removal of the 14α-methyl group of lanosterol in the biosynthesis of ergosterol. Inhibition of CYP51 across many species is believed to lead to undesirable side-effects, and hence a need for very selective drugs against this enzyme is desired.

Several reports have shown that azole-based antifungal agents inhibit CYP51. A number of these antifungal agents block ergosterol biosynthesis depleting its availability while causing excessive accumulation of lanosterol and other 14-methylsterols. A recent pharmacophore-based investigation of derivatives of 1-[(aryl)[4-aryl-1H-pyrrol-3-yl}- methyl]-1H-imidazole by Tafi et al. identified the following geometrical features required for CYP51 inhibition: (a) an aromatic N-atom with an accessible lone pair, (b) a di(arylmethyl) moiety at the azole N(1) position, (c) a second aryl group containing two coplanar aromatic rings. The alignment of these geometrical features with the template antifungal agent and the most-active ligand in the dataset used for the study. Similar pharmacophoric features were identified in the 4D-QSAR study reported by Hopfinger and co-workers.

Although current understanding of the influence of CYP enzymes in drug metabolism is well known and characterized, there remain areas that research has yet to shed light on. Questions such as (a) to what extent a given drug will induce or inhibit a specific CYP enzyme, or (b) to what extent are specific CYP enzymes responsible for drug metabolism of specific drugs remain unanswered. Thankfully, research to shed light into these areas is ongoing. Recent reports indicate that clinical efficacy of a drug as a function of ADME-Tox properties has undergone some dramatic change in the past decade. Failures associated with poor ADME profiles of lead drugs have reduced from ca. 50% of all clinical candidates to ca. 10%. Conversely, challenges of drug selectivity and toxicities have increased from ca. 10% of all drug failures to ca. 20%, becoming one of the most-problematic areas requiring solution today. This chapter has attempted to provide an overview of the new paradigm, which leverages recent advances in computational algorithms and increased experimental data, to address these problems. Ekins et al. have proposed a workflow, where computational chemistry plays a central role in building virtual filters that can be applied to large virtual or real chemical libraries to eliminate ligand candidates that may potentially act as substrates or inhibitors for many of the drug metabolism enzymes. The pruned outputs from these in silico filters can be used to further refine these models to make them even better in clinical candidate evaluation. In closing, clinical efficacy of lead candidates can also be improved if (a) the candidate can be metabolized by more than one CYP enzyme, (b) its metabolism is not dependent on a CYP enzyme with a significant genetic polymorphism, and (c) the candidate does not significantly inhibit any of the CYP enzymes that mediate oxidative pathways of drug metabolism, i.e., 3A3/4, 2D6, 1A2, 2C19, and 2C9/10. Drug candidates meeting all of these conditions have a greater chance of making it through the clinic and ultimately into commercial viability.

5

Clinical Practice

The discipline of pharmaceutical medicine has borrowed for itself the principal element in the scientific foundation of therapeutics - the controlled randomised clinical trial - because new medicines must be proven to be therapeutically effective and safe before being licensed for prescription in clinical practice. Indeed, the precise regulatory requirements on evidence needed for a product licence (marketing authorisation) stimulated pharmaceutical companies to adopt existing principles and procedures for evaluating medicines and, more significantly, to develop and refine them. As a consequence, a high proportion of therapeutic research is nowadays not only sponsored by pharmaceutical companies, but their staff contribute greatly to the design, conduct, analysis and reporting of clinical trials. Pharmaceutical and biotechnology companies, although sponsors of a clinical trial, may decide to contract part or the whole of a clinical trial to a contract research organisation (CRO), in which case the obligations placed on the CRO staff are the same as those placed on the staff from the pharmaceutical company. The responsibility and accountability upon clinical and scientific staff is codified in regulations and guidelines clearly stating the sponsor's and investigator's obligations. There is also a statutory requirement for complete and accurate information on all human exposure to a new medicine to be provided in a marketing licence application for a new medicinal product. Thus, the improved standards of therapeutic research owe much to these regulations and to the efforts to fulfil them. Pharmaceutical medicine not only borrowed the clinical trial, but in many ways has made it the fundamental tool of drug evaluation.

Concept of the Controlled Clinical Trial

The concept of the clinical trial is relatively recent. It stemmed in part from the availability of more effective treatment modalities in the last 50 years or so. The main stimulus arose from the recognition of the possibility that by chance a patient's spontaneous improvement could coincide with the administration of a remedy and that this recovery could be attributed to the remedy when in fact the remedy was valueless. Therefore, some structured approach was necessary.

Efforts to evaluate different treatments began in the 1930s. The design of these early clinical trials leaned heavily on agricultural experiments, where randomisation had been employed to reduce bias by confounding factors (soil characteristics, moisture, sun, wind) and to reduce observer bias. This work by RA Fisher in the 1930s led many, including Sir Austin Bradford Hill, to adopt similar experimental designs in clinical trials. These really took on greatest importance in the 1940s and the "British trial" evolved and was widely acknowledged as a template in clinical trial methodology. The other fundamental reason for organising clinical trials before a new medicine is licensed for wide-spread clinical use is that the effects of the medicine must be thoroughly assessed in patients with the illness that it is intended to treat. Because the response varies between individual patients and is affected by the situations in which the medicine is used, it is desirable to evaluate the medicine in groups of patients who represent a range of circumstances and to deduce from these trials the overall response. The word "control" means that the potential new medicine under investigation is compared with a "control" group. The control may be placebo, no treatment, active control or different doses of the drug under investigation.

Types of Clinical Trial

Clinical trials should be conducted and analysed according to sound scientific principles, with due regard to ethical considerations, in order to achieve the trial objectives. Trials must be reported fully and objectively, and results must be accessible to those who need them. Clinical trials as part of drug development aiming towards marketing authorisation must ask important questions and be designed to give answers that are as clear and unambiguous as possible. This is a tough challenge for an individual trial and more so for a complete clinical development programme.

There are a number of ways of classifying clinical trial designs. The most frequently used is according to the phases of clinical development. Clinical development is conventionally divided into four phases, which are a logical and progressive sequence of a continuous expanding process starting with very few subjects observed closely under laboratory conditions and proceeding into tens, hundreds and eventually thousands of patients as the licensing dossier is compiled. The concept in this classification is that results from one phase will inform the design of the next. The classical phases are:

1. *Phase I* Clinical pharmacology in small numbers (tens) of healthy non-patient (or patient) volunteers to assess tolerability, preliminary safety, pharmacokinetics, and pharmacodynamics where practicable (i.e. biological effect using surrogate endpoints [see later] or, rarely, therapeutic effect)
2. *Phase II* Frequently divided into IIa and IIb:
   (a) *IIa* Clinical pharmacology in patients with the target disease (small numbers - tens to 100-200) to assess pharmacodynamics, pharmacokinetics, and dose-(or concentration-) effect responses for preliminary efficacy and safety, and to validate surrogate endpoints
   (b) *IIb* Larger scale (several hundreds) trials in patients to formally assess the dose-response relationship and continue to expand the efficacy and safety databases
3. *Phase III* Formal therapeutic trials (randomised, controlled, in hundreds or thousands of patients) to determine efficacy and safety on a substantial scale; comparison with existing drugs; usually includes three or more doses of test drugs; usually international programme
4. *Phase IV* Postlicensing studies in the target population, with widening of entry criteria to broaden experience in clinical practice; study objectives may be marketing, further formal therapeutic and comparator trials and surveillance for safety.

Although the logic and simplicity of these divisions is appealing, drug development is rarely as straightforward as this account implies. There are interactions, overlaps between phases and often redundancy in the process. The use of population pharmacokinetic screening to investigate more extensively the plasma concentration-effect relationship, to establish the variability in dose response across different age ranges, disease states and ethnic groups, and to focus on sex differences, has been integrated into Phases II and III of many clinical development programmes. These so- called "*population approaches*" to assess variability in drug response and to refine the efficacy-safety relationships are complementing or replacing the "*special risk*" group trials.

A complementary approach, and one geared more to the construction of a regulatory application, is to classify the trial according to its objectives. Studies conducted for socioeconomic purposes are frequently included in a regulatory application, but may continue to be conducted during marketing. There has been an impetus for the manufacturer to include these data because negotiations on the pricing of a new medicine, particularly its reimbursement, and the evolution of managed healthcare mean that, at the time of product launch, the manufacturer needs to have some evidence of the value of the product in terms of quality of life of the patients and for the patients' healthcare costs. Therefore, in the later stages of product development and extending into the immediate postmarketing period, clinical studies are likely to incorporate pharmacoeconomic measures, either as a satellite programme or as an integral feature. There is a continuous debate on which clinical studies provide the best evidence, which, in turn, raises the question "evidence for what?" In broad terms evidence from clinical trials is required for five purposes:

1. To move a drug through a development programme
2. To gain marketing authorisation
3. To select one drug rather than another for addition to a therapeutic formulatory and inform a health policy
4. To treat the individual patient
5. To investigate specific aspects of the drug, for example incidence of an adverse event.

The debate about quality of evidence most frequently ranks large randomised controlled trials as the gold standard, at least for efficacy, with controlled observational studies in the middle, and uncontrolled studies and opinions at the bottom. The evaluation of therapeutic benefit and risk is, in fact, never ending because clinicians will subject marketed medicines to comparison with other existing or new medicines, and they will experiment with alternative dosage schedules and combined use with other treatments. Clinicians are not necessarily convinced by one comparative clinical trial, even though it is scrupulously designed, conducted and analysed and regulatory authorities require and expect specified numbers of randomised clinical trials (RCTs). The controlled clinical trial aims to demonstrate that an observed effect is not the result of chance. But statisticians will argue amongst themselves about the representative validity of evidence in a population sample, and most will broadly agree that it is often equivocal. Added to this uncertainty, clinicians realise that the clinical trial adopts a specific framework of study, subject selection and assessment, which may be different from routine clinical practice. Therefore, one clinical trial is one piece of evidence on therapeutic value. The medical community will judge it, both formally, for example by the UK's National Institute for Clinical Excellence (NICE) issuing guidelines, and informally, and decide whether one treatment is more suitable than another in a particular subject.

In common but serious and multifactorial diseases such as cancer or heart disease, even small treatment effects can be important in terms of their total impact on public health. To expect dramatic advances in these diseases may be unreasonable, and small effects should be sought. Thus, the classical dilemma is whether to identify a high-risk subject who has a significant chance of responding to a given drug, or to expose a large number of study subjects knowing that only some will respond, but without being able to predict response. Advances in pharmacogenetics are expected to assist in predicating individual subject responses. Amassing sufficient evidence to demonstrate small but valuable effects in wider populations from a number of trials uses the methods of systematic review; analysing the accumulated results using appropriate statistical methods is termed meta-analysis.

The principles of a meta-analysis are that:

1. It should be comprehensive, i.e. include data from all trials, published and unpublished
2. Only RCTs should be analysed, with study subjects entered on the basis of "*intention to treat*"
3. The results should be determined using clearly defined disease-specific endpoints.

There are strong advocates and critics of meta-analysis as a concept. Arguments advanced against it are as follows.

1. An effect of reasonable size ought to be demonstrable in a single trial.
2. Different study designs cannot be pooled.
3. There is a lack of accessibility to all relevant studies.
4. There is a publication bias (“*positive trials*”).

In the development of a new medicine the manufacturer controls the programme, and the structuring of the data from initial recording to electronic capture is decided by the sponsor. The meta-analysis of a series of clinical trials that share such commonality, would be easier. Rather than using as the unit of observation a single study or a subgroup of study subjects, collecting and merging data from the individual subjects could address not only the general benefits of a treatment, but the management of the individual subject.

Finally, a randomised comparative trial with one alternative marketed medicine can only address the choice between the two. Other comparative trials with other treatments build up a picture of overall therapeutic benefit and risk, and these trials may help to define groups of study subjects who differ in their response from the general population.

Observational Studies

A controlled clinical trial is an experiment and, as just mentioned, it deliberately alters the fabric of routine management of study subjects. It does so in two ways. First, it directs which treatment modality will be given to a particular subject, usually by randomised allocation without the doctor or subject knowing which treatment they will receive out of the two or three chosen for the trial. Therefore, a subject may not receive the conventional treatment that the clinician might otherwise have chosen. Second, the selection and investigation of subjects distorts routine clinical practice by excluding some subjects by virtue of certain characteristics, usually because of disease complications or other disorders or treatments that might make it difficult to distinguish the factor that really contributed to any improvement or deterioration. Thus, the selection of study subjects and the treatment allocation are fundamental features of a comparative clinical trial.

However, it is important, once the product is generally available, to identify if possible what is happening in routine medical practice and to do so without disturbing it. Ideally one wants to look down as if from a helicopter and to observe without intruding. More specifically, the decision to treat or not, and then the choice of treatment, must remain inviolate. The observational study is an important epidemiological (pharmaco-epidemiological) tool and in pharmaceutical medicine it can provide unique surveillance of a medicine's actual usage compared with its recommended usage, its clinical efficacy, and, in particular, its safety in those circumstances. The side-effects can be distinguished from untoward effects of the disease being treated, of other concomitant disorders and of effects caused by other medicines taken by the subject or by another cohort of subjects receiving an alternative remedy. Observational studies may be prospective as well as retrospective.

Global Implications

Researchers in the pharmaceutical industry have realised that there are limits to the availability of economic and human resources in the development of new drugs. The costs of research and development can only be recovered if the whole global market is used. However, this approach has, until recently, been difficult because of contrasting requirements for new drug application approvals from the key regulatory authorities of the three main regions. To register a new drug worldwide, the pharmaceutical companies were required to repeat studies just to satisfy different national requirements. Even within the requirements of Good Clinical Practice (GCP), several guidelines and regulations could apply to each individual country. Some guidelines would meet the requirements of the most rigorous regulatory agencies (for example, the US Food and Drug Administration [FDA]) but others relied on the investigator's interpretation of some vague recommendations. Drug regulatory harmonisation, such as that driven by the International Conference of Harmonisation (ICH) and in Europe by the new Clinical Trial Directive, has considerably reduced these national and regional variations. At present, the concept of the global dossier or common format for the preparation of the technical documents is being pursued. The dossier will contain sufficient information on the new drug to support product approval in most parts of the world. Needless to say, the concept of global studies cannot remove the ethnic variations in pharmacokinetics and pharmacodynamics, or social and dietary differences between regions. So called "*bridging studies*" may be required to allow extrapolation of "foreign" clinical data in a different region to that where the clinical development took place.

There are other advantages of conducting global studies. There may be a greater pool of suitable investigator sites and study subjects for a particular indication. The multicentre trial produces results faster by achieving quicker recruitment. It is also more likely to provide the critical power to the trial when trying to show small differences within acceptable confidence limits.

Whether the study is multicentre in one geographical region or truly global, it will require the utmost effort in planning. Frequently, two tiers of organisations are formed, one with the overall control of the study and one specifically relating to a particular district or country. Communication should be considered paramount in ensuring uniformity of procedures and the removal of local variations.

Good Clinical Practice (GCP)

The procedures for assuring quality of clinical trials have evolved over the past 30 years, culminating in several published guidelines. There are three key GCP documents - the GCP guidelines of the International Conference on Harmonisation of Technical Requirements for the Registration of Pharmaceuticals for Human Use (ICH), the Code of Federal Regulations (21 CFR) of the United States, and the Declaration of Helsinki. In today's global climate, the pharmaceutical physician should work to ICH GCP, of which the Declaration of Helsinki is the foundation.

Apart from a few minor differences, the FDA has adopted the ICH GCP guidelines. The contents of the FDA Code of Regulations with reference to the protection of human subjects, Institutional Review Boards and Investigational New Drug Applications provide information for new study drugs that will need to be registered in the US. Most potential new drugs will be marketed in the US in order to reap a financial return. Two other documents are relevant to clinical trials: the World Health Organisation (WHO) Guidelines for Good Clinical Practice for trials on pharmaceutical products, still used for clinical trials in some parts of the world, and the new EU Clinical Trial Directive,

Declaration of Helsinki

The principles of medical research are based on the Declaration of Helsinki. The general assemblies of the World Medical Association (WMA) have, since 1964, made recommendations for guiding physicians in clinical research involving human subjects. Although not legally binding, the Declaration forms the foundation of all other significant international documents on the ethical conduct of biomedical research.

The Helsinki Declaration covers all the important ethical considerations, such as the involvement of a qualified physician in any clinical trial, putting the well-being of the study subject before science and society, the use of scientific principles in the design of the study, the need for informed consent and a review by an ethics review committee; in fact, all areas covered by the ICH GCP.

In October 2000, the latest revision of the Declaration of Helsinki was approved by the WMA. The new version is very different from previous versions, with more detail on how clinical trials should be conducted. It requires that study subjects should have access to the best treatment identified by the study once the study has been completed. It also recommends that local participants in a study should be able to benefit from the study results, whether they are positive or negative. These principles were approved to avoid the exploitation of economically poor countries. In addition, the Declaration requires greater transparency regarding economic incentives involved in clinical research.

ICH GCP

In the middle part of the last century, drug development experienced several events that gave weight to greater harmonisation within countries initially, and then, internationally. In the US, a terrible mistake in the formulation of a children's syrup in the 1 930s forced the American government to initiate the creation of a product authorisation system under the FDA. The thalidomide tragedy in Europe alerted many regulatory authorities to the dangers as well as the benefits of new synthetic drugs. Safety considerations in addition to efficacy became paramount in new drug treatments. With the public expectation for new drugs to be both safe and effective came an escalation of the cost of research, and an ever- increasing healthcare bill for governments.

Global harmonisation was felt to be an acceptable solution in reducing costs by avoiding unnecessary duplication of clinical trials in humans and to minimise the use of animal testing. Hence in 1990, drug regulatory authorities of the EU, Japan and the US got together with representatives from the pharmaceutical industry to try to reach a consensus on the safety, quality and efficacy requirements authorising new medicinal products. This was the beginning of ICH.

At that time, the methodology for conducting clinical trials was very variable and there were a considerable number of guidelines from regions and countries relating to the conduct of clinical trials. Global directors of pharmaceutical companies would have a shelf full of the various versions of GCP guidelines, many of them country specific. With the advent of ICH GCP, a more uniform process of conducting clinical trials has been achieved globally. Many countries have modified the format of ICH GCP to the local conditions, but in general, the principles of ICH GCP have been observed.

EU directive

A new Directive has been authorised by the EU to cover clinical trials undertaken in the EU. Each country will be required to adopt the Directive by 01 May 2004. Before the Directive was approved, there were variations between EU countries both in the legal requirements and, in some cases, the actual procedures adopted for conducting clinical trials, some countries adopting more vigorous ethical and scientific methodologies than others. For example, the GCP inspectorate in the UK had to be "invited" to conduct most inspections since there was no legal basis for normal routine inspections. The Directive is designed to simplify and harmonise the administrative provisions governing trials and will apply to both commercial and non-commercial studies including healthy volunteers (Phase I) studies. Only non-interventional trials, where the assignment of the patient to a particular therapeutic strategy is not decided in advance by a protocol are excluded from the scope of the Directive. In non-interventional trials, the treatment of the subject falls within current practice and the prescription of the medicine is clearly separate from the decision to include the subject in the study. No additional diagnostic or monitoring procedures will be applied to the subject.

The Directive covers:

1. National authority approval
2. Study subject benefit and risk
3. The use of children and adults who are unable to give consent
4. Establishment of ethics committees in each member country
5. Establishment of inspectorates to verify GCP standards
6. European database to be set up for all member states with clinical trial information (to limit unnecessary trials)

7. Good Manufacturing Practices (GMP) for study drugs and the provision for a manufacturing licence for investigational medicinal products (IMPs), and labelling requirements
8. Pharmacovigilance standards
9. Gene therapy trials and xenogenic cell therapy.

Basic Ethical Considerations

The basic ethical questions of clinical research should never be underestimated. The pharmaceutical physician will need to be aware that failure, intentionally or because of misguided enthusiasm, to protect the health and well-being of each study subject can have very serious consequences. In an age where the medical profession is constantly under scrutiny, the drug industry is heavily criticised and the communication industry extremely active, mistakes in clinical trials are punished. Therefore, before a study is commenced, a review should be made that the scientific approach is current, the motivation is clear, the processes are unambiguous, and there should be sufficient data to judge the safety and effectiveness of the interventions proposed. There needs to be a clear distinction between *medical research* and *medical practice*. In medical practice, the sole intention is to benefit the *individual* patient who is consulting the clinician; it is not to gain knowledge of general benefit, although such knowledge may incidentally emerge from the clinical experience gained. In medical research the primary intention is to advance knowledge so that patients in general may benefit in the future; the individual study subject participating in research may or may not benefit directly.

Medical research is not the same as a medical experiment or, for that matter, innovative treatment. Medical research is a systematic series of related and controlled investigations to establish facts, to create general knowledge and to deduce principles. One experiment will rarely achieve that level of understanding. On the other hand, a *medical experiment* is a single procedure chosen with the hope and expectation of succeeding and with the aim of seeing what happens. The medical experiment needs in turn to be distinguished from *innovative treatment*, where a clinician selects for an individual patient a treatment that is outside conventional medical practice. The sole motive for innovative treatment is choosing the best possible course of action in the particular and unique clinical circumstances of the patient's illness. Unfortunately, innovative treatment can masquerade as medical research, especially as doctors apply the term loosely, and can evade the necessary constraints. If the purpose of the treatment is the acquisition of information for the benefit of future patients, especially if it is repeated, the treatment must be regarded as medical research and be subjected to the necessary controls. There is always a risk that a speculative new treatment or procedure will be adopted, especially where no treatment has previously been effective. This evasion of rigorous and critical testing can expose patients to suboptimal and even valueless treatment.

Clinical trials can be divided into those that may result in some benefit to the participant, and those trials where no benefit can conceivably be expected. The most obvious example of the latter is the trial involving the healthy non-patient subject. Such trials are frequently called non-therapeutic. Therefore, therapeutic studies are those from which the subject may derive benefit from exposure to the study drug. This is an oversimplification. For example, a Phase IIa dose-ranging study in study subjects with the target disease will include some doses which may be ineffective, or which prove to be too high. The length of the treatment may be too short and the design of the trial (for example, crossover design) may be inappropriate to determine a therapeutic response within the confines of the study. Thus, therapeutic trials tend to occur in the later stages of clinical development at Phases III and IV.

Clearly there is an ethical question as to whether the foreseeable risks and inconveniences to a study subject or patient participating in a clinical trial are outweighed by the anticipated benefits to that patient. Even more critical is the question of whether the risks being undertaken by the healthy volunteer are considered acceptable when the volunteer will not benefit medically.

Most people recognise the need for better medical treatments. However, there are many examples in modern history where the risks to the individual study subject have outweighed any benefit to either the subject or society. Society is rightly wary of medical research involving human study subjects.

Peer Review of Proposed Biomedical Research

Modern medical research expects the proposed procedures and protocols of clinical trials to be submitted for peer review and that the human study subjects involved are provided with trial information before freely consenting to participate in that clinical trial.

Modern review boards or independent ethics committees (IECs) are required to act on behalf of the community in deciding whether the proposed research is justified on ethical grounds. They also act on behalf of members of the community in ensuring that there are sufficient safeguards to protect those individuals who directly participate in the research, and, for both the study subjects and those not directly participating, that confidentiality of participant's medical information will be maintained.

The independence of the review board is an essential feature. It is felt that those initiating and performing medical research should not be the sole judges of whether the research conforms to accepted codes of practice and, furthermore, that scientific or medical colleagues, if arbitrating alone, cannot be entirely independent, even though they are not directly involved. As researchers we must recognise that fallibility in ourselves and in others. We all like to think that we fulfil our moral duty to other human beings, but ethical aspects can be easily overlooked, usually unwittingly, in our enthusiasm for the aims of the studies or, more commonly, in our commitment to the precise scientific design of the work planned. In the same way our conviction that the study is justified might lead us to understate risk, discomfort or inconvenience when inviting subjects to participate. We have already made our value judgement and if one adds in the tendency for clinicians to be paternalistic towards patients and for colleagues to exert some peer pressure on each other, it is evident that patients, colleagues and students might feel that they ought to "rally round". Today, an ethical review is an essential part of the biomedical research process. IECs provide ethical guidance on research protocols and ensure the protection of research participants. In the US, similar bodies called *institutional review boards* (IRBs) have a similar role to that undertaken by IECs in the rest of the world.

In Europe generally, considerable variation in composition and in procedures occurs between IECs. Membership frequently depends on individuals who are willing to give their time without payment. Also, suitable members for this type of review board often have limited time. The new Clinical Trial Directive should provide the incentive for greater uniformity. A single IEC will give an opinion on a multicentre study within 60 days. The preparation of the documentation for a review by the IEC should be of a high standard and the precise requirements of that particular committee followed.

Informed Consent

In all studies, informed consent should be sought from the subject or, where special situations occur, from his/her representative. The precise nature of this consent depends on the study design, procedure and the country where the study is being conducted. Increasingly, some clinical trials will involve study subjects that are mentally handicapped, children or subjects who, because of the medical condition (for example trauma or stroke), are unable to give proper consent. Under these circumstances, the IEC and the pharmaceutical physician need to provide a framework, with additional safeguards to the vulnerable subject.

ICH GCP provides detailed guidance on the information and structure of both the subject information sheet and the informed consent form (ICF). Some IECs provide alternative requests to the international requirements, perhaps in an effort to reduce the length of the information sheet or to simplify the information. Some pharmaceutical companies provide too much information, particularly with reference to possible adverse events, to provide (debatably) protection from litigation.

Essentially, the ICF must be a document that can be understood by the study subject. Where required, the ICF should be translated into the subject's native tongue. In addition, the informed consent process should never be purely a signing of a form. The investigator should discuss with the subject (or his/her representative) the contents of the information sheet/ICF before the ICF is signed. The investigator will need to have a clear understanding of the difference between providing information and offering advice to the subject. Where possible, the advice to the subject should normally come from the personal physician, if different from the investigator.

Notification to the general practitioner

Where Phase II, III and IV studies are conducted in a hospital or contract research environment, it is strongly advisable to inform the subject's general practitioner (GP) in writing of the nature of the study and to obtain the GP's agreement, preferably in writing. This is essential for Phase I studies in non- patient volunteers, and it is routine practice in all Phase I clinical pharmacology units. However, increasingly, particularly in mainland Europe, study subjects will be found not to have a personal physician or, if they have, that their last visit to the physician could be a considerable time ago.

It is also advisable to tell the study subject that the GP will be informed about the clinical trial. Difficulties occur when the clinical trial is for an indication of a socially unacceptable condition such as a venereal disease. Rightly or wrongly, the subjects have fear that knowledge of the illness may not be safe with the "family" doctor. In these exceptional circumstances, the IEC should decide whether the GP should be informed only with the agreement of the study subject.

Confidentiality

All information generated during the course of the study with regard to the subject's state of health is confidential, and the subject's agreement must be obtained before disclosure of such information to a third party. The actual name of the study subject should never appear on any documents relating to the clinical trial that leave the investigator's site and, as far as possible, the anonymity of the study subject must be maintained throughout any clinical trial. Normally, the study subject is informed both verbally and in the ICF that certain other individuals besides the investigator site staff will view his/her medical records. In clinical studies sponsored by pharmaceutical companies or institutions, the monitoring and quality assurance (QA) personnel from the sponsors and CROs, and inspectors from a regulatory agency will review the medical records of the study subject.

All the medical records of the subject should be available for comparison with the data recorded in the case report form (CRF). In the past, physicians have not allowed medical records to be available for the so-called "*source verification*" by non-physicians since they felt that this broke the strict confidentiality of the study subject's medical records. However, frequent mistakes in transferring important clinical data to the CRF, the recruitment of subjects who do not meet the inclusion and exclusion criteria, and the occasional blatant fraud has led to an insistence by sponsors and regulatory agencies for sponsor's review of study documentation. Indeed, verification of source data cannot take place without access to the medical records of the study subject by the sponsor's staff.

Modern clinical research requires considerable co-operation and partnership between the investigator, the sponsor and the regulatory authorities. In consequence, the investigator will need to treat certain "outsiders" with the same amount of trust that is shown to nursing staff and fellow physicians. Violations of confidentiality of subjects are rare from sponsor staff and certainly no more frequent than that experienced from hospital staff.

The ICF should provide sufficient information to the study subject to comply with the EU Directive on the protection of personal data. The ICF should provide information on which company or institution is sponsoring the study, the purpose of processing the clinical data, the categories of the recipients for whom the data may be disclosed, and an explanation of the right to access the data of the subject by the subject. If this EU Directive on the protection of personal data were to be taken literally, most clinical trials would cease, particularly where clinical data were transferred outside the EU. Of the non-EU countries, only Switzerland and Hungary apparently meet the requirements of the Directive at the present time! Other countries such as the US, Canada, Australia and New Zealand apparently fail to meet the requirements of the Directive when handling personal data and therefore, in theory, European data cannot be processed in these countries. Fortunately, the so-called "Safe Harbor" scheme allows clinical data to be sent to defined organisations in the US that comply with the Directive's principles. It is anticipated that similar agreements will be set up to overcome these legislative hurdles so that global studies driven by European pharmaceutical companies and institutions can be undertaken without problems.

Pharmacogenetics

With the advent of pharmacogenetics in drug development, genetic markers introduced at a very early phase may be used. For example, to assist in the prediction of variability in drug response, it may be feasible to measure expression of the mRNA or a protein level.

A good clinical trial is designed to take account of the variability in response (either efficacy or adverse event) that is expected when a new active is tested. This response depends on an individual's genetic make up, and on a number of environmental factors, such as disease state, other drugs, and age. The size of the trial and the selection of study subjects are carefully determined to reduce the variability in response to a minimum (i.e. to maximise the sensitivity of the trial) so that the trial endpoints can be determined with as much certainty as possible. Pharmacogenetics is the study of the differences among individuals with regard to clinical response to a particular drug, be that response efficacy or safety (adverse reaction). It is to be distinguished from pharmacogenomics, which is the study of differences among a number of compounds with regard to the gene expression response to a single (normative) genome. Pharmacogenetics is not a new science; what is relatively recent is the advent of genomic technologies (in particular, rapid screening for specific gene polymorphisms and knowledge of genetic sequences of target genes, such as those coding for enzymes, ion channels, and other receptor types involved in drug response) that have permitted the identification of polymorphisms in genes linked to drug effects and then to phenotypic responses. This has led to the concept of "the right medicine for the right study subject". The use of pharmacogenetics in clinical trials has been introduced for certain drug development programmes in Phases I to III. These have been focussed on drug disposition, pharmacodynamics, and adverse drug reactions. Significant advances have been made in the understanding of pharmacogenetics of drug metabolism enzymes, and a comprehensive listing of genetic polymorphisms influencing these enzymes that are of potential clinical relevance has been compiled. Significant examples which have implications for clinical trials include anti-HIV compounds that are potent inhibitors of metabolism mediated by cytochromes P450. Future trials may also need to take account of potential consequences of genetic polymorphisms in other pharmacokinetic processes. For example, in subjects who lack a functional protein (enzyme or transporter) the "normal" doses of a given drug may evoke a different effect. In addition, or alternatively, such subjects may not be able to activate a prodrug or may not be able to eliminate drugs (for example, by renal excretion) so efficiently. However, it must be stated that the current evidence for the clinical importance of genetically determined variability is not impressive; it is important to read the original source literature with a critical eye. Furthermore, enthusiasm for knowledge of genotyping alone cannot account for pharmacokinetic behaviour in most cases. The pharmacokinetic consequences of the activity of a polymorphic enzyme will also depend on, for example:

1. Whether it mediates metabolism of the parent drug, primary metabolite or both
2. The overall contribution to clearance from the affected pathway
3. The potency of competing pathways of elimination
4. The potency of active metabolites.

In turn, whether significant pharmacokinetic differences arising from the polymorphisms translate into relevant alterations in pharmacodynamics (and clinical efficacy) depends on the operating region of the concentration- response relationship, therapeutic index and utility, and whether kinetic variability is outweighed by variability in receptor sensitivity or number, or in the turnover of the natural receptor ligand. An understanding of the pharmacogenetics of pharmacodynamics is probably less advanced than that of pharmacokinetics, but inherent variability in pharmacodynamics may be greater than in pharmacokinetics. In turn, whether pharmacokinetic-pharmacodynamic variability translates into clinically relevant differences in drug response depends on further clinical and operational issues, such as compliance, and doctor/patient perception of efficacy and side-effects. To date, there are few solid examples, shown in replicated well controlled trials, for associations between genotype or other nucleic-acid derived data and pharmacodynamic responses to a drug. Current thinking on the contribution of pharmacogenetics to dynamic responses (both efficacy and adverse events) has been assisted by classification of responses into type I and type II. Though not entirely separable, type I pharmacogenetics relates to genotype variants in pharmacological receptors and other processes that contribute to a disease or syndrome. Hence, unrecognised or undiagnosed disease heterogeneity provides one explanation for different drug responses. Type II pharmacogenetics represents genotypic variation that influences the response to a drug that is not related to the pathogenesis of the disease (i.e. to interindividual variability). Both types may contribute to a variable extent and to help explain variable responses to a drug in a multifactorial disease such as essential hypertension or asthma.

The impact of these considerations on study subject selection, sample size, and endpoint measures will need to figure in future clinical trial designs.

Studies in Special Groups

Clinical trials may need to be conducted in certain study subject groups that are often either not included or are poorly represented in "standard" clinical development programmes. These include children, the elderly, and in particular, the very elderly and frail, and ethnic minorities. Moreover, it may be necessary to consider specific studies in women of childbearing age for drugs other than those specifically designed for them, for example the oral contraceptive. Another consideration is the applicability of data generated from one ethnic group to the regulatory dossier for a country in which a different ethnic group predominates.

Studies in special groups pose similar ethical problems to those in healthy young adult subjects, but there are additional concerns, for example, with trials in children and the very elderly. The ICH has done much to gain a commonality of approach to drug development in those groups, and many are also in line with Committee for Proprietary Medicinal Products (CPMP) guidelines.

Paediatrics

The scientific basis for development and clinical usage of drugs for children, with some notable exceptions, lags sadly behind that in adults. There are a number of reasons for this, the most important of which are lack of commercial incentive, practical and ethical difficulties in trial conduct, and an historical perspective that children are "*small adults*". There are two significant consequences: first, there has been a lag phase before medicines with suitable indications used in adults become available for use in children. An example is treatments in asthma. Secondly, many drugs for paediatric prescribing are used either "off label" or are licensed for another indication. However, the situation is rapidly improving, with publications, symposia and regulatory guidelines making their appearance.

In Europe, the adoption of the ICH EII guideline, based on the existing EU CPMP guideline, is in place. In the US, the FDA introduced in 1997 the "stick and carrot" legislation whereby extra market exclusivity for six months for the whole product range is granted following an agreed and executed clinical trial programme in a paediatric population. The FDA also has stipulated under the Pediatric Rule (1998) that a development plan for a new or marketed product will include a paediatric programme, unless the FDA specifically waives or defers studies.

An important step in the development of paediatric medicines has been the practical, if arbitrary, age and developmental categorisation as follows: preterm newborn infants, term newborn infants (0–27 days), infants and toddlers (28 days–23 months), children (2–11 years), adolescents (12 to 16–18 years, depending on the region). Whilst studies may not be required in all age bands, and, indeed, it may be agreed that some bands are too wide for certain diseases, at least this approach gives a framework for a continuous clinical development programme in which the pharmacokinetic and pharmacodynamic characteristics can be related to physiological chronology.

The guidelines on development of paediatric medicines advise that the need for a paediatric component must be considered on the basis of the seriousness of the indication and the lack of satisfactory alternative therapies. It recognises three main categories:

1. Medicinal products for diseases predominantly or exclusively affecting paediatric patients, when a full development programme, with the possible exception of initial safety and tolerability, would be required at an early stage
2. Serious or life-threatening diseases occurring in both adults and paediatric patients where there are currently no or limited therapeutic options – the paediatric component should be started early after initial proof of safety and of concept has been generated in adults, and the paediatric studies should form part of the marketing application
3. For medicinal products intended to treat other diseases, studies in children would be less urgent and started only when results of adult Phase II/III trials were known to be reassuring. However, companies should have a clear plan, giving reasons for timing.

The types of trials to be undertaken demand a flexible approach, and depend on the seriousness of the disease, other therapeutic options, and the pharmacokinetics at different ages. For example, if the disease process and efficacy endpoints are similar in adults and children, then an extrapolation from adult efficacy data, together with pharmacokinetic studies in the appropriate paediatric age range, together with safety studies, could form the basis of a successful application. Likewise, it may be possible to extrapolate efficacy from older to younger paediatric groups, with pharmacokinetic and safety studies in the relevant younger study subjects. Where there is no known correspondence between efficacy and blood levels, then clinical or pharmacological effect studies in relevant age groups would be expected. Finally, where the course of the disease or outcome of therapy in paediatric study subjects is similar to that in adults, but the relation to blood levels is unclear, then a "pharmacokinetic–pharmacoydnamic" approach may be possible. This would be combined in the application with safety studies and clinical effectiveness studies in adults linked to these pharmacokinetic/pharmacodynamic studies in children.

For novel indications or where the disease course and therapeutic outcome are likely to be different in adults and paediatric subjects, then clinical efficacy studies would be needed. Other important considerations in studies of paediatric subjects are:

1. an appropriate formulation that is palatable

2. consideration of the volume of blood to be taken in a study for the pharmacokinetic time point analysis
3. the need for monitoring long-term follow up in postmarketing surveillance and safety assessment of marketed medicines studies to determine effects of the drug on physical functions and development, such as bone maturation, growth and sexual development.

Ethnic factors in clinical trial development

The influence of ethnic factors on drug responses in clinical trials is important in two contexts. First, the regulatory application should contain data that is generated from subjects whose ethnic mix is in proportion to that in the population where the medicinal product will be used. Second, an applicant may wish that data generated in one country with one ethnic predominance should be used to gain marketing approval in another country where the ethnicity of the population is different.

The ethnic factors that may affect drug responses can be classified as intrinsic or extrinsic. Intrinsic factors are either genetically determined, such as polymorphisms in drug metabolism and genetic diseases that could influence response, or physiological and pathological, such as age, major organ function and diseases peculiar to the geographical region. Some intrinsic factors, such as height, weight, body surface area and receptor sensitivity, that govern kinetics and dynamics may have influences by both mechanisms. Extrinsic factors (environmental) include climate, culture (educational status, socioeconomic factors), medical practice (especially other medicinal products) and differences in regulatory practice, methodologies (especially subjective endpoints like rating scales) and endpoint measures. Factors like smoking, food habits and alcohol intake influence drug responses probably by both intrinsic and extrinsic mechanisms.

The scientific methodology for the influence of ethnic factors on efficacy responses (with a few exceptions) is not well advanced. It is probably fair to say that too much anecdotal information has been put forward to suggest that ethnic differences exist. It is probable that ethnic differences are no more likely (and maybe less likely) to contribute to the variability in responses than are inherent differences in an unselected population drawn from the same ethnic population. However, as stated above, it would seem prudent to ensure that at least the major ethnic groups in whom the drug is to be used should be represented in a clinical development programme. Some properties of a medicinal product that might be sensitive to the effects of ethnic factors include: non-linear pharmacokinetics, a steep dose–response curve for efficacy and/or safety, a narrow therapeutic dose range, significant metabolism through a single pathway subject to polymorphism, low bioavailability, and the likelihood of multiple (and varying) co-medication.

Data predominantly generated in one ethnic group to be used for registration in another may be acceptable in their entirety, or "*bridging studies*" may be required in the second ethnic population to determine if differences exist. The need for bridging studies depends on whether the medicine is "*ethnically sensitive*" or "insensitive" on the basis of the criteria discussed above. For example, if the product was metabolised through a route that displayed no genetic polymorphism, had a wide therapeutic index, a shallow dose–response curve and there were universally agreed endpoints to determine efficacy and safety, then no bridging studies would be needed. Where the fate of a major development programme rests on foreign data, it is wise to discuss their acceptability with the appropriate regulatory authorities at an early stage.

Elderly population

Many drugs will be used in elderly subjects, and certain diseases, for example Alzheimer's disease, are associated with the ageing process. Clinical studies to test the efficacy and safety of medicinal products in elderly subjects need to take account of the following.

1. Will the drug be used predominantly or entirely in that age group?
2. How might age affect the pharmacokinetics or dynamic responses (tolerability and efficacy) of the drug under test?
3. To what extent can results be extrapolated from younger populations?
4. To what extent are the effects of age separable from those of deterioration in specific organ function (especially kidney and liver)?
5. Are there special ethical issues involved in the development of this drug?
6. Can some important questions concerning development and clinical use of this drug in the elderly be answered by a "*population screen*" approach or will specific elderly study subject trials be required?

Definition of "elderly" is arbitrary and it is obvious that chronological ageing does not necessarily correspond with physiological or pathological decline. As the populations of Western cultures are ageing, it is becoming increasingly recognised that experience of drug usage, either in preregistration or surveillance studies, in the frail and very elderly will become increasingly important. ICH guidelines on studies in geriatric pateints adopt 65 years and over as the cut off point, but recognise that older age ranges should be studied. They also point out that it is important "not to exclude unnecessarily study subjects with concomitant illnesses". Again, this raises ethical dilemmas. Trial endpoints need to be given particular consideration in the elderly. For example, health questionnaires that include practical outcomes, such as ability to walk further or rise unaided from a chair, may be more appropriate in the elderly than measures of surrogate dynamic effects. Correlations between changes in rating scale and clinical outcomes are particularly problematic in the elderly, and the duration of Phase III comparative efficacy studies needs careful consideration. Another issue is whether to conduct Phase I safety and tolerability studies only in elderly subjects if the drug is specifically for use in that age group. It may be argued that it is unethical to conduct such studies in young healthy volunteers if such an age group will never receive the drug.

Compensation and Insurance

Should a study subject suffer any deterioration in health or well-being caused by participation in a study, the sponsors of the clinical research must provide appropriate compensation without regard to the question of legal liability. A statement to that effect should be present in the protocol. Frequently, the insurance policy of the sponsor includes the pharmaceutical industry, clinical investigators and the institution where the clinical study is being undertaken. There is considerable variation between countries concerning the type of insurance and compensation that is required for a clinical trial. These differences need to be considered before starting any multicentre clinical trials in different countries. Increasingly, the medical profession and some governments, particularly in Europe, are recommending moves towards no-fault compensation to reduce the huge costs of litigation.

In the UK, the information sheet provided to the consenting study subject in a clinical trial sponsored by a pharmaceutical company will usually contain a reference to the Association of the British Pharmaceutical Industry's (ABPI) clinical trial compensation guidelines. It is not included in the information sheet of non-commercial studies. Study subjects taking part in clinical trials are not usually paid, unless it is a non-patient volunteer study. However, it may be necessary to compensate participants for out-of-pocket expenses such as travel, and this should be stated in the protocol and in the information sheet/ICF. Financial incentives for study subjects should not be the main reason for entering a study.

Use of Placebo

The new version of the Declaration of Helsinki has highlighted concerns in the use of placebos in clinical trials. The Declaration states in its 29th Ethical Principle that the "effectiveness of a new method should be tested against that of the best current prophylactic, diagnostic, and therapeutic methods." Although this principle does not rule out the use of placebo, IECs and some regulatory authorities are going to be more vigilant when a placebo treatment arm is used. At least one government agency (the FDA) believes that the placebo comparison is preferable to an active agent because it is a fixed and reliable reference point. However, in studies in which life-threatening disorders are being treated, comparisons will always be done with agents, if they exist, that may have a favourable effect on the disorder.

Preparation for Clinical Trial

This chapter aims to provide sufficient information for the pharmaceutical physician to prepare and support effectively a clinical trial. However, clinical trials come in many forms and what is appropriate for a single-centre non- sponsored trial is totally inappropriate for a multicentre global study sponsored by a big pharmaceutical company or institution. Similarly, a Phase I non-patient volunteer study is very different to a Phase IV study. The types and classification of individual clinical trials, and the purposes to which the results are put, have been broadly described in the introduction.

The principles should be the same for any clinical trial:

1. The protection of the study subject, with the involvement of all parties - the investigator, sponsor, IEC and the regulatory authorities
2. Sufficient results from preclinical and human studies to indicate that the study drug or procedures are safe, the results being assessed by qualified experts
3. The design, conduct, and analysis of the trial comply with scientific principles
4. The clinical study objectives should be part of a development plan for that study drug or procedure.

Clinical Trial Design

Preparation for the clinical trial

Whilst an individual clinical trial needs to "stand alone" in the sense that each trial is set to answer specific questions, and that its objectives, design, conduct, results and conclusions are interpretable in their own right, most trials in clinical drug development are part of a series. Design needs to be considered on two levels. Included in the first level is an understanding of the context in which the trial will be conducted, extending through a series of steps to anticipating the outcome and deciding on consequential action. The second level of design is more focused and concentrates on selecting the optimal manner in which the trial will be conducted, choosing from various options in order to obtain the best plan. This section will deal with design, both in the broader and narrower sense, although it will not be possible to give a detailed account of individual design strategies, for which the reader is referred to other excellent texts. Too many studies are conducted for the wrong reason or the true

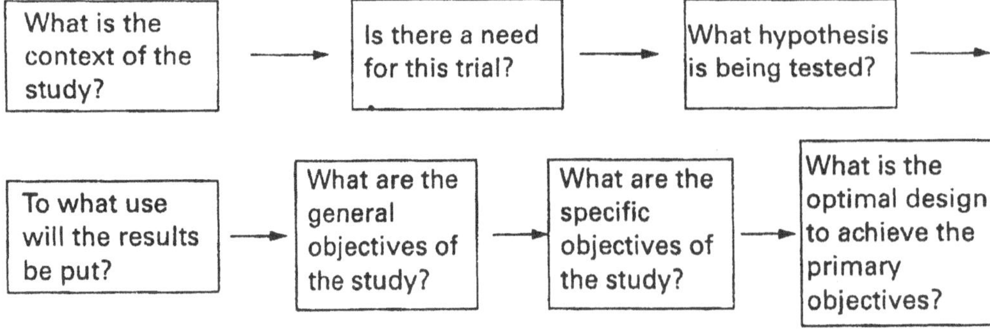

Fig. 5.1. Reasons for conducting a clinical trail.

purpose is obscure. The purpose should be clarified at the time the clinical development plan is formulated, when the clinical trial in question is put in the context of a series of human studies and clinical trials as part of an agreed strategy for evaluating a new medicine. This process of stating the reasons for conducting the trial is assisted by considering a series of questions.

Creating a hypothesis

A hypothesis is a proposition assumed for the sake of argument; it is a theory to be proved or disproved by experiment. In the context of the clinical trial, it is a statement of expected outcome to the study, which will provide a clear and interpretable answer to a realistic question. In that sense, hypothesis creation is about biological phenomena. Take for example the hypothesis that drug A will have a greater effect on blood pressure than will drug B. It is convenient to set about testing the hypothesis by assuming that the treatments are equally effective (or ineffective), as the case may be. This is the "no difference" or null hypothesis. Thus, when two groups of study subjects have been treated, or each subject has had a course of each drug, as in a crossover study design, and it has been found that one drug produces improvement more frequently than the other, it is necessary to decide whether this difference is due to a real superiority of one drug over the other, or whether the result could have arisen by chance. This decision is reached by the application of tests of statistical significance. The correct significance test will establish how often a difference of the observed size would occur due to chance (random influences) if there were, in reality, no difference between the treatments. In a second example, the hypothesis might be to show that two drugs are equivalent or that one is not inferior to the other. A different set of statistics will be needed to test this hypothesis.

Response variables

Efficacy endpoints

Efficacy variables are chosen according to the objectives of the trial. They may be the therapeutic effect itself (for example, irradication of infection, healing of peptic ulcer) or a factor related to the therapeutic effect or some surrogate effect.

There is a considerable literature on surrogate endpoints. From a practical point of view, the physician working in the pharmaceutical industry needs to be precise in his use of the surrogate endpoint.

The characteristics of an "ideal" surrogate endpoint for use in Phase I-IV trials would depend on whether the emphasis is on the efficacy or the safety evaluation of the potential medicine. The characteristics of an ideal surrogate endpoint would include:

1. A plausible biological link to the therapeutic endpoint
2. A parameter that can be determined repeatedly and reproducibly on different occasions and by different investigators
3. Simple to perform, and robust
4. Economically viable
5. Acceptable degree of specificity and sensitivity
6. Preferably non-invasive
7. Applicable across a wide range of patients
8. Sensitive to dose-related effects
9. High predictive value for therapeutic or clinical endpoint.

The last point (i.e. a high level of validity) can only really be confirmed in Phase III or IV, when a sufficient number of study subjects have achieved a therapeutic response that can retrospectively be correlated with the change in surrogate marker. Thus surrogate markers, in this context, are most valuable for selecting second-in-class or follow up drugs, when validity has already been tested with the first compound. This is a particularly important point and is often glossed over in debates with regulatory authorities as to whether a suppogate endpoint is an indication in its own right.

In the evaluation of pharmaceutical products, commonly used surrogate endpoints include:

1. Pharmacokinetic measurements, for example plasma (serum) half-life, concentration–time curves of parent drug or active metabolite
2. An *in vitro* or *ex vivo* measure of drug effect, for example mean inhibitory concentration (MIC) of an antimicrobial against bacterial culture; inhibition of ADP-induced platelet aggregation with a fibrinogen receptor antagonist
3. An *in vivo* marker of effect related to the pharmacology of the drug, for example hypoglycaemic response to an antidiabetic agent; change in concentration of a "serum marker of disease" such as C-reactive protein with antirheumatoid agents
4. The *in vivo* antagonism by the potential drug to an exogenously administered agonist, for example inhibition of weal and flare response to subcutaneous serotonin by 5-hydroxytryptamine $(5HT)_3$ antagonists; the inhibition by a leukotriene LTD_4 antagonist of bronchoconstriction induced by inhalation of LTD_4
5. The investigational appearance of tissues or organs, for example endoscopy findings of a peptic ulcer; the radiological appearance of joint erosions.

Surrogate endpoint data can be used for a number of purposes. These include:

1. 'Proof' of physiological/pharmacological effect
2. Determination of dose–response relationship prior to Phase III trials
3. Confidence in Phase I and IIa trials that further evaluation of a pharmaceutical product is warranted
4. Assistance in choosing between several compounds in the same biological or chemical class for progression to Phase II
5. Yielding comparative effect or safety data between two drugs with a similar mechanism of action
6. To register a drug for an indication.

In recent literature, the concept of surrogate endpoint has become inextricably linked to the term "*proof of principle*" or "*proof of concept*" study. There is nothing fundamentally new in this idea. It is an attempt by sponsors to design, execute and interpret "*small scale*", preferably short- term trials at the exploratory phase of development in which a selected surrogate (or surrogates) is determined as the "go/no go" decision point for continuation or termination of a development programme. The overall objective is to reduce the increasing costs of clinical development, having recognised that the majority of novel substances that enter Phase I will not reach the marketplace. Only time will tell whether this new emphasis will be successful.

Safety endpoints

Safety variables are broadly of two kinds: those related to the unwanted pharmacological effects of the drug and those that are unpredictable. The first require specific questions or investigations to be included in the trial at time points related to the pharmacodynamic and pharmacokinetic characteristics of the drug. For example, in vulnerable subject groups, such as the elderly or those with renal or hepatic disease, or during long-term studies when drug or metabolite accumulation might occur.

Non-specific safety questions are usually addressed in three ways.

1. A standard set of haematological and biochemical investigations is included before, during and after the trial. These investigations should be comprehensive, but not exhaustive, otherwise they will generate a large volume of data that will need processing and that may, by chance, throw up findings that are not related to drug effects.

2. Study subjects are asked about their response to treatment using an open question such as "How has the medicine suited you?".
3. An adverse event form should be provided by the sponsor, which will have clear instructions as to what constitutes minor, major and serious adverse events, how these are to be recorded, and what action is required as a consequence.

Patient population in trials and in clinical practice

The indication (or indications) for which a new drug is designed is the prime determinant of the population in which it will be used in clinical practice. For some drugs, the indication is clear at the start of the clinical development programme, for example a "me-too" cyclo-oxygenase inhibitor or a novel delivery system for insulin. However, for many drugs, particularly those that interfere with one or more pathways in a complex series of biochemical or immunological steps, the final indication(s) may be less clear, for example anti-TNF (tumour necrosis factor). Furthermore, serendipity may come into play during the course of the trial programme, as was the case with the phosphodiesterase 4 inhibitors which are now in use for male erectile disorders, but were originally designed for the treatment of heart failure. Finally, if the aspirations of pharmacogenetics are realised (the right medicine for the right patient), then indications will be defined not just by disease, but also by population characteristics.

For the present and immediate future the general path of subject selection for clinical developmental trials will tend to follow the pattern of moving from highly selected and well defined subject groups to an ever-broadening and less selected population, up to and beyond granting of a marketing authorisation. Inevitably, this will include study subjects who may or will not respond, but this knowledge must be balanced against the need to create a comprehensive safety database at the time of marketing against which future safety can be judged.

Trial elements

Eligibility criteria

The defined population for the clinical trial will be chosen on the basis of a series of inclusion and exclusion criteria, which together constitute the eligibility criteria. Inclusion and exclusion criteria are of two kinds: general and specific. General criteria include age, sex, race, weight, previous medical history, previous and concurrent medication and status of major organ functions (for example, hepatic and renal function). Specific inclusion criteria are of two kinds. The first set applies to trials testing therapeutic or surrogate endpoints. For example, in a trial of an antihypertensive drug, specific entry criteria for the level of systolic and diastolic blood pressure, measured over a stated number of visits, in a particular position, and with a specific piece of apparatus, would be stated. The second set of specific inclusion criteria applies to trials of drugs in special groups, such as early phase studies in healthy normal volunteers to assess tolerability, safety and pharmacokinetics, or kinetic and metabolic studies in study subjects with renal or hepatic impairment who may respond differently to the drug.

Bias

Bias is the introduction of a systematic error or series of errors that distort the data obtained, and which may affect the analysis. Bias is distinct from random error that occurs by chance. During the design and execution phases of the trial, bias may occur in the selective sampling of subjects for the trial, in allocating the treatments, in measuring the critical endpoints and in recording safety and tolerability data. Bias may be introduced consciously or unconsciously by sponsor, investigator or study subject through a prejudice the individual may hold or through ignorance about one of these aspects in the trial design or execution.

Bias is best avoided by anticipation. Aspects of clinical trial design that are introduced to avoid bias include stratification of subjects, randomisation of treatments, double-blind design and using prospective, rather than retrospective observational, cohort, case-controlled or uncontrolled designs. A statistician must be consulted during the protocol design stage, as many biases have a statistical basis that may not occur to those not trained in that discipline. Bias in execution of trial manoeuvres can be avoided by choosing objective rather than subjective assessments wherever possible, by employing validated instruments (such as questionnaires) and by using standardising techniques, for example the questions about adverse events and the order of undertaking a series of tests. Digit preference is a recognised problem in recording numerical data, for example in the recording of blood pressure, and special instruments have been introduced to set the baseline at random so that the true recorded blood pressure is obtained by subtraction of this baseline from the observed reading.

Bias in subject selection may not be avoided simply by randomisation. Randomisation will avoid weighted allocation to one treatment regimen rather than another, but it will not avoid selection of the wrong kind of subject in the first place, which will subsequently affect the degree to which the data can be extrapolated. Thus, an investigator may have a preconceived idea about the safety of a drug or about its effectiveness in a particular subset of subjects who nonetheless meet the entry criteria. This prejudice may be avoided by stratification of subjects for defined risk factors before randomisation, so equal numbers will be allocated to the treatment regimens.

Choice of trial design

There is no generally accepted classification of trial design because each aspect of a design (for example, dose ranging, blinding) can be used in combination with almost any other. It is simpler to describe the various design aspects from which one can select a combination that meet the trial objectives.

Pilot trials

There is no succinct and universally accepted definition of a pilot trial. It is usually open in design and small in scale. Its use sometimes implies some degree of uncertainty either about the safety (for example narrow therapeutic ratio) or efficacy of the medicine, or doubt about testing it in a particular context or indication. Pilot studies may examine feasibility (i.e. examine in one small-scale study the sense and practicability of testing a hypothesis so that large resources are not committed without some gain in confidence; for instance, the chosen endpoint may not be suitable or sufficiently sensitive). Pilot trials do not imply "quick and dirty" research or a sloppy approach. They demand as much planning as other types of trial. They can be performed during any phase of drug evaluation, but are most frequent as a vanguard trial early on. Sometimes pilot studies lead to or are converted into definitive trials, and this possibility should be discussed with a statistician in advance of starting the pilot trial. Pilot trials can use many aspects of trial design: double blind, parallel or crossover.

Pivotal studies

Strictly speaking, pivotal (as with pilot) does not imply a particular design aspect, but rather the use to which the trial will be put. By convention, such trials will result in important decisions being made about the medicine (for example, designing the dosage schedule or comparing it with a benchmark comparator) or a pivotal trial will be crucial in defining efficacy and safety. As such, the trial will be subjected to comprehensive QC and QA, and will attract a higher than usual degree of scrutiny by sponsors and regulators. Pivotal studies can occur at any phase in a drug development programme. In regulatory terms, the pivotal trials are those identified by the sponsor for the regulatory authority to judge the efficacy and safety of the drug.

Blindness

The term "blind" refers to a lack of knowledge of the identity of the trial treatment. The aim of blinding is to avoid bias in trial execution and interpretation of results, and it is achieved by disguising the identity of the trial medications. The simplest method is to use formulations that look identical, which is frequently possible with tablets or capsules, but is more difficult for oral solutions that look and taste different. Alternatively, blinding can be achieved for the testing of two non-identical active comparators by the use of the "*double dummy*" technique, whereby each active agent has a matched placebo and study subjects in each limb of the trial take two sets of tablets: one active and one placebo. Special considerations for blinding have to be given for studies involving suppositories, eye drops, skin patches or more esoteric treatments.

There are various levels of blinding, extending from open or open label, where all concerned with the trial are aware of the identity of the trial medicine, to the other extreme of total blindness, in which everyone who interacts directly with the study subject or who comes into contact with the observations or data is unaware of treatment allocation; statisticians, efficacy review committees, pathologists and experts invited to interpret objective endpoint criteria are unaware of treatment identity. In between there are various combinations of blindness, for example single blind (subject unaware, but physician informed) and double blind (both subject and investigator unaware of treatment allocation). The latter is most frequently used and it is generally regarded as generating the most reliable data for interpretation. Increasing levels of blindness bring increasing complexities, higher costs and longer time penalties to trials. The protocol author must bring common sense to bear on occasions. For example, when a drug and placebo are to be given intravenously and samples need to be made up fresh for each administration, is it really necessary for the pharmacist to be "blind" to the preparation of the material? In multicentre trials in which mortality or significant morbidity is the endpoint, it is common practice to have a blinded "*efficacy endpoint*" committee, but an unblinded "*safety review*" committee.

There is much controversy over the use of open or open-label studies. It is a golden rule of clinical trial design that, wherever practicable and possible, open studies should never be conducted, but there are circumstances when they can or must be used.

Rules governing the unblinding of the trial must be given in the protocol. In the normal course of the trial, this occurs at the end of a stated period, although subjects may be maintained on "open" observation for a further period of time. The "breaking of the blind" is a serious matter, as it can spoil part or the whole of the trial. The occurrence of a major adverse event is the most frequent reason for unblinding and, in most circumstances, requires a discussion between sponsors and investigators.

Controlled trial

The word "controlled" in the context of clinical trial design has two meanings, one broad and one specific. In the broad sense, it relates to adherence to a tightly designed protocol in order to reduce the variability of factors and the biases that might influence the outcome. In the specific sense, control refers to the comparator treatment and/or "population" used in the trial. By custom, the term "*controlled trial*" has come to be equated with "*comparative trial*". Contrariwise, uncontrolled can mean a study which loosely adheres to entry criteria and procedures or, more specifically, to a design feature which does not include a comparator treatment or population group (non-comparative trial). Specific control groups are included in the clinical trial so that the medicine under test can be compared. If no comparator control group is included, then the effect of the drug is compared with baseline or historical data. Sometimes comparisons are made with both baseline and comparator groups. The types of control groups used in clinical trials include:

1. Concurrent placebo
2. Concurrent active medication
3. No treatment
4. Different dose of the same medicine (dose-ranging studies)

5. Concurrent use of usual or standardised care
6. Historical comparison of data obtained from the same subjects on no therapy, the same therapy or different therapy
7. Historical comparison of data obtained in other subjects on no or some different therapies.

The principle behind establishing a control group as opposed to a control treatment is the selection of a population as similar as possible to the group receiving the medicine under investigation. Whenever possible, a prospective rather than historical control should be used.

The choice of treatment control depends on a number of factors, including:

1. The phase of the drug development programme
2. The specific objective of the trial (for example, dose–response, comparison with active comparator)
3. The placebo response
4. The ethical position of use of placebo or active drug in serious conditions, for example epilepsy
5. The availability, choice and applicability of active comparator
6. The length of the study.

The major purpose of a control group is to allow discrimination of outcomes caused by the test treatment from outcomes caused by other factors, such as the natural progression of the disease, observer or subject expectation, or other treatments.

Placebo

A placebo is an inert medication (or procedure) that is used in conjunction with the double-blind technique to reduce bias in the population samples and in the treatment responses (subjective and objective). Placebo usage is useful to:

1. Distinguish the pharmacodynamic effects of a drug from the psychological effects of the act of medication and the circumstances surrounding it, for example increased interest by the doctor, more frequent visits
2. Distinguish drug effects from the fluctuations in disease that occur with time and from other external factors
3. Avoid false positive or negative conclusions.

The value of the placebo-controlled trial in the early evaluation of a new potential medicine cannot be overemphasised. It is particularly valuable when there is no accepted standard therapy in common use. There are many examples of prescribed drugs in different therapeutic classes that have never been subjected to controlled placebo trials. Other scientific arguments in favour of the inclusion of placebo arms in trials include the following.

1. No standard medical treatment exists.
2. Standard medical treatment has been shown to be ineffective.
3. The drug under trial is innovative in terms of mechanism and/or administration.
4. The standard treatment is inappropriate as comparator (for example, route of administration, choice of dose).
5. The response can only be measured by subjective endpoints.
6. A positive placebo response (particularly a large one) is well recognised in the condition to be treated.

There are a number of arguments against the use of placebo treatment that need to be considered.

1. It is unethical to withdraw an active treatment that is known to be beneficial, for example in epilepsy and tuberculosis.

2. There is no suitable placebo available or it is impracticable to attempt a true placebo comparator group, for example in a trial comparing an intravenous with an oral formulation.
3. Previous studies have convincingly defined the placebo response rate, and the study is designed to test dose response or activity against a positive control.

Although some of these arguments against the use of a placebo involve questions of ethics, the use of a placebo treatment is often preferable to the continued use of treatments of unproven or dubious efficacy or safety. Some old remedies that are still in current use have never been subjected to a placebo-controlled trial, and the opportunity to include them in a placebo comparison may only be with the discovery of a new medicine.

Some disease states or trial conditions militate in favour of a high placebo response rate and lend support for the inclusion of placebo in a comparative trial. These include long treatment periods, previous treatments and response to them, innate characteristics of the study subjects (for example, social class, educational level and personality type), influence of medical staff, environment and supervision during the trial, appearance and taste of trial drugs, and presence (or absence) of unwanted pharmacological effects. Some conditions may permit the use of placebos for short periods (for example, 2–6 weeks in chronic heart failure) but thereafter an active comparator would have to be introduced either routinely or on an "as needed" basis. Declaration of Helsinki has the following statement:

"The benefits, risks, burdens, and effectiveness of a new method should be tested against those of the best current prophylactic, diagnostic and therapeutic methods. This does not exclude the use of placebo, or no treatment, where no proven prophylactic, diagnostic or therapeutic method exists."

Section 29 was introduced to help to protect people in poorer countries from being used as research subjects for the benefit of those in developed countries, when they themselves may derive no immediate or future advantage, for example in the testing of new anti-HIV drugs. This is a laudable aim; however, such is the awe in which the Declaration is held that over-interpretation of it in order to challenge or even exclude the use of placebos in drug development in developed countries would have dire consequences for decision making on drug safety and efficacy that would affect drug developers, regulatory authorities, healthcare professionals and patients. Among the many arguments in addition to those listed above for the retention of placebo-controlled studies in the right context as opposed to only active comparator trials are the following.

1. Placebo-controlled trial of a new active medicinal product, if positive, means that the trial was capable of detecting a difference, and that the test treatment is, at least, more efficacious than placebo. This achieves two outcomes: provision of an internal validity check of the trial methods, and provision to regulatory authorities of a basis on which to judge the difference between a statistically significant but clinically inadequate effect that would probably lead to the drug not being licensed.
2. If only active comparator trials were available, then the trial objectives would have to be very precise from the beginning of a trials programme as to whether superiority, equivalence or non-inferiority is being tested. Demonstration of non-inferiority in turn depends on designing a trial with sufficient sensitivity, as it has to rely on indirect evidence that a trial is capable of showing a difference, without prior availability of placebo-controlled data.

Comparator medicines

Active comparators are included to act as a "*bench mark*" or "*gold standard*" against which the new drug is to be compared. The selection of comparator depends on the specific objectives of the trial. The main considerations are as follows.

1. Is the comparison to test pharmacological or therapeutic effect?

2. What dose or doses will be chosen?
3. Will one active comparator serve for all countries in which the drug will be marketed?
4. Is it possible to "blind" the study?
5. Is the active comparator the standard medication the study subjects will be receiving and how realistic is it to standardise dose and re-randomise into a clinical trial?

In practice in Phase II or III, the control or comparator group most frequently receives the medicine that is most widely prescribed, in a dose that has been established by regulatory approval and clinical experience to represent the optimal for that medical condition.

In some clinical disease states, a treatment regimen that has become standard represents the best practice, and may involve three or more drugs with different mechanisms of action. The potential new medicine will need to be tested against a regimen of therapies rather than a single agent. It may still be feasible and ethical to conduct a placebo-controlled parallel-group study on top of the standard regimen, but there is an added level of complexity to this approach. For example, for patients who have survived an acute myocardial infarction, the treatment regimen may include aspirin, an angiotensin-converting enzyme inhibitor, a lipid-lowering drug and a fibrinogen receptor antagonist. Selection of study subjects and analysis of surrogate endpoints need to be carefully thought out. There are three specific objectives of comparator trials: to show equivalence, superiority or non-inferiority of the new active substance. Each is governed by statistical and regulatory guidelines.

An extension of the concept of testing the null hypothesis of equal efficacy in the setting of large complex studies is the equivalence trial. There are two main categories of equivalence trial: bioequivalence and clinical equivalence. In the former, certain pharmacokinetic variables (C_{max}, AUC and $t_{1/2}$) of a new formulation have to fall within specific (and regulated) margins of the standard formulation of the same active entity. Proof of clinical equivalence can be much more difficult to demonstrate, but situations where it might be of interest are when the standard therapy has been shown to be beneficial but the innovative treatment is easier to use, has fewer side-effects or is less costly. This study design may be of value when investigators seek to establish that a mechanistically related compound achieves clinical results similar to those of the standard therapy.

Superiority trials of one active compound over another provide the second most convincing proof of efficacy after placebo-controlled studies. The reason for selecting this design rather than placebo has been alluded to already, i.e. it is ethically unjustifiable to use a placebo or (less convincingly) marketing requirements. Non-inferiority trials are more common than equivalence trials in Phase III drug development. In these, the objective is to show that a new treatment is no less effective than existing treatment. It may be more effective or equivalent, but using the confidence interval approach,

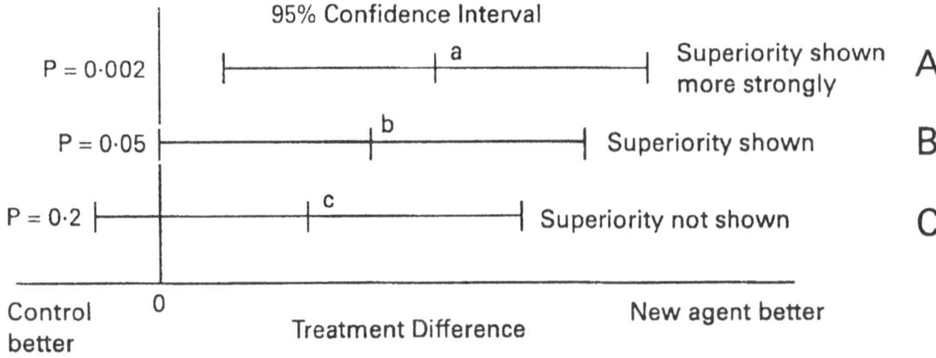

Fig. 5.2. Relationship between significance tests and confidence intervals for the comparison between a new treatment and control.

the only interest is a possible difference in one direction. Hence the 95% confidence interval should be entirely to the right of the point estimate for superiority and other trials.

Parallel or crossover design

Most clinical trials for clinical drug development select two groups of study subjects. In a parallel design, subjects are randomly allocated to one of the two treatments and remain on it until the end of the trial. In a crossover design, every subject receives each treatment allocated in random order, changing over at a halfway point. The response of each subject can be compared for both treatments, but in a parallel design the response of each group of subjects is compared.

The advantages and disadvantages of crossover and parallel group designs have been subject to extensive debate. Generally speaking, crossover designs are selected in the early phases of drug evaluation, particularly for the first dose-ranging trials in stable diseases. Parallel designs are frequently adopted for the definitive dose-ranging studies and for therapeutic efficacy trials.

Crossover designs are susceptible to carry-over effects, i.e. the treatment effect from the first period has not worn off at the time of conducting the second period. Tests of analysis can detect carry-over effects, but it is too late then to modify the design. Similarly, period effects may confound the interpretation of cross-over studies i.e. the order in which one treatment occurs in a sequence compared with another, influences the response to early treatment. Randomisation usually, but not always, precludes the effect.

Dose selection

In clinical practice, the optimal dose is the smallest that will result in the desired therapeutic response. Inherent within that statement is the concept of individualisation of dose for each given study subject, as it would not be unreasonable to expect considerable variation in response, depending on many factors such as body size, efficiency of the metabolising and excretory pathways, race, age, state of disease and so on. In practice, it is not possible for a sponsor to investigate more than a few doses, and frequently only one or two doses for registration of a given indication. It is often in clinical practice that adjustment (most frequently, downwards) to final regimens occurs. The impact of pharmacogenetics on individual dose has yet to be shown.

Dose-response relationships, potency and efficacy

An understanding of the dose-response relationship is fundamental to successful clinical drug development and to therapeutic practice. The pharmacological effect of a drug is related to the concentration of the drug at its site of action: within certain limits the higher the concentration, the greater the pharmacological effect. The relationship between the concentration of a drug at its site of action and the intensity of the pharmacological effect is called its dose-response curve. The shape and position of the curve describes the potency of the drug. A steeply rising and prolonged

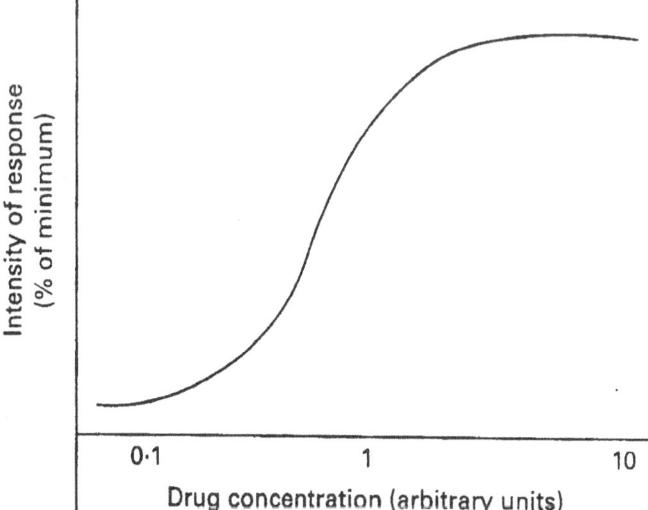

Fig. 5.3. The shape of most dose (or concentrations) response curves is sigmoid in which the rate of rise of the response eventually flattens off despite increasing concentrations.

curve indicates that a small change in dose produces a large change in drug effect, for example a loop diuretic. By contrast, the dose–response curve for the thiazide diuretics plateaus at lower doses, and increasing the dose produces no additional diuretic effect. The term *potency* is frequently used imprecisely and is often confused with efficacy.

It is important to distinguish between the two when designing and interpreting clinical trial results. Potency is the amount of drug in relation to its effect. For example, if weight for weight drug A has a greater effect than drug B, then A is more potent than B, but the maximum therapeutic effect obtained may be similar with both drugs. By increasing the amount of drug B, it may be possible to achieve the same response. Thus, the difference in weight of the drug that has to be administered has no clinical significance unless it is great.

Pharmacological potency is a measure of the concentration of a drug at which it is effective. It refers to the strength of the response induced by occupancy of a receptor and has to be further qualified for agonists and antagonists. Efficacy has both pharmacological and therapeutic definitions. Pharmacological efficacy refers to the strength of response induced by occupancy of a receptor by an agonist. It describes the way in which agonists vary in the response they produce, even when they occupy the same number of receptors. Therapeutic efficacy, or effectiveness, is the ability of a drug to produce an effect, and refers to the maximum such effect. Thus, if drug A produces a greater therapeutic effect than drug B, regardless of how much of a drug B is given, then drug A has the higher therapeutic efficacy.

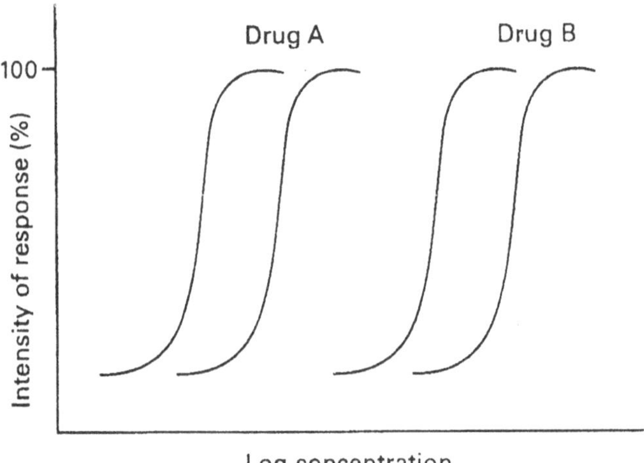

Fig. 5.4. Dose-response curves for two drugs; B is less potent then A. The curves under A and B represent theorised positions of efficacy and toxicity relations. The distance between the individual pairs represents the therapeutic ratio.

Drugs have both unwanted and wanted dose–response curves. The shape and position of the unwanted dose–response curve in relation to the desired effect describes the toxicity of the drug. Drugs that have steep dose–response curves for both wanted and unwanted effects are likely to have the greatest toxicity. For a consideration of the relative positions of these two curves, the concept of the therapeutic index has arisen. This is the maximum tolerated dose divided by the minimum effective dose. In practice, such single doses can rarely be determined accurately and the index is never calculated this way in man; "effective" doses are rarely available or determinable in sufficient subjects. However, the concept embodies a useful concept that is fundamental in comparing the usefulness of one drug with another, i.e. its safety in relation to its efficacy.

The application of the principles of dose–response relations to Phase II and III clinical trials focuses on the practical aspect of determining which doses will be selected for these trials and which will be taken forward to registration. Each subject in a clinical trial will have his/her own efficacy and safety dose–response curve for a given drug. The shape and position of these curves will be determined by individual subject characteristics – age, gender, genetically determined metabolism and so on – so that the dose–response (or concentration–response) curve from each trial represents an average, with a measure of variability that describes that population.

Dose schedules

By the end of a dose-ranging programme of studies, the sponsor should be able to define the following:

1. The therapeutic dose range in the core population who will most frequently receive the drug
2. The dose that is tolerated in the majority of the defined population
3. The minimum effective dose(s)
4. The maintenance dose range (when relevant)
5. The therapeutic dose range in "at-risk" groups, for example the elderly, the hepatically impaired, etc.

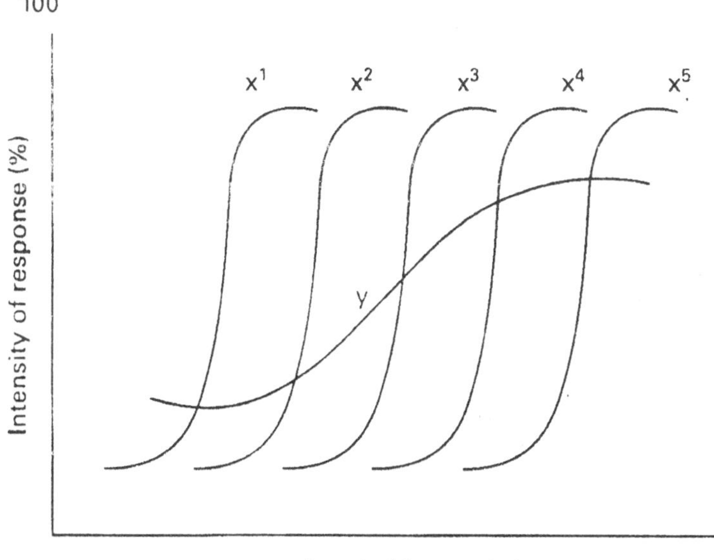

Fig. 5.5. X^1-X^5 are individual dose-response curves; Y is the average dose-response curve for the population.

Dose selection for exploratory studies requires knowledge of the pharmacology, toxicology, metabolism and kinetics in animals and man. Dose selection for Phase II and III studies depends on a number of factors. These include:

1. The pharmacokinetic characteristics of the parent compound and any active metabolites; in particular, the area under the concentration–time curve, clearance, plasma half-life and bioavailability of the formulation; on the basis of these data it should be possible to decide on the dosing frequency for the study, the range of doses to be used and to establish a relationship between the dynamic response and the plasma concentration of drug (or metabolite) achieved
2. The chances of detecting differences between intermediate doses based on the primary endpoint responses
3. The number of study subjects (and centres) available for inclusion
4. Whether a therapeutic or a surrogate endpoint is chosen as primary response measure.

Dose titration and concentration–response designs

Dose titration studies involve starting study subjects at a predetermined dose, which is increased incrementally until the desired therapeutic effect is achieved. Interpretation of such studies is complicated by the difficulty in distinguishing between the effect of the dose increase and the increased duration of exposure – continued maintenance at a smaller dose may achieve the same effect. Dose titration studies for antihypertensives have received adverse criticism by FDA regulators because they have resulted in higher doses being recommended for clinical use in some instances. However, more recently, Sheiner and colleagues have revived an interest in this design, taking account of the potential for period effects and period-by-dose interactions. They have suggested modification of the design (for example, inclusion of a randomly assigned placebo arm for the duration of the study) and analysis (use of a parametric subject-specific dose–response model). Using complex dose–response models, they showed that dose titration designs could perform better overall than a parallel group design for the model considered in the simulation, and slightly worse than a crossover design.

In a concentration–response design, subjects receive either a fixed dose (or dose range) of a medicine and their plasma concentrations are determined, usually at steady state, or various doses of a medicine are titrated until a predefined plasma concentration is achieved. In both designs, plasma concentrations are plotted against clinical response in order to determine if a relationship exists. These designs are only suitable for a selected group of drugs (for example, short-acting intravenous anaesthetic agents); their application to a wider use is limited by the difficulties in extrapolating from plasma concentrations to effective oral dose.

These new designs are attracting considerable attention, but their place in standard dose–response studies has yet to be evaluated.

Study subject compliance, tolerability and acceptability

Poor adherence to the schedule of taking the study medication will obviously confound interpretation of the efficacy and safety of the drug. There is usually good compliance in clinical pharmacology studies, especially those conducted in units where drugs are administered by the staff. However, in clinical research trials adherence to medication may be poorer.

Poor adherence to medication may be suspected from the assessment of compliance (for example, tablet count, biological marker) or from a low efficacy response and/or low adverse event reporting rate. Poor compliance may result from a problem with the trial or with the medication. Features of trial design that lead to low compliance include frequent and inconvenient visits, poor relationship between the investigator and study subject, and general lack of interest in the study. Problems with the medication can arise from poor acceptability (bad taste, pills too large or awkward shape), complicated design regimen (too frequent, too many medications) or perceived or real adverse events (low tolerability). These issues can frequently be addressed in subsequent clinical trials and improvement in compliance can be expected.

During the course of the trial, compliance may be improved or assessed directly by:

1. Observing the subjects taking their medication
2. Taking blood or urine or other biological samples to measure parent drug or metabolites
3. Including in the medication a biological marker that is non-toxic, inert, chemically stable and easily detectable in biological fluids (such markers include riboflavin, phenol red and small quantities of digoxin)
4. Making spot checks on the subjects at home.

Indirect methods to improve compliance include questioning the subject, assessing the biological response, making pill counts. The latter is not a reliable way of assessing compliance, although it is the most frequently used. It is easy to cheat, by throwing away pills or, worse, by taking a large number just prior to the clinic visit. The use of electronic counters in the cap of specially designed medicine bottles, which record the exact day and minute each time the container is opened, is possible. Obviously, it is no guarantee of ingestion, is expensive and could not be used in large trials. Subjects may obtain their clinical trials tablets from the pharmacist and not the investigator, and the former keeps a record of number dispensed and returned. There is some evidence that this improves compliance, as subjects seem reluctant to cheat a third party dispensing the drugs.

Assessment of compliance in a trial leads to the question as to whether the data generated from those who fail to comply should be included or excluded from analysis. The general principles that apply are that they should be excluded from Phase II (explanatory trial approach), but not from Phase III or IV trials. The reason for exclusion from Phase II is that these studies are designed to determine efficacy under well-defined eligibility criteria, and so non-compliers will dilute the efficacy response. Their data are usually included up to the point at which they discontinue, but the principle of "last observation carried forward" should not be applied in the statistical analysis. However, the safety data from subjects up to the point of withdrawal must be included. The reason for including subjects in a Phase III trial is that the objective in these studies is to evaluate medicines under conditions that are close to clinical use in the target population. Under these circumstances, analysis is conducted on the "*intention to treat*" principle, carrying forward the last observation to subsequent periods. Nevertheless, gross non-compliance throughout the trial by individual subjects warrants their exclusion. The rules governing the inclusion or exclusion of data from non-compliant subjects need to be determined during the protocol design phase.

The degree of study subject tolerability to a drug should be assessed in conjunction with the laboratory safety and efficacy data, so that an overall risk to benefit assessment can be made. Poorly tolerated drugs, however efficacious for use in self-limiting non-serious diseases, are unlikely to become successful medicines. On the other hand, study subjects with serious illnesses such as active rheumatoid arthritis are frequently quite prepared to put up with poorly tolerated drugs (for example, intramuscular gold injections or intra-articular steroid injections) if efficacy is good and the alternatives are no more attractive.

Experimental error

Errors in recording, transcribing, analysing or interpreting data are discussed elsewhere. Experimental errors are those inherent in the design or execution of the experiment; they are not due to bias, may be random or consistent, and may occur as a result of the instrumentation being used or in the calculation associated with the data they generate.

Equipment employed for the measurement of critical efficacy and safety endpoints should be sensitive enough to record what is demanded in the protocol and robust enough to record the information within the time-frame expected and with requisite accuracy and repeatability. It is pointless expecting to detect blood pressure differences of less than 5 mmHg if the instrument chosen cannot accurately record differences down to that level. Equipment needs to be validated against standard instruments at regular intervals and these facts should be checked by the clinical monitors.

The investigator needs to be realistic about the accuracy of and the consistency with which the human eye can record certain observations. Unrealistic expectations and tedious repetitive recordings can lead to random errors; these can frequently be anticipated by working through the study execution on a "dummy run" with the investigator.

Sample size

A major decision is how many study subjects to recruit because this affects planning throughout the study. The sample size refers to the number of subjects who finish a trial, not to the number who enter it. The number required should be the minimum that will fulfil the objectives and test the hypothesis. For all trials, the required number of subjects is chosen on the basis of:

1. The magnitude of the effect expected on the primary efficacy endpoint – for between-group studies, the focus of interest is the level of difference that constitutes a clinically significant effect; note that this may not be the same as a statistically significant effect
2. The variability of the measurement of the primary endpoints, i.e. the mean and the standard deviation of this primary outcome measure
3. The power or desired probability of detecting the treatment difference with a defined significance level – for most controlled trials, a power of 80% or 90% (0·8–0·9) is frequently chosen as adequate, although higher power is chosen for some studies.

The general rule is that the smaller the difference in effect to be detected between the two treatment groups, and the greater the variability in the measurement of the primary endpoint, the larger the sample size must be. Figure 5.6 gives an example of power curves, or statistical normogram, that relate sample size to size of effect to be detected. Including too few subjects in a study can result in missing a difference between two treatments when one exists, or, conversely, in declaring a difference when one does not exist. The latter is referred to as a Type I error (α), and may be viewed as the significance level necessary for the statistical test to detect a difference between treatments that is conventionally defined as significant (for example, $\alpha = 0{\cdot}05$). The former is referred to as a Type II error (β) and is the probability of not detecting a difference when one is present (i.e. the chance of missing a real effect). The power of the study ($1 - \beta$) is the probability of detecting this difference.

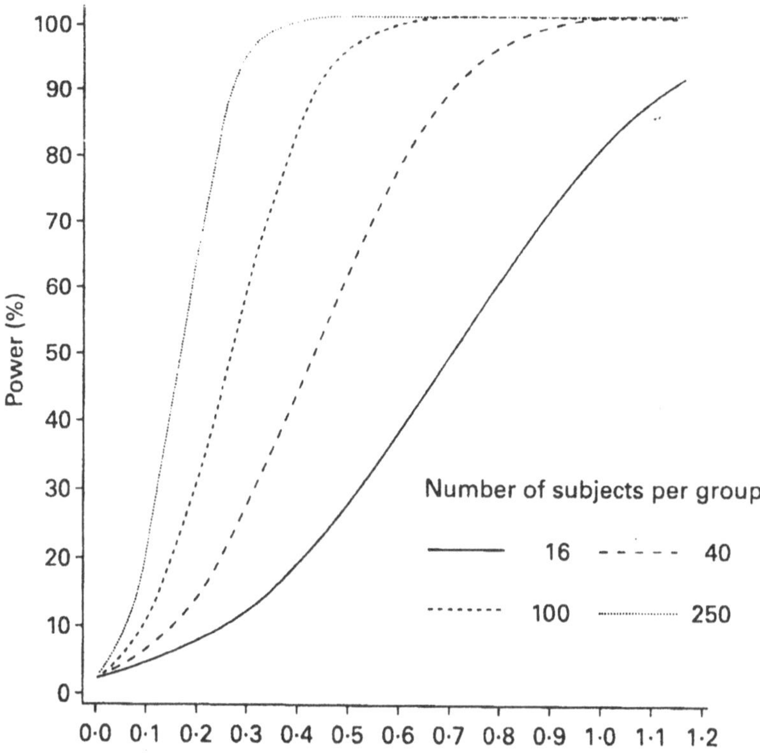

Fig. 5.6. Power curves: this is an illustrative method of defining the number of subjects required in a given study.

The aim of any clinical trial is to have small Type I and II errors and sufficient power to detect a difference between treatments, if it exists. Of the three factors in determining sample size, the power is arbitrarily chosen. The magnitude of the effect can be estimated with more or less accuracy from previous experience with drugs of the same or similar action, and the variability of the measurements is often known from published experiments on the primary endpoint, with or without drug. These data will, however, not be available for novel substances in a new class and frequently the sample size in the early phase of development is chosen on an arbitrary basis. Many clinical trials designed to show a difference between the two drugs must be very large; for example, studies to improve mortality and morbidity after myocardial infarction or coronary artery bypass surgery involve tens of thousands of study subjects. These are major undertakings for the sponsors and require a determined commitment at the highest management levels. Conditions in which there is a high placebo response rate usually require large sample sizes, and whilst the literature may help in determining this placebo response rate, it often turns out to be quite different in a new trial. In order to reduce the number of subjects on placebo in a clinical trial, some investigators employ an unequal randomisation technique, whereby fewer subjects receive placebo than receive active comparator. For example, the ratio of 1:2, or 1:3 may be chosen in a large clinical study. Some statisticians, however, insist that if this design is chosen, then all subjects must have an equal chance of receiving all medications. Thus, in a 2:1 randomisation of active versus placebo, the randomisation would actually be 2:1:1.

Subsidiary assessments

Clinical trials generate vast quantities of data, most of which are processed by the sponsor. Assessments should be kept to the minimum that is compatible with the safety and comfort of the subject. Highest priority needs to be given to assessment and recording of primary endpoints, as these will determine the main outcome of the study. The power calculation for sample size should be based on the primary critical endpoint. Quite frequently trials have two or more evaluable endpoints. It must be stated clearly in the protocol whether the secondary endpoints are to be statistically evaluated, in which case power statements will need to be given, or are simply descriptive. The temptation to include additional investigations, which is particularly easy when automated analyses are conducted in laboratories, should be avoided unless they add significantly to the trial. However, in long-term trials, it may be necessary to arrange extra visits at which critical trial data are not recorded but the subject is assessed for general well-being, and to maintain good relationships between the doctor and study subjects and compliance with treatment.

Statistical analysis of clinical trials

It is not the intention to give a detailed assessment of how to choose the correct statistical test and apply it for a given clinical study. Rather, some general guidelines to the use of statistical analysis will be provided.

The majority of studies designed and analysed by sponsors must have a significant input from a statistician. The protocol author and statistician will work together at the draft protocol stage and pay particular attention to the design strategy, avoidance of bias and the sample size. They will want to determine what size of effect they wish to observe in the trial, with what degree of statistical significance (usually at the 5% or 1% level) and with what degree of precision (usually at least 80% chance of detecting the defined useful target effect within narrow confidence intervals).

It is also necessary to decide how the primary endpoint variables will be analysed, what factors will be taken into account and how the result will be expressed. This most frequently involves analysis of variance or covariance. Predetermined comparisons of two or more treatments or doses can be made at specific time points, (for example, each visit or selected visits) or may be assessed over time, giving an "area under the time curve" analysis which will avoid multiple time-point analyses. How the baseline measurement will be used in relation to the critical evaluable endpoints must be determined before analysis. Comparison of two or more treatments usually takes into account the differences between baseline values between treatment groups at the point of randomisation. The way in which the analysis will influence the report and publications needs to be decided, as some regulatory authorities have their own statistical criteria that need to be observed (for example, for bioequivalence studies).

Interpretation

The interpretation of the results from a clinical trial or series of trials denotes the process of discerning their clinical meaning or significance, or providing an explanation for the data under evaluation. The importance of interpretation lies both within the clinical trial and beyond it in the use to which the results will be put. Within the context of the trial itself, correct interpretation of the results will determine whether the objectives of the trial have been achieved and whether the hypothesis is proven. Interpretation beyond the immediate clinical trial concerns comparisons with other studies, extrapolation to different populations and the impact on medical practice.

Efficacy data

The efficacy endpoints defined in the protocol will be primary or secondary, and each of these may be a therapeutic or a surrogate endpoint. For each of these there is a statistical and a clinical interpretation of the results.

Statistical data

The statistical significance relates strictly to the conditions under which the trial was conducted and will tell how often a difference of the observed size could occur by chance alone if there is, in reality, no difference between the treatments. The most widely accepted level of probability in therapeutic trials is set at 5%, which indicates that if the no-difference or null hypothesis is true, a difference as large as that observed would occur only five times if the experiment were repeated 100 times. This is then acceptable as sufficient evidence that the null hypothesis is unlikely to be true (but not impossible): in other words there is a real difference between the treatments. Any level of significance can be set for a given test; for example, at the 1% level, the chance of the null hypothesis being true would occur only once if the experiment were repeated 100 times. Such findings are generally said to be "statistically highly significant" ($P = 0{\cdot}01$) compared with "statistically significant" ($P = 0{\cdot}05$).

Confidence intervals

The statistical tests of significance determine whether an outcome could have occurred by chance. If the result of the test is that the observed difference is unlikely when there is truly no difference between treatments, it is necessary to know what degree of assurance or confidence can be placed in the power (or precision) of this estimate. For this, the confidence interval needs to be calculated. It reveals the precision of an estimate, showing the degree of uncertainty related to a result, whether or not it was statistically significant. For example, a result from a trial showing that a drug reduces systolic blood pressure by 2 mmHg may well be statistically significant, but it may be clinically meaningless. Doctors are interested in the size of the difference and the degree of assurance or confidence they can have in the precision (reproducibility) of this estimate. Confidence intervals are expressed as a range of values within which one can be 95% (or other chosen percentage) certain that the true value lies. The range may be broad, indicating uncertainty, or narrow, indicating a higher degree of certainty. Confidence intervals are thus extremely useful in the interpretation of small studies, as they show the degree of uncertainty related to a result, whether or not it was statistically significant. Indeed,

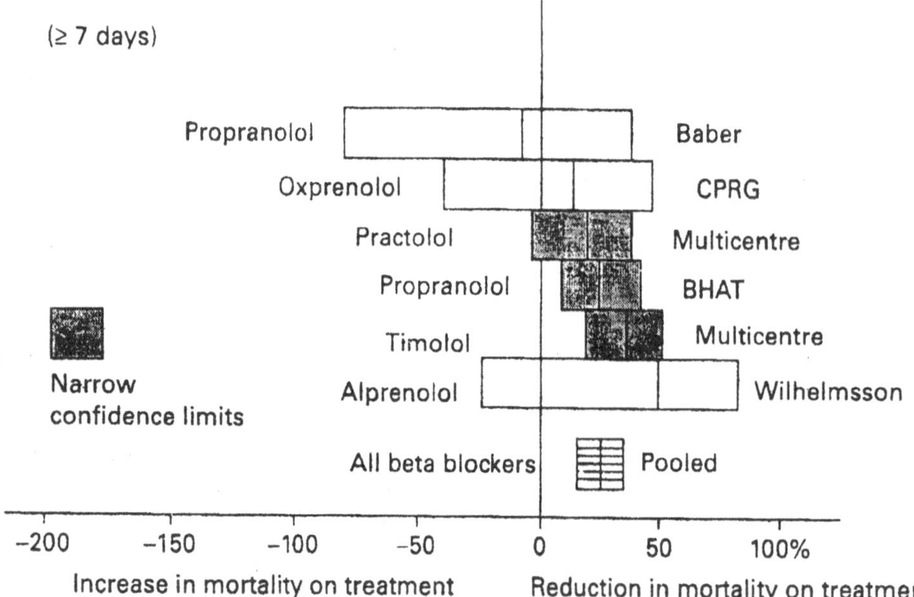

Fig. 5.7. Effect of beta blockers on postinfarction mortality. Difference in mortality rates is expressed as a percentage of control rate in six controlled trails of beta blockers.

a finding of "not statistically significant" can only be interpreted as meaning that there is no clinically useful difference if the confidence interval of the result is also stated and is narrow. If the confidence interval is wide, a real difference may have been missed in a trial of a given size. Inevitably, this means that the sample size was too small.

Errors

Therapeutic experiments can yield one or both of two kinds of error related to the efficacy endpoints.

1. The Type 1 error finds a difference between treatments when in reality, none exists.
2. The Type 2 error fails to find a difference between treatments when in reality they do differ, to an extent that might have clinical relevance.

The confidence intervals provide information on the likelihood of falling into one of these errors. However, the person interpreting the efficacy results must decide, as a guide for action, what target difference and what probability level (for either type of error) he or she will accept when using the results. The statistical significance test alone will not provide this information. It does not prove that a difference is due to one treatment being better than another (or not better); it merely provides the probabilities of the event. The significance findings and the interpretation of the position of the observed effect in relation to the zero point in the confidence interval can be combined to permit an interpretation of the clinical importance to be placed on the findings.

Although a "*statistically significant*" result of observed differences between treated groups may be achieved (say, narrow 95% confidence intervals which do not include zero), the difference observed may still be clinically unimportant. The setting of the target difference, and achieving a narrow confidence interval about that difference, will certainly help, but it is finally up to the clinical judgement of the sponsor and investigator to decide on the clinical relevance of the finding.

Use and extrapolation of efficacy data

The effects of treatments on efficacy endpoints can be used for several different purposes. They may be used to set a new hypothesis in further clinical studies. This is particularly the case for unexpected findings, such as a negative result despite a well conducted trial, or a positive result which is difficult to interpret, such as failing to show a difference between several doses of a drug, despite there being an overall difference compared with placebo. In Phase III, it is unusual for one clinical study to be conducted in isolation. Regulatory authorities require a minimum of two pivotal trials and the sponsors would probably undertake two studies in order to be sufficiently confident to proceed. These two pivotal trials are usually planned at the same time, but the results from one may be awaited in order to help design the second. The sponsor will wish to use the efficacy results from Phase II and III studies to make a therapeutic claim. The interpretation of the efficacy data will determine the target population for whom that claim is made, and whilst sponsors may wish this to be as wide as possible, the claim must reflect the trial population that has been studied. This will, of necessity, involve an interpretation of safety data in conjunction with efficacy results.

Once registration is granted, a new medicine will be compared both formally, within clinical trials, and informally, by clinical usage, with currently available medicines. Company representatives, both medical and commercial, will draw to the attention of potential prescribers the results of the major registration trials in published literature (sponsored or peer reviewed), in advertisements and at meetings. The key question for the individual physician with regard to the new drug will be "How large a response in the most important efficacy variables is necessary to convince me that the new therapy is worth using in my patients?". This will be supplemented by other questions relating to safety and, in turn, the risk:benefit ratio, the effects on quality of life, patient acceptance of the new medicine and costs of treatment. The wise clinical practitioner will scrutinise the results of the major efficacy trials and compare the study subject populations studied therein with his own patients. Because clinical trials are designed to reduce the variability of response, early disappointments with new drugs used in medical practice frequently arise from circumstances outside the control of clinical studies. For example, usage in the home environment compared with hospital-based clinical trials or constant use of self-prescribed medications in clinical practice may confound interpretation of results if outside the clinical trial environment.

Recent publications on major clinical trials whose implications will involve a recommendation to change clinical practice have included summary statistics that quantify the risk of benefit or harm that may occur if the results of a given trial are strictly applied to an individual patient or to a representative cohort. Four simple calculations will enable the non- statistician to answer the simple question "How much better would my chances be (in terms of a particular outcome) if I took this new medicine, than if I did not take it?". These calculations are: the relative risk reduction, the absolute risk reduction, the number needed to treat, and the odds ratio.

Interpretation of efficacy data at a healthcare level

Within the last 20 years or so, three major features of controlled clinical trials in particular have permitted significant advances in deciding whether treatments are of value or not: randomisation, systematic review and meta-analysis, and the concept of the large-scale, simple (to understand and conduct) randomised trial in areas where only moderate benefits can be expected. All of these elements are likely to underpin future trials for purposes of regulation, pharmacoeconomics and healthcare policy. Yet there is no room for complacency or allowing standards to slip. Systematic reviews of some of the hundreds of thousands of trials published since 1948 are revealing that, in many trials, inadequate steps were taken to control biases, and insufficient numbers of participants were studied to yield reliable estimates of effects, i.e. much effort, money and subject participation has been wasted. The pressure to give greater public access to types of, and results from, clinical trials is to be applauded on one hand, but the quality of those trials and their interpretation must be carefully investigated.

Preparation of Documentation for the Clinical Trial

Single-centre Studies

There are considerable advantages in conducting single-centre studies when considering the early stages of the development of a new study drug. Most Phase I units using non-patient volunteers are single centres that have a population of volunteers, the expertise and the intensive monitoring required.

In the past, Phase I units were seldom subject to the regulatory scrutiny experienced by sites used at later stages of drug development. Similarly, investigator-instigated research and non-commercial research failed to follow the GCP guideline and were not subject to the same Directives as those used in commercial research. The new EU Directive has changed this situation since it covers all such studies. The clinical pharmacologist involved in these types of studies should be aware of the pitfalls that are often present. Resuscitation procedures and equipment are often unsatisfactory and the appropriate guidelines are not followed. Staff training in resuscitation is often inadequate and resuscitation trolleys poorly equipped or maintained. The trial protocols are changed to cater for changes in doses and number of subjects without amendments being approved in advance by an IEC, and failure to report serious and unexpected adverse drug reactions has been common.

Single-centre studies are used where new devices are being developed. For example, the development of devices releasing local anaesthetic or analgesics will require various diverse skills including engineering, surgery and pharmacology. If quality of life instruments (questionnaires) are being used in a study, they need to be validated and, if appropriate, copyright permission obtained before the start of the study.

Probably, the most frequent use for single centres is where a particularly uncommon indication is treated, for example Turner's syndrome, or a technique is practised, for example artificially induced bronchial spasm, where there are sufficient appropriate subjects for meaningful analysis and where there is sufficient experience and knowledge to minimise the risks to the study subjects.

Multicentre Studies

Improvements in medical treatments have been substantial, so much so that benefits of recently introduced medicines over existing ones are smaller than when these standard treatments were originally developed and compared with remedies that existed then. The mean difference in some clinical efficacy endpoints between treatments may be less than 20%. This requires a large population sample in clinical trials in order to achieve sufficient power to detect a difference, if it really exists, with confidence.

Most medical conditions (for instance, peptic ulcers) present rather infrequently at any single hospital centre and it would therefore be impossible to recruit 200 or 500 study subject subjects in a reasonable period of time. If instead one invites several investigating centres to recruit study subjects and to pool their findings, this constitutes a multicentre trial. Thus, one reason for conducting a multicentre trial is to increase efficiency. The advantages can be offset by differences in procedures, often resulting from differing interpretation of instructions. These mistakes, when coupled with other errors made in each centre, mean that the multicentre trial could turn out to be even less reliable than the single-centre trial in terms of quality of data.

It is therefore essential to incorporate procedures that will ensure not only that the clinical data are collected in a uniform and similar manner at each investigating centre but that they are also handled and analysed in an identical manner. Measures such as the use of compatible validated computer systems and similar databases will allow the merging of data. At each centre, critical efficacy data should be determined with identical procedures and, where appropriate, these should be specified in protocols and monitoring conventions. Standard operating procedures (SOPs) should be prepared to ensure that investigators at each site are carrying out the more common methodologies, such as blood pressure measurements, blood sampling, radiograph measurements, in a similar manner.

Obviously it is desirable to use one centre for the central collection of data, but that requires sufficient resources and close liaison with the person(s) monitoring the trial. Pharmaceutical companies have learnt that it is simpler and more efficient if they became custodians of the data, using their own computing facilities for data capture and their monitoring staff to bring in high-quality records. The transfer of the data to the sponsor allows the pharmaceutical company to hold all the data electronically, not only data for a particular clinical trial but data from all the clinical trials relating to the development of a specific study drug. When regulatory submission takes place, agencies like the FDA can "interrogate" the clinical data in order to establish the validity of the analysis and interpretation. Computer- assisted new drug application (CANDA) is the frequent form of application in US. Without doubt, the use of paper applications will decrease in other regions of the world when global standards for the electronic transfer of regulatory information have been established and computer systems are properly validated.

Multicentre trials have thrust pharmaceutical companies into the role of coordinating the design, conduct, analysis and reporting of all trials on a new medicine, and given them a real incentive and the resources to do so. In a similar manner some of the collaborative groups running large-scale intervention trials, which often span several countries and several thousand study subjects, adopt similar procedures. However, if the multicentre trial is being conducted independently of a pharmaceutical company or large institution, clinical data should not be analysed by each individual centre. The clinical data should be sent to one centre to be entered into a common computer database for analysis. If possible, the coding for the whole trial should be done by the same individual. It would also be wise to employ sufficient expertise in statistical analysis of clinical trials and suitably trained computer staff, as well as a validated computer system.

Sponsored Therapeutic Trials

The main sponsors of therapeutic trials are the pharmaceutical companies. Therapeutic trials are needed for regulatory approval of new medicinal products. Indeed, the manufacturer holds the investigational license and controls the supply of the trial medication. The medical department of the pharmaceutical company will be responsible for preparing a plan of development, which may be subject to alteration as the clinical data accumulates. The medical department will decide on the design and objectives of the clinical trial, prepare the protocol, select the comparative medicines, and select the investigators. Their decisions are crucial if the clinical data obtained are to convince the regulatory authorities to grant a marketing application.

It is only comparatively recently that the quality of therapeutic trials sponsored by pharmaceutical companies has become adequate. However, with the advent of a more active monitoring role by the sponsor, and audits with the global framework of ICH GCP and other guidelines, this situation has changed. Frequently, the standards are higher than those conducted independently by individual clinicians.

Postmarketing trials of recently licensed medicines can provide an opportunity for a pharmaceutical company to familiarise a doctor with a new product. These studies have more to do with the marketing department of the pharmaceutical company than with serious research. Although regulatory authorities do not encourage such studies, there are undoubtedly several therapeutic issues that remain to be answered at the time when a new medical product is licensed and marketed. These studies are termed postmarketing surveillance (PMS) and safety assessment of marketed medicines (SAMM) studies and are usually carried out at the request of the regulatory authorities. Large sponsored clinical trials are required for the investigation of postmarketing safety issues. The clinical trial should involve treatment of study subjects under normal clinical conditions rather than the more specialised environment of a clinical trial. In other cases, postmarketing clinical trials involve combination therapy or medicoeconomic benefits of the treatment to be evaluated.

Ownership

In the past, various individuals and organisations have claimed to own the data produced from a clinical trial, including the state, the sponsor, the investigator and, in some cases, the patient or study subject. It is certainly true that with the advent of the EU Directive on Data Protection, the claim of ownership to his/her data by the patient or study subject has been strengthened. Unfortunately, there is no clear ownership of clinical data except that of society. Even then, society needs to respect the wishes of individual subjects who have been clinical trial participants. Is there a difference in ownership between data produced from product-driven research to that produced in policy-driven therapeutic research?

In product-driven therapeutic research, the pharmaceutical company must satisfy the regulatory and government agencies as well as the prescribers that the new product is effective, safe and meets the qualities required of GMP. The institutions that will pay for the drug - an insurance company or a government health authority - will need to be convinced that the product is good value. In return, the pharmaceutical company may, at some time in the future, recoup sufficient profit to pay the shareholders but also to pay for the development of the product. In the past, pharmaceutical companies avoided their results being made available for inspection. The ownership of the clinical data was clearly that of the pharmaceutical company. However, the ever-increasing requirements of the regulatory authorities and the creation of inspectorates to enforce these requirements mean that the majority of pharmaceutical companies will provide all the data obtained from a clinical trial if requested by an appropriate authority. This has been reinforced by the new Declaration of Helsinki, which requires the publication of both negative and positive results. and ICH GCP, where clinical trial reports need to be provided whether the clinical trials are completed or not.

Fundamental healthcare issues may also be involved in the situation of policy-driven therapeutic research. The future investment of society in health may require a large-scale and national clinical trial to answer questions relating to the prevention of disease or premature death. This type of clinical trial will not simply relate to one manufacturer's product. As such, it is preferable that the trial is organised on a national level, not necessarily with the exclusion of the company(s) involved. An independent data-monitoring committee (IDMC) should oversee the clinical trial with as much support from the pharmaceutical company as possible. The clinical data collected belongs to the state and should be treated with the same quality standards as any pharmaceutical company sponsored study.

Preclinical Investigations

There is a requirement to provide the investigator in a Phase I study with as much information as possible concerning the probable pharmacokinetic and pharmacological profile of the study drug. The investigator will need to decide the initial safe dose for the clinical trial and identify parameters for clinical monitoring of potential adverse effects.

Study Master Files

This term is generally used to denote the administration file kept for each trial and each investigation centre. Once the study has started, other documents will be added, including completed CRFs, ICFs and subjects' medical records, and other documents directly involved in the study. Some documents have to be kept specifically at the sponsor's office or the controlling centre. Separate files will contain financial and budget-related documents.

Protocol

This document describes the objectives, design, methodology, statistical considerations and organisation of a trial. Other information should be present such as the background and rationale for the clinical trial. It is a document key to any clinical trial, but is consistently prepared badly. There should be a logical approach to preparing a protocol.

Approach to construction of the protocol

Most pharmaceutical companies will have their own format for a protocol. Independent investigators will adopt their own or their institution format. All should follow the elements describe in the ICH GCP guidelines.

Frequently, the format for the protocol will be to "cut and paste" from a previous protocol, which may or not be a similar study to that being written. Certain sections may be the same, but care needs to be taken to avoid specific information relating to some previous study suddenly appearing in the text of the new protocol.

Several individuals may be involved in preparing the protocol. In a pharmaceutical company, it is usually left to a senior member of the medical department to coordinate the contributions, which should include those of the pharmaceutical physician, the statistician and sometimes the senior investigator involved in the study. Input from the principal investigator at an early stage in the development of the protocol is important. He/she can often contribute on practicalities (for example, selection of subjects) and primary endpoints. The protocols for independent studies may be prepared by the investigator but should always involve the advice of an experienced statistician familiar with clinical trials. Whether the protocol is for a commercially sponsored or an independent study, vigorous proofreading and review should take place. Reputable pharmaceutical companies will have protocol review boards with representatives from QA, data management as well as the pharmaceutical physician and statistician. A respected and disinterested colleague should review the protocols for independent studies.

When each new draft is produced, whether it is in development or considered final, each page must have "footers" indicating the version and the date of preparation. This will help to reduce confusion about which draft is being reviewed or used. In addition, pages become detached and mixed up with other versions. The final draft should be signed off by a very senior representative of the medical department sponsoring the clinical trial, the statistician involved in the preparation of the protocol and perhaps the senior investigator or medical advisor specialising in the indication or procedure. These signatories are confirming that the content of the protocol is their professional responsibility. In addition, each individual investigator involved in the clinical trial will sign off the so-called signature page present in each protocol, thereby agreeing to follow the protocol exactly.

Unfortunately, amendments to the approved protocol are frequent. These will require the same sign off/approval of signatures as required for the original protocol. If the amendment has any impact on the clinical trial, either medically or statistically, it will need to be approved by an IEC. The following questions must be answered before the final version of the protocol is ready.

1. Does the protocol make sense? It is recommended that someone other than a physician read the protocol. In the case where there are many investigator sites, the individuals reading the protocol will be tired and overworked! Also, laypersons such as those present on IECs will need to understand the document.
2. Is there a flow diagram of the essential elements of the study procedure?
3. Has the document been word processed? There should be no spelling mistakes, the contents page should match the pagination, and the presentation should be professional.
4. Is there a statement that the clinical trial will be conducted in compliance with the protocol, GCP, and the applicable regulatory requirements?
5. Is there a clear description of what source data will be recorded directly into the CRF and what will be recorded in the medical records? Normally, the protocol identification number, the date of consent, the date of commencement of the study, the visit dates, the start and finish dates of the administration of study drug and/or treatment, concurrent medication, adverse events and key efficacy parameters should be in the medical records. However, these items are the absolute minimum.
6. Are there clear instructions for reporting of adverse events and serious adverse events (SAEs)? There should be full instructions for the reporting of SAEs (including addresses and fax numbers), with time limits. The investigator does not always report SAEs that occur to a subject who has finished a study. All SAEs that come to the knowledge of the trialist should be reported unless the protocol provides guidance or time limit when the authors can justify that the occurrence of the SAE could not be related to the treatment received in the clinical trial. In a blinded study, there should be clear instructions when and by whom the code for a particular study subject should be unblinded in an emergency.
7. Does the protocol state that personal medical data obtained from the clinical trial will be made available to monitors, auditors and inspectors from regulatory authorities?
8. Does the protocol clearly state that the study cannot begin without approval of the IEC or IRB? This section should describe the consent process and state when informed consent should be obtained.

Informed consent by the subject must be obtained before he or she participates in the clinical trial. Only in special circumstances when the subject is unable to give informed consent can other arrangements be made. In the simple protocol, a review by the investigator of the medical history of the subject will establish the subject's suitability to enter the study. The patient should be given sufficient time to read the information sheet, discuss any concerns with the investigator, personal physician, partner, family or friend before giving consent and entering the study. Before the subject gives written consent, no invasive procedure (such as blood sampling or radiological examination) should be performed in deciding the suitability of the subject for the study. In addition, no drug, even if it is known to be a placebo, should be administered to the subject before written consent is given, unless it is part of an ongoing treatment for the indication that the subject suffers from. In some clinical trials there is a "wash-out" period when the subject is not allowed to take his or her routine medication: again, this must not take place until the subject has given written consent. In the more complex protocols, guidance must be given as to when consent should be obtained. Some data may already have been acquired from routine medical procedures undertaken for that particular indication and it may be inappropriate to repeat the procedure, for example radiological examination, after the subject has entered the trial. In volunteer non- patient studies, consent should be obtained from the volunteer before conducting screening tests to establish the volunteer's suitability as a potential subject in a Phase I study. The consent process is then repeated with a different information sheet/consent form before the volunteer enters a specific trial.

Informed consent form

Consent should be a four-stage process:

1. Verbal discussion between the investigator and the stuay subject
2. Review by the study subject of the ICF
3. Consideration by the subject
4. Signing the ICF.

This can be an oversimplification, particularly if the study subject is not in full health or is in a state of mind that does not fully appreciate all the implications. The investigator may be advised in situations like these to consider whether the study subject should be in the trial at all, particularly if they may drop out later. A copy of the ICF should be provided to the study subject.

The ICF consists of two documents - the information sheet and the actual consent form. They must be considered as a pair of documents, not separate entities. Normally a "core" ICF should be present in the appendices. The core ICF may need modifications to comply with local regulations. It is the responsibility of the sponsor/institution, or in an independent study the investigator, to prepare an ICF that meets the requirements of ICH GCP and any additional requirements of the local regulatory authority.

Several areas are usually done badly in the preparation of ICF.

1. The version number, date and page number (i.e. x of y pages) should be on each page. Without these features, new versions of the ICF will be mixed with old versions in the wrong page order in the "bustle" of the investigator site.
2. IECs and the institutional authorities often modify the core ICF. Local conditions, customs, interpretation of words and regulations may require some changes to the ICF. It may be acceptable to describe Alzheimer's disease as memory loss; however, removal of the section informing the study subject that other individuals besides the investigator will review his/her medical records is not acceptable since it is fundamental to ICH GCP.
3. The ICF should be written in a language that can be understood by the average study subject. Simple words should be used wherever possible: for example, "stop" instead of "discontinue", "avoid" instead of "abstain" and "cause" instead of "induce". Many study subjects will not understand technical words such as "placebo" and "erythema". Measurements of volumes should be described in domestic measurement such as teaspoonful or cupful rather than in millilitres.

4. Many ICFs lack any description or mention of alternative procedures or courses of treatment.
5. There should be consistency between the possible adverse events described for the study drug in the protocol, investigator's brochure and ICF.
6. Most countries have specific requirements for their ICF. It is essential that the requirements are known when the country-specific ICF is prepared. These examples could easily have changed by the time the reader is checking an ICF. In the UK, reference should be made to the ABPI Clinical Trial Compensation Guidelines. In other countries, for example Ireland, the study subject is allowed a specific length of time to decide whether to enter the study.
7. Mention has already been made of the new Directive on the protection of individuals when processing personal data and on the free movement of such data. At this time, the manner of how this Directive will be applied to data from clinical trials is still under review. However, the ICF needs to state the rights of the study subject. The subject will be told who controls the confidential data relating to him or herself, the purpose for which it is being collected and who will receive the data. In addition, apart from reinforcing the confidentiality of the data, the subject will be told that they have a right of access to check that the data relating to them are correct.
8. If the ICF is to be translated into another language, then someone fluent in that language should do the translation. Expensive translation agencies often provide a grammatically correct translation but in archaic language. The translator should provide a translation certificate stating what was translated and when, and the translator's name, status and appropriate qualifications. The translator should state that the translation was carried out to his/her best ability, and the statement should be signed and dated. A different person should then translate the translated ICF back into the original language. The latter document will then provide confirmation that nothing was left out in the original translation.

In studies where subjects are mentally or physically unable to give proper consent, special arrangements will need to be made. Where appropriate, the ICF will be read to the subject in the presence of a witness, or consent will be provided by the next of kin or the subject's representatives. Studies in which the study subjects cannot provide informed consent will become more frequent as more difficult indications, for example trauma, stroke, dementia, and handicapped or very young children become the focus of clinical trials.

Investigator's brochure

The investigator's brochure provides more detail than the protocol in relation to the background to the study, and should help to facilitate a better understanding of the rationale for the protocol, and its key features. In an ideal world, the potential investigator will receive the investigator's brochure before deciding to participate in the study. The brochure should provide the investigator with sufficient information to decide if the proposed study is justified and, together with any published papers, allow the would-be investigator to answer any questions that arise from trial personnel at the site and the IEC. There will be contributions to the brochure from specialists such as toxicologists and pharmacokineticist, and possibly from pharmacists if details of the study drug are included. A pharmaceutical physician should review this document carefully.

As more information becomes available concerning the study drug or treatment, new versions of the investigator's brochure should be prepared. Any thing that might alter the perception of the trial and its risks, such as a serious finding, must be communicated in writing, but a new version of the investigator's brochure should be distributed as soon as practical so that all concerned with the study have the facts. In any case, it is expected that a new version of the investigator's brochure will be prepared on an annual basis unless there is minimal new information. All documents should have the version number and date in the "footer" to avoid confusion between different versions. Receipts will be required from the investigator when a new brochure is received, and old brochures should be recalled and accounted for. The investigator's brochure is a confidential document and its security should be entrusted to the principal investigator.

Reference should be made to ICH GCP Guidelines when preparing an investigator's brochure. The recommended format includes the following elements: physical, chemical, pharmaceutical properties and formulations of the study drug, non-clinical pharmacology studies, pharmacokinetic and metabolism in animals, toxicology, effects on humans, summary of data, and guidance for the investigator, which includes details of how to recognise and treat a possible overdose or adverse reactions caused by the study drug or treatment.

Case report forms (CRFs)

The CRF (sometimes known as the clinical record form) is the partner to the protocol and to some extent they should be prepared together. The CRF should be designed and printed in such a way that all information on each trial subject is collected in a sequence and manner dictated by the protocol. It also acts in part as a checklist. The data to be collected extend from the study subject's demographic data, to the endpoint measures and adverse events observed. In replying to a series of questions, the investigator will record the study subject's response, sometimes by marking prepared squares. For example, in a bronchitis study the squares will characterise the cough, its frequency, precipitating factors, and quantity and appearance of sputum. The CRF will contain objective measures (for example, routine blood pressure readings and absence or presence of critical physical signs), and most endpoint measurements (for instance, peak expiratory flow readings). Most of these items may not be recorded in the medical records so the CRF is the only source of the data. The investigator or his/her co-investigators should sign that such items were correctly measured according to the protocol and accurately recorded in the CRF. Most CRFs have accompanying explanatory and guidance notes to assist the investigating team, together with a summary of the trial activities, including the timing and key actions at each point (for instance, taking of a blood sample).

The protocol should clearly indicate the data that should be present in the medical records as well as in the CRF. For some types of source data, the CRF is accepted by regulatory agencies as the source document. However, much information will be transcribed from other original documents (for example, radiological report, medical correspondence, laboratory results and the medical records).

Frequently, sections (sometimes known as modules) that have been used in other trials are collated together. This procedure has the advantage that ambiguities and mistakes found in other trials have been removed but, unless good QC is in place, sections will be left in that have no relevance to the present study. There should be "*field testing*" of the CRF by colleagues and even investigators before the start of the study. The CRF must be easy to understand, and the correct questions must be asked. The study statistician should be involved in the review of new CRFs to ensure that the questions asked meet the requirements of the statistical plan.

Depending on what will happen to the CRFs when they are completed, data managers should also be involved. The clinical data will need to be coded and then entered into a database before being further checked for completeness and correctness. The next step will be the analysis of the data. The manner of presentation of the data in the CRF will avoid some of the mistakes that occur during data entry, particularly if it is entered manually rather than by electronic transfer.

Each page of the CRF should include investigator identification, study subject number, protocol number, subject initials, and visit and/or study day. All pages are numbered as x of y pages with the version and date of CRFs in a "footer". Each appropriate section requires the signature from the investigator and a final sign off.

Practical considerations are often forgotten. The preparation of the CRF will take time, particularly if guidance notes are interspersed with individual pages. For example, in an endoscopy study, the site of lesions and other features can be recorded on a diagram. If study diary cards are used, they should be prepared at the same time. The printer's proof should be checked for accuracy before the printing is performed. The transfer of the final format to "no carbon required (NCR)" paper in order to create immediate copies will prolong the process in preparing the CRF. NCR paper should be of high quality whatever the budget for the study, otherwise only the top copy will be readable.

Source documents

Source documents are original documents such as medical records, laboratory report sheets, subjects' diaries or evaluation checklists, pharmacy dispensing records, recorded data from automated instruments, magnetic media and radiographs. The concept of what source documents are required in a clinical trial is often obscured by folklore. It has been said that inspectors from regulatory agencies have insisted that all data in the CRF is repeated in "*medical records*". This has resulted in the copying of the original CRF and calling the copies the source documents. This procedure gives little credit to inspectors and none to the investigators. The question that needs to be asked is why there is a need for source documents and, in particular, clinical trial information in the permanent medical records.

The protocol should specify what should be recorded directly into the CRF and what will also be recorded in the medical records. The CRF will contain all the pertinent data associated specifically with the clinical trial but some will be repeated in the medical records, for example, the protocol identification number, date of consent, date of commencement of the study, key baseline medical findings, visit dates, start and finish dates of the study drug/placebo or treatment, concurrent medication, adverse events and key efficacy and any unscheduled or scheduled actions or interventions (such as escape medication).

There are obvious benefits to any future consulting physician to know something of the medical history of a study subject, including any significant data obtained from a past clinical trial that might affect future medical care. In many cases, knowledge of the medical history contained in the medical records will decide whether the study subject meets the inclusion or exclusion criteria for the study. Additional information obtained from biopsy reports, radiographs and similar documents will provide confirmation that the data in the CRF are recorded correctly.

Some investigators and sponsors provide specific checklists for a clinical trial, which they claim are an alternative to the medical records. Information relating to medical history will be copied from the permanent records onto these checklists and most of the key parameters required to be recorded in the CRF will also be present on these checklists. However, monitors, QA auditors and inspectors need to see all the medical records available to the investigator. Some investigator sites, in particular those in outpatient departments, have no available medical records for individual subjects. The study subject may have not have a personal physician. In this situation, the subject may be the only person to provide any information about his/her medical history.

Storage of medical records

The investigator in the institution conducting the study should be aware of what happens to the medical records of study subjects who have participated in clinical trials. The medical authorities or the institution should have guidelines for the retention of records before they are changed into an electronic form by scanning, microfiched or destroyed. Usually when they are changed into another form, the medical records will be reviewed by administration staff and those items deemed not essential will be removed and destroyed. The investigator should be aware that complete medical records will be required for any future inspection by a regulatory agency. The medical record for each participating subject should be labelled on the front, stating that the record should not be destroyed without consultation with the investigator or before a certain date.

Study subject diary cards

These are small documents that form part of the source documents and are usually filled in by the subject during a study. They allow the subject to record on a daily basis any modest adverse event, for example headache, that occurs while taking the new treatment or an efficacy parameter, such as a change in their medical condition. Again, care should be taken in the preparation of the diary so that it is "user friendly". It should record days and weeks, not dates, use domestic time, not the 24-hour clock, and layman's terminology.

Alert card

The use of an alert card is not a specific regulatory requirement. However, in many clinical trials, it is appropriate that an alert card is given to subjects, particularly if they are outpatients. In an emergency, the alert card will identify that the subject is in a clinical trial and provide information on the nature of the clinical trial and whom to contact for information. The alert card should contain the sponsor's name and address (if appropriate), investigator's name, address and telephone number, with a 24-hour contact number (the contact should have knowledge of the study and not just be an "on-call" physician), the protocol number, the indication and the subject's name and address and identification number.

Standard operating procedures (SOPs)

SOPs are detailed written instructions designed to achieve uniformity in the performance of a specific function. Many pharmaceutical companies, hospitals and institutions have documents which they call SOPs. SOPs may provide guidance that can be applied to any clinical trial. The manner that blood pressure is taken, the storage of clinical trial material, or contractual or budgeting processes and documents may also be subject to SOPs. The local IECs will have SOPs concerned with the review of protocols and other documents. There are also specific SOPs used by an investigator and by the sponsor providing details as to how to conduct a clinical trial and in some cases, specifically for a protocol. These types of SOPs can be used to support the maintenance of similar methodology in a global multicentre study, for example unblinding procedures and the interpretation of data.

SOPs should be written so that they can be of use to new or experienced staff both for training and for information. Forms, templates and checklists should be referenced in the SOPs and flow charts should be used to illustrate the procedures being described. The SOP should be reviewed and, if required, updated on a regular basis.

Study Drug and Its Documents

The time taken to prepare, pack and label medications in accordance with regulatory requirements has delayed the start of many clinical trials. Not so long ago, the care and attention devoted to the preparation of study drugs was far from stringent. However, the regulators pointed out that it was illogical that experimental products were not subject to the controls that would apply to the formulations of which they are the prototypes. Nowadays, study drug material is produced according to GMP. A Certificate of Analysis and the documented assurance that the material has been produced according to GMP are required. The New Clinical Trial Directive will require the issuing of manufacturing licences for IMPs and labelling requirements. Manufacture of the study material should start as early as possible. Foresight is not easy, particularly when a series of related trials using the same medicine is being planned and scheduled to start over perhaps a two- year period. The enormity and uncertainty in the task are self-evident.

Manufacture

Manufacture of the study drug may be by the pharmaceutical company sponsoring the clinical trial or may be contracted out. The primary and secondary manufacture of clinical trial medications requires a long run-in period, probably six months or longer. It is affected by other manufacturing commitments and the state of technical development of the study drug. A decision should be made as early as possible that the formulation being used in early studies could be used in the marketing form. In particular, delays will be encountered if several formulations are tried with different dissolution rates. In this situation, the extent and timing of the clinical response could vary between formulations. If such variation is potentially significant, a clinical comparison of the formulations (bioequivalence study) may be required and, if the differences are marked, it could throw doubt on the medical meaning of the clinical trial(s) already performed.

The size of the order for clinical trial medication can be immense, equalling the order for start-up stock for the product when it is eventually launched. It is therefore a major undertaking if the whole requirement for the clinical development programme is ordered at one time; however, this is more efficient than placing smaller orders for supplies at irregular intervals. It is also sensible to anticipate the clinical trial needs after the launch, as other comparative trials may be sponsored or independent investigators may ask for trial stocks.

Comparative Medication

Apart from manufacturing placebo formulations, the company may need to approach the manufacturer of an already marketed product for clinical trial supplies if their medicine is chosen as a comparator. The precise requirements (such as similar size, colour and no identifying features) can be difficult to meet. Any approach may be met with some hesitation for valid reasons, but equally the reaction may be obstructive, asking for unreasonable access to information. It is customary to provide a copy of the protocol, or at the least an outline of it, with clear indication of the material needed and the time-frame for its supply.

Faced with difficulties in obtaining supplies directly from a rival manufacturer, the sponsoring company may decide to elect for a "***double-dummy***" technique or to mask the identity of the marketed comparator and to simulate the appearance of the new medicine. In doing so it must be realised that the absorption characteristics of the comparator might be changed (for instance, by a shellac coating) and it is essential that the bioavailability of the modified and the original formulation is checked beforehand.

Presentation

The clinical trial material must be suitably packaged for the purposes of the trial, meeting the optimal pack size dictated by the period of medication and the intervals between visits when trial prescriptions are renewed. For instance, a built-in excess of tablets or capsules is customary, partly to meet a possible delay in renewing stocks of study drug, particularly in a long-term trial. Another reason for an excess of study drug is to provide the subject with a known amount of study drug that is more than they need. A count of the "returns" will later reveal compliance, whereas if the number of tablets given was the exact requirement, the participant might be tempted to throw away those not taken, thus disguising their non-compliance.

The material must be appropriately labelled, giving a batch number and the medication code number. The latter must accord with the randomisation schedule. The necessary steps must be put in place and monitored in order to give the correct randomisation code for the study drug, comparator (if there is one) and placebo, and thereby ensure that each subject receives the correct allocation. Quality control steps in the packaging and labelling must be arranged and checked. The dosage instructions must be clear, and the identity of the investigator centre and of the sponsor given on the label. Where the study drug is being used in a blind study, it is essential to establish any differences between the test drug and the comparators in smell, appearance, consistency to touch, and taste. Many blind studies have been unblinded by such basic characteristics.

Shipping and Importation

The transport of medication to the investigating centre requires forward planning, particularly if it is abroad. In that instance, there will be a need for importation documents and if it is a research medication, waiving of custom's dues, and certification that its use has been approved, usually by an investigational licence. The local company staff may be the recipients at the point of importation, often signing for and collecting the medication. Alternatively, the principal investigator may be the direct recipient and must be provided with the necessary documentation to give accreditation and clearance of the trial material. Local company staff will be able to advise on the procedures, the usual delays and the necessary documents.

The registering and checking of these supplies at the investigating centre is equally important as all material received, used and returned must accounted for. In the majority of investigator sites, the pharmacy will play an important part in the storage and accountability of the study material. In some countries, the local regulations insist that a pharmacist supervises the storage and allocation of the study drug. Occasionally, there is no pharmacy at the site or the investigator makes his or her own independent arrangements with the sponsor. In these circumstances, the investigator will be responsible for the practical arrangements of storing and administering the study drug without the involvement of a pharmacist. The study drug should be stored in a secure facility free from pests and vermin, whether it is the hospital pharmacy or the consulting rooms at the investigator site. The environment where the study material is kept should be monitored and controlled for temperature and humidity.

Study Drug Documentation for the Master Files

Documentation should be available showing what is stored in the pharmacy or investigator's study drug cupboard, what has been administered to the subject and what has been returned in the form of leftover study drug or empty containers. In addition, there will be other documents giving more details of the nature of the study drug, codes for unblinding subjects in a blind study in case of emergency, and perhaps import licenses. These documents will be found in the investigator and pharmacy master files and/or in the sponsor's or coordinator's office.

Shipping documents

The manufacturer of the study drug should provide a standard request form for the investigator or sponsor to use when ordering supplies. Well-designed forms help the person completing the form to provide critical information. Each shipment should be accompanied by a document listing the contents of the shipment. Particular attention should be given to the dates when the study drug was dispatched from the supplier and when it arrived at the study site. A long interlude implies that the study drug may have been stored in an unsuitable area on the way to the site (for example, on the runway in high summer). The investigator should acknowledge receipt of the shipment by completing a copy of the form and returning it to the supplier. There should be an indication of when the study drug reaches its expiry date. Ideally, the expiry date should be given on the label of the study drug.

Frequently, in early trials of a new study drug, the expiry date is extended as more stability data become available. Any additional labelling by the sponsor or by the investigator should be documented fully and, where possible, a second person should QC the process. The labelling should always meet the GMP regulations applicable in the location. Drug accountability at investigator sites is often inadequate. Unless there are specific instructions in the protocol to the contrary, there should be a clearly documented trail of the drugs supplies that came in, what was administered to the subjects and what was returned by the subject in terms of unused medication. Any relaxation of drug accountability, as is seen sometimes in a multicentre study of many thousand subjects, can cause problems in monitoring the correct formulations and dosages given to the subjects. The significance of the results in such a trial may then be called into question.

The amounts and dates of departure of the study drug from the pharmacy should match that of administration of the drug to the subject, unless the drug is being transferred to a hospital clinic for short-term storage. A similar procedure should take place if the study drug is being stored within the clinic, either all the time or temporarily. The investigator, pharmacist or their staff should always check any returned study drug. What is actually present in terms of number of capsules, tablets or pills in the returned containers from each individual study subject should match what is recorded in the CRFs, and on the dispensing and returns records. There should be destruction certificates if unused study drug has been destroyed by the pharmacy. Alternatively, there should be documentation that states clearly what was returned to the study drug supplier and acknowledgement from the supplier that they have received the unused drug.

Sealed codes used for unblinding a study subject

Sealed codes are usually sealed envelopes, "advent" sheets or sealed label covers on the study drug containers that, when opened, will indicate which treatment the subject has been administered in a blind study. Their purpose is to provide the information the investigator needs for treating a subject for a SAE in an emergency. Only in a life-threatening situation (for example anaphylaxis) should the blind be broken by the investigator. Normally, the investigator should contact the sponsor for them to unblind the subject if necessary, thus improving the chances of maintaining the blinding of the whole study. There must be adequate arrangements to be able to unblind a subject in emergency outside the normal working day, and the sponsor or the investigator should provide a 24-hour helpline that can provide the necessary information concerning a particular protocol.

The sealed codes should be provided with the study treatment, and a blinded study should not start until the sealed codes are available at the site. Investigators sometimes unblind their own study subjects out of curiosity when the study has been completed at their site. Investigators should be informed that this must not happen. All sealed (and unsealed) codes should be checked and returned to the supplier at the end of the study. Unblinding of a study should never take place until all the study subjects, including those subjects at other sites, have completed the study and then should only be done by the appointed statistician in a controlled manner.

Running of the Clinical Trial

Before the Start of the Study

The previous sections have described how a clinical trial is designed, the documentation that must be prepared, and the preparation, documentation and dispatch of clinical trial material. None of these areas should be carried out in isolation and need to be addressed long before the first study subject is recruited. The pharmaceutical physician cannot be responsible for all these tasks unless he or she is carrying out independent research. Even then, he or she should seek expert help in the design of the study in relation to the statistical analysis and how the data will be collected and entered onto a database.

Selection of the investigator

The selection of investigators is critical to the success of a clinical trial. Unless there are very special circumstances, the principal investigator should have previous experience of clinical trials and qualifications that reflect experience in the indication involved. Exceptions can be made when a study drug is being investigated in general practice. In this situation, not every practitioner will be trained to undertake clinical trials or have special knowledge of the disease being treated. The sponsors should overcome any deficiencies by providing training and good monitoring. However, many of the most relevant criteria of sufficient and suitable staff support, facilities and study subject population will be determined in the so-called prestudy visit.

The pharmaceutical physician may wish to conduct his/her studies as an investigator or may be part of a sponsor organisation selecting investigators for a trial. The considerations may be different but the outcome will decide if an appropriate investigator is taking part in a study.

Considerations before becoming an investigator

The pharmaceutical physician as perhaps the physician in charge of the potential site will need to decide whether it is feasible for clinical trials to be carried out in his/her facilities. Similarly, the independent investigator should be honest with his/her self as to the practicalities needed before starting clinical research. The most important considerations are of time and resource. The physician should seek information about the sponsor: whether the reputation of the sponsor is known, both for adequate monitoring and support, and the use of user-friendly protocols and CRFs. The potential investigator should ask him/herself what is the motivation for doing the clinical trial. It is often financial, perhaps to provide additional funds for new equipment or staff, it may be scientific curiosity, or desire to improve patient treatment with a research drug, or it may be a desire to improve an individual's professional status by publication.

Considerations by the sponsor in selecting suitable investigators

There are various ways to select good investigators but none is foolproof.

1. Investigators found to be satisfactory in previous studies may be selected. However, circumstances do change, supporting staff leave, enthusiasm wanes, or other studies demand attention. The best investigator of a previous study, recruiting all study subjects requested and providing the cleanest clinical data, may fail in the next study.
2. There will often be a need for one or two opinion leaders to be involved in the study. They may have helped in the design of the study and contributed to the protocol and will contribute to any future publications. Their influence amongst their peers may help later to promote the use of the product. Often, but not always, they will wish to actively participate in the study although often most of the clinical trial work at their site will be delegated to a more junior physician. It should never be assumed that an investigator with high professional standing in his/her field will necessarily be a good investigator. Often the opinion leader is called a "principal investigator". However, the term is often used loosely and can equally be applied to an investigator in charge of several co-investigators or subinvestigators at an individual site and having little influence on the design of the study.
3. Sometimes pharmaceutical companies are familiar with suitable investigators in a therapeutic area with which they have previous experience. The opinion leaders themselves may know individuals suitable as investigators. Young investigators with some clinical trial experience may have suitable study subjects for a particular trial, and the ability and patience to cope with the considerable recording and documentation required in most clinical trials. However, recommendations that originate from the marketing department of pharmaceutical companies should be treated with caution. A physician who is a good customer for company products may not have the qualities required by an investigator.
4. There are now several commercial organisations that can provide a list of "suitable" investigators for a particular indication. Any assumption that the individuals are in fact suitable should be based on an independent assessment.

Prestudy visit

It is no longer sufficient for the pharmaceutical physician of a pharmaceutical company to meet a potential investigator in a restaurant and, with a handshake, discuss and agree on any future involvement by the investigator. Experienced senior staff of the sponsor should always visit the investigator site before a new clinical trial starts, even if the investigator has been involved in previous studies. Most pharmaceutical companies have checklists and SOPs of the requirements of an investigator site.

Key questions will need to be answered relating to staff support and the present work-load of the site. The competence of the staff to conduct any procedures, the maintenance, calibration and QC of any equipment to be used and whether other clinical trials demand too much resource are all questions that need answers. In addition, the facilities should be inspected to establish whether the site could store and archive securely the large amounts of documents and study drugs that will be present. The pharmacy may play a major role in the study and therefore the facility and the pharmacist should be visited.

Questions should always be asked about the site staff's understanding of GCP and whether the investigator appreciates the need for informed consent, ethical approval and the review of highly confidential documents by outsiders. Finally, the sponsor will need to explore with the investigator the protocol, which may be still in draft form at this stage. The investigator will need to know what will be required of him or her and the site staff and whether the procedures in the protocol are acceptable to him/her. When the protocol is finalised, the investigator will need to follow the protocol exactly. Other interests (for example other clinical trials) of the investigator at the site may interfere with any participation in the study and the site may not be able to provide sufficient suitable study subjects.

At the time of the prestudy visit, and certainly before any study subjects are recruited, other activities will need to take place. The medical management will need to select the laboratories to be used, and organise QA auditors to check any software houses involved in the production of software for the clinical trial. The software used (for example, in electronic diaries or interactive voice response technology [IVRT]) will need to be audited to establish that validation procedures are in place. There should be plans for QA auditors to visit any plants involved in the distribution of the study drug. Only in very exceptional circumstances do the qualifications and experience of the pharmaceutical physician warrant their involvement in these exercises. He or she should understand that these activities need to be undertaken and the contribution that each activity will make to the study. Team cooperation at the sponsor site is essential for the future success of the study. However, the pharmaceutical physician will be involved if part of the clinical work is to be delegated to a CRO or site management organisations (SMO) or they are part of a strategic team planning the clinical trial. Some of these entities are explored below.

CROs and SMOs

There is a growing reliance by sponsors on contracting out part or all of the work of the clinical trial to a subcontractor. Manufacturers often find that they cannot organise every clinical trial that they require. The reasons are many, but commonly reflect limited staff resources, pressures of time, and inability to identify and organise investigators, especially into a collaborative group (for instance, general practitioners in one locality). In independent studies by investigators, additional expertise may be needed in statistical analysis or data management and similar areas. Subcontractors offer different services, from large CROs capable of conducting an international clinical trial with minimal contribution from the sponsor, specialised groups for data management, safety monitoring, auditing, or a single consultant for statistical analysis or medical writing.

A recent development has been the emergence of SMOs which are really CROs involved at the sharp end of clinical trials, i.e. the investigator site. Nearly half of all delays in clinical development occur with the setting up and initiating of studies at investigator sites. These delays result from obtaining IEC approval, study subject recruitment or the training of staff. Individual SMOs should be able to identify investigators capable of conducting the trial and have access to a large number of suitable study subjects. In addition, time can be saved by the sponsor through having a single contact for contract and budget negotiations, and having investigator sites familiar with GCP and the requirements of the local regulations. SMOs are usually regional or national business enterprises with one or more locations. Several varieties of SMOs exist, some specialising in particular indications perhaps attached to an institution focused on that indication, some providing support for independent investigators and some being totally independent business enterprises.

The pharmaceutical physician should be involved in the selection of CROs and SMOs. He/she is often best qualified to judge the professional competency of the physicians involved in any contractual work. There needs to be a clear understanding as to who will provide medical advice to the investigator and to the non-physicians in the clinical trial teams, who will be responsible for the assessment of the medical significance of adverse events, serious adverse events and safety issues in general, and who will be conducting any medical coding. The responsibility for custody of the clinical data should be clearly defined at each stage from initial recordings to the final analysis. It is essential to define the roles and responsibilities of the sponsor, including the sponsor's medical expertise, those of the contracted organisation, as well as of the investigators, who will always have ultimate responsibility for their study subjects and their safety.

Technical Considerations

Before a clinical trial starts, the use of technical aids such as IVRT, remote data entry, and electronic diaries has to be considered. In the section on Monitoring Visits, mention will be made of the use of electronic tracking system that provide status and monitoring reports. All these systems utilise computer systems that must be validated. Double and McKendry described computer validation as the process that documents that a computer system reproducibly performs the functions it was designed to do. The document "Guidance for Industry - Computerised Systems used in Clinical Trials" published by the FDA in 1999 gives clear recommendations of what is required.

Interactive voice response technology (IVRT)

The use of IVRT can improve the efficiency of various procedures carried out at the investigator site. Investigators and their staff interact with the electronic technology by pressing the appropriate keys on their touchtone telephone in response to a recorded voice request. In a typical example, when a new subject is recruited to a clinical trial, the subject randomisation number can be allocated in return for demographic information such as subject initials, eligibility criteria, age, sex and weight. In addition, IVRT can be used to track clinical trial material and ensure that the correct allocation of study drug is provided to each subject. Batches of study drug will prepared in lots of two, three or four, etc - each lot ensuring that an equal number of subjects at a site receive study drug, comparator and placebo.

Remote data entry

Remote data entry is the process where data are entered into a laptop or personal computer rather than onto a paper CRF. Normally, this process will take place at the investigator site. The computer screen provides a so-called electronic CRF (eCRF), which, like the paper CRF, will require a series of answers or parameters to be recorded. The system provides screen prompts and checks. These remind the investigator to complete responses and can immediately draw attention to any inconsistency between responses. Not all the data can be recorded directly into the eCRF and, as with the paper CRF, key elements will still need to be recorded in the study subject records.

The internet provides a modern solution for the transmission of data to the sponsor office. Web browsers provide a point-and-click interface that allows data to be downloaded to a remote server. Monitors can review the data from the sponsor's office and instruct the investigator in any corrections required. This procedure has the potential to provide higher quality data through earlier interventions. In addition, analog signals from physiological parameters such as ECG and blood pressure monitors can be routinely downloaded onto the internet and transferred for remote analysis, before the findings are entered into the clinical trial database. Security of the internet has been an issue but can be better ensured with the use of electronic signatures and encrypted data transmission.

Electronic subject diaries

Paper subject diaries are notoriously poor in their legibility, completeness and accuracy. Electronic diaries are small, portable devices that can present text and graphics to the subject. They allow the subject to record and store responses, which can be time-stamped for each entry made. The data can then be downloaded directly into the clinical trial database. The main drawbacks include the need for training of the subject in the diary's use, possible errors in local time settings and the logistics of distribution, maintenance and recovery of the diaries.

Clinical laboratories

Traditionally, the local hospital pathology department was used to provide laboratory safety data for clinical trials. Increasingly, sponsors are using central laboratories to which some or all the laboratory samples for a multicentre study are sent. Central laboratories provide standard methodology, which reduces variation between investigator sites and where a single and well-established reference range is used. In addition, all the laboratory results can be transferred electronically to the main database, thus avoiding the opportunities for mistakes to occur in the copying of data from the laboratory report sheet onto the CRF and then entered manually into a database.

However, there are drawbacks as well as advantages. Clinical trials for certain intensive care indications, for example trauma and acute myocardial infarction, will require frequent monitoring of certain laboratory parameters, and the use of quick results as provided by a local laboratory is essential. In other situations, investigators will sometimes obtain laboratory data from two sources - local and central - from the same sample. This may be due to poor training but frequently reflects the investigator's mistrust of data from an unfamiliar and perhaps foreign central laboratory. The protocol must be very clear about which results will be used in any safety analysis. The regulatory authorities will not accept an arbitrary selection based on favourable or unfavourable results that may bias any future safety analysis. Some laboratory parameters of the samples, for example mean cell volume, prothombin time and microbiology, may need to be measured quickly at the local laboratory. Blood samples for the estimation of drug or metabolite levels may need to be analysed quickly, before degradation takes place. In addition, the central laboratory selected may be in a different part of the country or even in another continent and samples will need to be sent by courier.

A good central laboratory will provide adequate packaging and arrange the courier service. The International Air Transport Association (IATA) regulations for the transport of biological samples across national borders need to be observed. Most blood samples will fall into risk group II. Further information can be obtained from the IATA website. Staff responsible for the packaging of the samples for dispatch will require appropriate recognised training.

Study subject recruitment

In the past the recruitment of study subjects has been highly dependent on the activities of the investigator and which study subjects were attending his/her clinic. Recommendation of a studv subject by the treating physician is still the preferred method for recruiting study subjects. However, advertisements for suitable study subjects are being used increasingly. These may be placed on notice boards in clinics, in the local press, and on television and radio. The most recent development has been the use of the internet, particularly for studies where recruitment is difficult.

However tempting it is for the pharmaceutical physician, investigators and sponsors to use advertising, they should be aware that there are certain guidelines and regulations to observe before embarking on any advertisement for a clinical trial.

1. An IEC should review the advertisement or the recording of the proposed video or audio message before it is publicised.
2. Only limited information should be presented – the name and address of the clinical investigator, the purpose of the research and, in summary form, the eligibility criteria for the study, a precise description of any benefits to the subject, the time or other commitment required by the subject, the location of the research and the person to contact for information.
3. No claims should be made, either explicitly or implicitly, that the drug or device is safe or effective for the indication.
4. Terms such as "new drug", "new medication" or "new treatment" should not be used without an explanation that the study drug or treatment is experimental.
5. Advertisements should not promise "free medical treatment" when the intent is not to charge for taking part in the investigation. The key aspect is that subjects should not enter clinical trials purely because they cannot afford to obtain medical treatment for their illness.

Training of the investigator and site staff

The competence of the investigator and the site team is clearly the responsibility of the institution or employing authority, and at a practical level, of the investigator. The sponsor cannot train them in the medical, scientific or technical aspects of procedures related to study subject investigation or care. The sponsor, the institution or the independent investigator will need to ensure that the basic procedures required in the clinical trial are explained. At a practical level, all staff involved in a clinical trial will be required to undergo training in both the basic principles of ICH GCP and in the key elements of the specific clinical trial. Inspectors from regulatory agencies will expect fully documented training. A long-term training programme for each member of the clinical management team should be part of any responsible sponsor terms of work. The training of site staff will be carried out at initial visits to the site and at investigator meetings.

Investigator meetings

Some investigators view investigator meetings as an opportunity to enjoy luxury hotel accommodation and food at the expense of the sponsor, usually a pharmaceutical company. Investigator meetings differ from site visits and are an essential part of the preparation for a site before recruitment of subjects for a clinical trial. Pharmaceutical physicians should view investigator meetings as an important part of the process of meeting investigators and learning about problems before they occur.

Investigator meetings can be single-centre or multicentre meetings and may have global representation. Meetings should be attended by the investigators, their staff, and key individuals from the sponsors. They should always occur before a study starts and before a clinical trial commences at a particular site. Sometimes investigator meetings take place during a study to update investigator site staff and train new investigators to the study. They should include sections relating to GCP and safety aspects, drug accountability and administration, recording of data, and a detailed review of the protocol. If the actual meeting is well structured and planned, it is an opportunity to ensure uniformity of procedures and the resolution of any misunderstandings.

Use of the independent data-monitoring committee (IDMC)

The pharmaceutical physician may be asked to serve on an IDMC. It is an independent committee that may be established to assess at intervals the progress of clinical trials, with particular respect to the safety data, and critical efficacy endpoints. The members of the committee are mainly physicians who have the power to recommend the continuation, modification or stopping of a clinical trial. When working with a "blind" study, some of the members may sometimes be unblinded and great care needs to be taken not to unblind the other members. Another use for IDMC is to provide an independent pool of experts to evaluate a particular parameter of efficacy in a multicentre study, such as the size of a growth in a radiograph. This provides some degree of uniformity when many different physicians and specialist at individual sites are measuring many radiographs.

Ethics committee application

The investigator is normally responsible for obtaining ethical approval for a clinical trial through the Local Research Ethics Committee (LREC), which is usually based at the institution or within the employing authority (university or hospital). The investigator will be responsible for the application to the LREC to conduct the clinical study at his/her site and provide the appropriate documents (for example, protocol, ICF, subject recruitment procedures, investigator's brochure and any new safety information, information on payments and compensation and the investigator's *curriculum vitae*) as well as notifying the IEC of any protocol amendments, which will also require approval. Annual or more frequent reports of the progress of the study and any safety issues, including serious adverse events, will need to be provided. The sponsoring company should provide assistance in obtaining approval from the IEC and prepare the appropriate reports for the investigator. At present in the UK, there are two principal types of IECs - the LRECs and Multicentre Research Ethics Committees (MRECs). The approval of the LREC needs to be obtained for each centre taking part in a clinical trial in a particular area. If a multicentre study is to be performed in five or more LREC geographical boundaries, then the approval of the MREC must be obtained first. The principal investigator will play a major role in the submission process. Recently, a new Central Office for Research Ethics Committees (COREC) has been established to streamline the work of research IECs in the UK. It has published new documents detailing a standards framework for the processing of research proposals.

Regulatory approval

Most clinical trials must be approved from the appropriate government agency before they start. There is considerable variation in the requirements of each country, although the new European Directive should make the process of regulatory approval simpler in the EU. For the US, an Investigational New Drug (IND) Application is made to the FDA using Forms 1571 and 1572, the latter giving details of the investigators, facilities, and IEC(s).

Budgets and contracts

The administrative aspects of clinical trials ought to be straightforward but often are not, mainly because of failure to clarify what each party expects. Responsibilities must be clearly defined.

Budget

The budget must be set, the means of payment agreed, and contractual arrangements for premature trial termination decided. In addition, the legal contract should include payments, if any, when a study subject drops out, or when it is impossible to evaluate an individual subject (for example, protocol violations by an investigator caused by blatant recruitment of subjects who do not meet the inclusion criteria). If these are not addressed at the outset, considerable annoyance and misunderstandings will arise. There should be a clear understanding of the costs and expenses that the site's institution or hospital will absorb and what the sponsor will pay for either directly or indirectly. Investigators conducting independent research must realise that they too have additional expenses when conducting research and someone will be picking up the bill. It is essential to have a written contract with the institution. In preparing it, one must identify other supporting services (for instance, laboratory investigations and the use of the pharmacy) that are effectively subcontracted by the clinical investigators, but are sometimes omitted as recipients even within their own institution. It is helpful to try to separate the cost of materials and equipment hire from the cost of the services provided by staff. In some cases, the institution where the investigator site is situated will demand a "*handling charge*" for handling the contract and dealing with the invoices. This may cover some or all the salaries of the site staff, the use of the facilities and equipment, and disposable supplies. Many larger pharmaceutical companies now utilise a contracts manager aided by someone skilled in purchase negotiations, otherwise trial costs can he absurdly high and unrealistic. In all financial matters concerning clinical trials, all costs and expenses must be clearly recorded.

Contract

The contractual basis should be outlined in a "letter of agreement". In addition to the undertakings relating to the particular trial, some standard provisions should be included either in the contract, in the protocol or in both. These include an indemnity statement, a study subject compensation statement, an inspection/audit understanding, and a publication statement. The investigators' responsibilities under ICH GCP guidelines and related procedures should be identified. Often most of these can be simply listed and it is recommended that industry-agreed procedures (for instance, ABPI guidelines) are adopted and quoted as these are widely accepted.

Financial disclosure

Globally, there is concern that biased results could be produced from studies conducted by investigators who own shares or other financial benefits in the pharmaceutical company sponsoring their trials. The Declaration of Helsinki (2000) requires that "sources of funding, institutional affiliations and possible conflicts of interest should be declared in any publication". All studies conducted on products that are likely to be part of a submission to the US FDA require the sponsor to make a disclosure of financial holdings of the investigators that participate in all studies. Any significant payments (US$25 000) that could influence the outcome of the trial, proprietary interest in the product under study or significant equity interests need to be declared by the investigator. Before commencing a study, the investigator should make a financial disclosure. Most future products will need to benefit from the potential sales of the US market. Even when there is a considerable financial interest in the success of the product, the financial disclosure will not necessarily rule out totally the investigator's role in the study. Most inspectorates are more interested in what is not declared than what is.

During the Study

Collection of the data

The expertise of the pharmaceutical physician when employed by a sponsor will be used to support the clinical trial team in four main areas during a clinical trial.

1. He/she will be required to support the monitoring staff and understand their function at the site. In particular, he/she may be required to give medical interpretation when inclusion and exclusion criteria are considered.
2. He/she will be required to understand the importance of and to review adverse events and SAEs. He/she will be required to have an overview of new safety issues.
3. He/she will be required to interpret the significance of the laboratory data in relation to the study drug.
4. He/she may be required to support the coding of medical terms before the clinical data are analysed.

Monitoring visit

One of the advantages of working with a large institution or pharmaceutical company is that the clinical trial should be properly monitored. Investigators conducting independent studies should be aware that a study nurse or another physician does not replace the role of the independent monitor or clinical research associate. The clinical trial monitor acts as a QC supervisor, usually covering several centres involved in the same trial, and so achieving uniformity in the checking and in the remedial actions taken. The monitor will help in the interpretation of the protocol or relay procedural instructions, which can reduce misunderstandings, and help to create uniformity across all investigating sites. The monitors are required to carry out source data verification, i.e. to compare individual subject's medical records and other supporting documents with what is recorded in the CRF and to check that the information in the CRF is complete, accurate and legible. Omissions such as concomitant drug treatment or development of a concurrent illness should be corrected. In addition, all missing visits and subjects failing to complete the study, and the reason for each failure, must be recorded. Informed consent documentation and the documents present in the master file at the site should be checked.

Both ICH GCP and the FDA require the monitor "to assure adequate protection of the rights of human subjects involved in clinical investigations and the quality and integrity of the resulting data". The investigator and the site staff will have primary responsibility for these aspects of clinical research. The regulatory inspectorates have, on numerous occasions, observed failures in both consent and ethical approval procedures, and in data recording, when there has been no or inadequate monitoring.

After each visit to the site, the monitor is required to record in the visit report the errors and the remedial action. These visit reports may be reviewed by the regulatory authorities. Repetitive errors will be highlighted in the monitoring reports, along with the status of each subject recruited at the site. In some pharmaceutical companies, the information in the report is recorded on an electronic tracking system. The system will provide rapid updates on the progress at a particular investigator site. These updates, together with others from other investigator sites, allow rapid assessment of the progress and status of the whole trial. Errors found in the CRF or in the documentation in the files are recorded in a convenient manner usually by tabulation in "*error logs*". These list the corrections required of the investigator and provide indicators where improvements are required. Efforts to produce high-quality, so-called "clean" CRFs at the site will be rewarded later when preparing the clinical trial database for analysis. Any queries and corrections that occur once the CRF has left the site will require the correction to be approved and signed off by the investigator. The clinical trial monitor is a temporary member of the site team. A good monitor will conduct scheduled visits, and the investigator and the site staff should provide sufficient time to answer questions and correct data in the CRF that has been transferred incorrectly from source documents. Often negative answers are left blank rather than answered and signatures are absent when required. The monitor will need space to work and should be provided with requested documentation, including medical records, for review.

Adverse events

There is considerable confusion in the use of terminology in this area. Edwards and Aronson proposed the following definitions.

1. An adverse drug reaction is "an appreciably harmful or unpleasant reaction, resulting from an intervention related to the use of a medicinal product, which predicts hazard from future administration and warrants prevention or specific treatment, or alteration of the dosage regimen, or withdrawal of the product".
2. An adverse effect is an all-encompassing term, to include all unwanted effects, making no assumptions about mechanism, evoking no ambiguity and avoiding the risk of misclassification. But it is an adverse outcome that can be attributed to some action of a drug.

3. "*Adverse reaction*" and "*adverse effects*" are interchangeable terms, except the former is seen from the point of view of the subject and the latter from the point of view of the drug.
4. An adverse event is an adverse outcome that occurs while a study subject is taking a drug, but is not necessarily attributable to it.

It is important to distinguish between event and reaction. In clinical trials, this acknowledges that it is not always possible to ascribe causality.

Types of adverse drug reaction

There are several classifications of adverse reactions, but the most commonly employed define two principal kinds (A and B) and three subordinate classes (C, D and E).

- Type A (augmented) reactions are due to the pharmacological effect of the drug, often in exaggerated form. They are dose related, predictable, and they can occur in anyone.
- Type B (bizarre) reactions occur only in some people and are not part of the known pharmacology of the drug. They are not dose related and are the result of unusual interaction of the study subject with the drug. These effects may be predictable where the mechanism is known (for example, the genetic polymorphism associated with some hepatic metabolising enzymes) or unpredictable (for example, due to immunological processes).
- Type C (continuous) reactions are due to long-term use of the drug (for example, analgesic nephropathy or peripheral neuropathy with reverse transcriptase inhibitors).
- Type D (delayed) reactions are teratogenic or carcinogenic responses.
- Type E (end-of-use) reactions occur with rebound withdrawal phenomena.
- Recently a Type F has been added: unexpected failure of therapy.

In Phase I and II studies, Type A reactions are by far the most frequent. Type B are rare, which is fortunate as some can be serious or even fatal. The problem is many orders of magnitude worse if the adverse reaction closely resembles spontaneous disease that has a background incidence in the population in the trial.

Reporting adverse events and establishing causality

An adverse event or experience is defined as "any undesirable experience occurring to a subject whether or not considered related to the investigational product(s)". Sponsors will have their own set of definitions and SOPs governing reporting of adverse events. The following account be generally applicable to most situations. Adverse events can be described as serious or non-serious. Under SAEs the ICH GCP includes an event that:

(i) is fatal
(ii) is life threatening
(iii) results in persistent or significant disability/incapacity
(iv) requires hospitalisation or prolongation of hospitalisation
(v) is associated with a congenital abnormality/birth defect.

The investigator has the responsibility to notify the sponsor immediately he/she has knowledge of an SAE. Where applicable, the IEC and relevant authorities should be also be informed either by the sponsor or by the investigator. This will allow the appropriate measures to be taken to safeguard the study subjects. Although the time-frames below provide more time than originally was required by regulatory authorities (for example, the FDA), the reporting of SAEs, whether considered alarming or not, should have priority over most other activities in a clinical trial. The ICH guidelines states that certain SAEs may be sufficiently alarming so as to require very rapid notification to the sponsors and appropriate authorities. Fatal or life-threatening unexpected SAEs require notification by telephone or fax within seven calendar days by the sponsor or investigator to the authorities. The telephone or fax report must be followed by a hardcopy report within a further eight calendar days. The report must include an assessment of the importance and implication of the findings, including relevant experience with the same or similar entities. All other serious unexpected SAEs that are not fatal or life threatening must be reported as soon as possible but within no more than 15 calendar days. Establishing a cause–effect relationship between an adverse event and the use of a drug is a serious and difficult problem.

With this kind of classification in mind, how can a sponsor (or anyone else interested) assess whether an adverse event is associated with a particular medicine? Broadly, there are two approaches – global introspection and use of algorithms. Both rely on the application of logic to the set of circumstances presented. Global Introspection is most frequently used and involves one or more experts considering the factors associated with the medicine and institution. The main factors to consider are:

1. Previous experience with the medicine, for example background incidence of reaction in this disease group
2. The study subject's medical history, for example more frequent in the elderly, hepatic and renally impaired; previous exposure to the medicine; presence of other disease
3. The characteristics of the adverse event, for example timing of event, plasma concentration of parent drug and metabolites, laboratory tests
4. Effects of rechallenge, dechallenge and response to treatment
5. Alternative explorations of adverse event, for example other therapies.

The risk of rechallenge has to be very carefully considered. Its use will depend on the severity of the reaction, availability of a specific antidote, ease and speed of reversing the effect and the subject's willingness to be exposed for a second time. Rechallenge is not infrequently undertaken in Phase I studies when an exaggerated response occurs and a smaller dose can be used. IEC approval must be obtained and consideration given to the use of active drug and placebo in a randomised double-blind administration.

Determining clinical significance of an adverse event

If an adverse event has been causally linked to the use of the drug in the trial, the sponsor, usually in conjunction with the investigator, will need to decide on the clinical relevance of the event and the action that needs to be taken. The issue is important to:

1. The individual subject
2. The rest of the subjects in the trial
3. Those about to receive the drug in the clinical development programme
4. The overall future of the drug.

The clinical significance (in both the narrow and wider context) of the adverse event will be determined by considering the following factors.

1. How serious is the event?
2. Will it reverse spontaneously and completely?
3. What specific therapy is available?
4. Are particular groups of subjects at risk and should clinical usage be restricted?
5. Are there any clinical or investigational factors that could predict who may develop the adverse event?
6. What is the benefit:risk ratio?
7. Is the drug a novel medicine in an otherwise poorly treated and severe disease?
8. Are alternative medicines toxic?

These deliberations may result in several outcomes. Clinical development may continue as planned, but additional vigilance with more frequent visits and special tests may be added. The dose may be reduced or certain "at-risk" subjects may be excluded from further trials. The drug may proceed to registration, but the authorities may stipulate that a postmarketing surveillance study be conducted. The drug may be withdrawn from further clinical development.

Council for international organization of medical science (CIOMS)

CIOMS is associated with safety, providing various forms such as the form normally used to report SAEs (CIOMS I) but also many other types of forms, for example CIOMS II for the international reporting of periodic drug-safety update reports. The council is active as a medium for international discussion on safety and bioethics.

Laboratory safety data

When the CRFs arrive at the data manager's office, questions will arise relating to laboratory safety data. Queries may occur at the investigator site and advice can be requested from the pharmaceutical physician at the sponsor associated with the clinical trial.

There are several different kinds of laboratory safety data that require interpretation. These include routine screening for study subject selection, diagnostic evaluation of the subject, identification of risk factors, monitoring the progress of the disease or treatment, detection of adverse reactions, determination of appropriate dosages for certain "at-risk" subject groups (for example, those with renal impairment).

In general, the interpretation of laboratory safety data is undertaken for the following reasons:

1. To identify trends in the data, even if the individual or mean values lie entirely within the "normal" reference ranges. Delta checking are "flags" that appear in a laboratory result printout for a parameter indicating inconsistency with previous results. The laboratory equipment has to be programmed so that significant changes will be flagged. They could indicate change in the subject's condition or a wrong specimen or reagent
2. To identify predictable or unpredictable laboratory abnormalities, which may need particular attention in further studies
3. To identify abnormal values in an individual study subject
4. To identify groups who are potentially at high risk
5. To establish a "*denominator*" for any problems that may occur in this or subsequent studies.

References ranges and sources of error

The trends in data or individual abnormal values are only interpretable if the reference values are known and the test is reliable. Reference ranges usually refer to the mean value and two standard deviations either side of the mean. Thus 95% of a sample population who are free of disease will fall inside this range, with 2.5% above and 2.5% below. The sponsor should know the source of subjects who provide this normal range, and most laboratories periodically update their ranges of reference values to reflect the population they serve. Reliability indicates that the test is consistent over time and a reliable test correlates highly with successive measures.

An individual study subject with one or more abnormal safety values in a trial may have responded adversely to the drug, but other causes should be sought. These include concurrent and intermittent illnesses, concurrent medications, alcohol or drug abuse, and progress of the disease. The careful follow up of the subject with repeated laboratory tests during and after treatment will usually resolve whether the observations arc attributable to the drug.

Some changes in laboratory values in groups of subjects, but remaining within the normal range, are more difficult to interpret. Seeking similar trend patterns in concurrent or subsequent clinical trials may help to confirm or dispel beliefs about attributing the abnormal findings to the drug. A not infrequent finding of this kind is a transient rise in liver transaminases or creatine kinase, but usually a careful history and follow up investigations will determine whether the enzyme changes are due, for example, to an acute viral infection or to exposure to the drug.

Laboratory safety data can be erroneous, and this must always be considered when abnormalities are reported. There are numerous sources of error, which may be related to the study subject (for example, self-medication, certain foods, undue exercise), sample collection technique, storage and transport, the analytical technique used (for example, high variability, inappropriate reference ranges, interfering substance in the sample), or to the report (for example, transcription errors). When there is doubt about the validity of the test, it should be repeated and, if necessary, at a different laboratory.

Action taken in response to abnormal findings

Individual study subjects may have to be withdrawn from the trial if abnormalities in laboratory safety data are confirmed and considered serious. Trends in laboratory findings in certain groups, for example the elderly, or in all study subjects may result in additional investigations being requested in subsequent clinical trials, for example measurement of hepatic transaminases. Further clinical trials will provide information as to how well the study drug is tolerated and whether the benefits revealed by laboratory safety and efficacy data outweigh the overall risk.

Data Management

The assembling of clinical trial data before analysis constitutes a major workload, dictated by the quantity and the quality of the data. If the quality is poor, the process is extended by remedial steps going all the way back to the investigator site. Therefore, all the preceding efforts to bring high-quality data from investigators are amply justified by the resources and time actually saved during the data management process. Computerised systems are essential for handling the quantity of the data, and for future interrogation. Organisations and pharmaceutical companies are still inclined to create separate databases for each trial, using different machines, different codes and different locations (for instance, different countries). In the drive to save time and money, it is essential to avoid this situation. IT specialists will reassure that, with a little programming, the merging of such data from many trials will be easy, but problems still frequently occur.

Two elements are features of modern data management: a validated computer system and highly professional specialist staff. Non-validated computer systems are unacceptable. The FDA documents "Computerised Systems Used in Clinical Trials" and the 21 CRF 11 Regulations should be followed when processing clinical data in any computer system, even if the results will never be required to be used in any US regulatory application. All indications suggest that the principles in these documents should be adopted globally for clinical trial work. Specialist staff should be responsible for handling of the clinical data. Nowadays, data management is a recognised discipline with professional associations and university courses. Trained programmers and statisticians support them. Any temptation to avoid use of trained staff but instead relying on secretaries, investigator site monitors or nurses could prolong the time of processing and may endanger the integrity of the results.

Computer systems in clinical trials

Because the use of computer systems in data management is so important, it is appropriate to have a basic understanding of what is required for a validated computer system. In simple terms, certain features distinguish the computer system from a non-validated system. The computer system has to be developed, implemented, operated and maintained in a controlled manner, from the design stage to its decommissioning. Each stage will need to be fully documented. Written functional specifications should be available. In many cases, the computer systems will be off-the-shelf commercially available systems and the vendor will need to have evidence that the product has been developed in a controlled environment. Often the QA personnel from an organisation using the particular system will visit the vendor to try to establish that accepted validation practises are being followed. They may be allowed to see test results that must exist of the development and installation. When any new software or hardware is used in the data management centre, so-called end-user testing should be undertaken. Also, if changes are made to the system or perhaps new versions of software introduced, then additional testing may be required and certainly the alterations or maintenance documented. There will be a need for written guidance documents, for example SOPs relating to the use of the system, proper backup of data and, most importantly, security to prevent unauthorised individuals entering the system and changing data. Finally, all staff using the system need to be trained in its use.

Process

The system reflects the process undertaken in many data management groups. Although the positions of some of the stages such as data entry and query generation may vary, as in the case of electronic data capture at the investigator site, the activities will be similar for all data management. The clinical data may arrive in various forms at the data management centre. CRFs can arrive by fax, post or courier, central laboratory data by email or by diskette, scans by courier, assessments by an expert panel via courier, ECG and Holter data by courier or post, etc. It is therefore essential that proper tracking systems are in place.

The data manager will need to liaise with the programming and statistical individuals to decide the structure of the database. The requirement of interim analyses may impact on the processes and is of major significance if a clinical trial is blinded. Separate staff will be needed for the interim analysis if the regular staff are to remain blinded for the final analysis. Other considerations include the coding of the data and the dictionaries to be used, when and how the SAE/adverse event data will be incorporated into the structure and how much of the cleaning of the data will be done electronically (i.e. diagnostic programming). If data entry is performed in several centres (for instance, different countries) the standards must be identical. A centrally based validation group will monitor that these standards are being maintained and will identify early any persistent problems so that these can be avoided everywhere. Once the majority of data have been prepared as draft tables, figures and listings and the final review have taken place, the database is "locked". Only by a controlled and fully documented process should the database be unlocked to allow changes to be made. Inevitably, "late" SAEs will cause additions to be made to the "unlocked" database.

Coding

The process of coding was originally used to refer to "data entry". Coding was required because the old databases had little storage and by the selection of a corresponding code (numeric, alphabetic or alphanumeric) to the word or phrase of medical terminology, the database storage space could be conserved and searches of the database were possible. With modern sophisticated databases, storage should not be a problem. However, the use of coding does allow more advanced medical terminologies to be used and facilitates data search and manipulation. It also provides reproducibility and standardisation. Many large data management groups have professionals who concentrate solely on coding. These personnel are usually medically trained and have a thorough understanding of the coding dictionaries. An important factor of having one central team performing the coding means that the coding is standardised and the clinical database is held in a central and uniform manner.

The pharmaceutical physician will have a role in ensuring that the coding has been carried out correctly. His/her medical training could easily be required to confirm some of the coding. Specific clinical data could be lost or misrepresented because a particular disease or adverse event was coded too generally. The opposite of this problem is coding that is too specific. A term can be coded in a

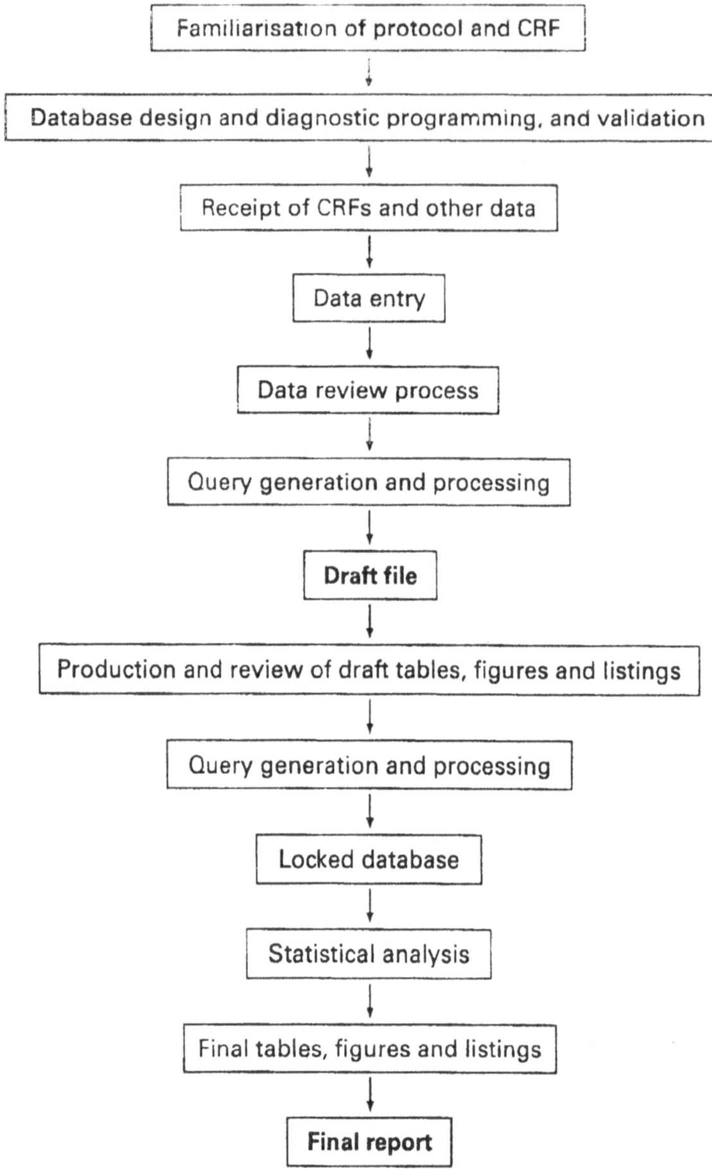

Fig. 5.8. Data management process.

way that fails to describe the disease or event because there is not enough flexibility in the coding. This can also cause problems when the clinical study report is written, when safety clinical data are being interpreted. Translation can cause problems during the coding process; it is important that the translation is done by a trained translator. There is a plethora of medical terminologies available but the Medical Dictionary for Regulatory Activities (MedDRA) has been adopted by the ICH as the standard medical terminology for regulatory communication.

Audit and data trails

A fundamental principle of GCP is that the records recorded in the CRF or in any of the accompanying documentation, for example copies of diary cards, cannot be changed without the agreement in writing of the investigator. Changes due to errors or missing data will have to be made to the computer files to produce "*clean data files*" (files free of known errors). These changes should be noted on the original CRFs or in error logs on to which written amendments are added, signed and dated by the investigator. Many individuals, including senior pharmaceutical physicians, have wanted to alter data on CRFs because "they know the data are wrong". However, an unauthorised change to any data supplied by the investigator is unacceptable. Once "clean file" is declared, any subsequent changes must be justified and authorised. Modern computer systems can provide a record of all the changes (i.e. audit trail) that have been made, by whom and why, a feature that could be required at any future regulatory inspection. Any changes, for instance to a classification of study subjects, must be justified and agreed by all concerned. Another important series of steps is extraction of data and, in a similar manner, a "data trail" should be established, showing how data were manipulated to create tables, graphs and data sets or lists for statistical analysis. It is crucial that the manner in which these were structured (i.e. rules applied, identifiers of data sets) is recorded so that they can be reproduced later, for instance, when more data from other trials are available. The statisticians will rightly ask questions about the database, essentially seeking assurance on the points outlined above. Their analysis can only be judged to be correct if it truly reflects the original CRF data. Understandably, the statisticians' confidence in the data presented to them is of paramount concern and their questioning of data should be regarded as legitimate.

Statistical analysis

Before the study starts, at the stage of the clinical trial design and the preparation of the protocol, a qualified statistician must be consulted and a statistical analysis plan produced. A summary of this plan will be included in the protocol but usually a more detailed document of the plan is prepared. The qualified statistician will have experience of clinical trials and ideally should be a chartered statistician or equivalent. It is essential that the statistical analysis described at the beginning of the study is used at the end of the study or reasons documented as to why it has been changed. Frequently, the results of the analysis are not as expected. It is tempting for some research workers to "massage" the data with statistics in an attempt to produce the results that they would like. The treatment of missing data, data for subjects who did not meet inclusion criteria and should therefore have been excluded, and missing critical or secondary endpoint data feature frequently in many revised plans. In addition, when there are protocol changes, the impact on the original plan is often underrated. The ICH has produced a number of guidance documents.

Data integrity

The institution, pharmaceutical company or independent investigator carry considerable responsibility as custodian of trial data and is potentially exposed to charges of bias, of suppression or even of alteration of data. Data may be modified in order to correct errors but all changes must be tracked. Quality control and assurance steps must be part of the process - not only carried out but also recorded.

The end of the study

The closing down of the clinical trial at the site after the last visit of the last study subject has finished and all the CRFs are completed is an important part of the clinical trial. The process of archiving the documentation, both at the site and at the sponsor office, needs to take place. These processes are usually neglected or treated as "Cinderella" operations to be carried out by the most junior of staff. It is only when the QA auditor or, worse still, the inspector of the regulatory agency wishes to see the documentation that failure to archive properly, with detailed inventories, becomes apparent. The clinical trial monitor should visit the investigator site and ensure that the appropriate arrangements have been made to archive, and officially close down the site. These documents will include nearly all the documents in the investigator's master file, the investigator's copies of the CRF and any records that are in the pharmacy associated with the study. The monitor will advise the investigator to try to prevent the medical records of the study subjects from being deleted or lost and check that all randomisation codes have been returned from blind studies without being opened except in a recorded emergency. Study drug, returned from subject use or unused, will be destroyed or sent back to the supplier. The final safety report will be sent to the IEC.

The investigator may wish to archive the site's documents at the site or may wish the sponsor to supply space. In this case, the documents should be sealed so that there is no opportunity for anyone but the investigator to see these documents. All the documents at the sponsor's office, whether paper or electronic, should also be archived. The length of time required to archive the documents is at least two years after the last approval of the marketing application or any contemplated marketing application, or at least two years after the formal discontinuation of clinical development. These requirements make long-term planning for archiving difficult because usually one does not know what the status of the study drug will be in six months' time, and certainly not in two or three years.

Regulatory inspections and quality assurance audits

The new European Directive has reinforced the need for European agencies, as well as those of the US and Japan, to conduct inspections of clinical trials. Sponsors, mindful of the implications of failed inspections, are carrying out audits by their QA units to try to ensure that standards at a particular site meet the regulatory requirements of GCP, and of any future regulatory inspection. Frequently, the inspections will occur two or more years after the end of the study.

Inspectors will visit the investigator site and may possibly wish to visit the sponsor's office. They will review the documentation of the study file. Approval documents of the IEC will be compared with any amendments made to the protocol or to the subject's information sheet/ICF. Consent forms for the study subjects will be inspected to establish who actually gave consent and whether this was before entry into the clinical study. A thorough source data verification of the CRF with the source documents, including the medical records, will be undertaken. Documentation relating to drug accountability will be matched with each subject's CRF. The facilities will be reviewed and the site staff interviewed. Further information can be obtained from FDA guidance manuals. Frequent questions asked include:

1. The whereabouts of original documents if only photocopies are available
2. Is there sufficient source documentation to indicate that the study subject existed?
3. Is the medical condition suffered by the subject appropriate for the study?
4. Did the subject attend all the visits or otherwise?
5. Who collected the trial data and was this appropriate?

In a similar manner, QA departments and consultants paid for by the sponsor will conduct audits of investigator sites. Again, like the clinical trial monitor, there may be some annoyance by the investigator and his staff that some person, who may not be a physician, should be appointed by the sponsor to review the clinical trial documentation at the site.

Preparation of the Clinical Report

The purpose of a clinical trial is to gain new knowledge that adds something to existing evidence and so it may, together with other trials, influence therapeutic decisions. If the knowledge is not written down, then it is unlikely to be known by more than a few individuals. This Section concentrates on the technical requirements of a clinical trial report for the registration of a pharmaceutical product. However, readers would be well advised to use the recommendations of ICH Guideline E3 on the preparation of such a report.

Many surveys have revealed deficiencies in published papers describing clinical trials, and some of these shortcomings are fundamental. For instance, there is no mention of protocol amendments, or steps to avoid selection bias, of checks for compliance by study subject, and of QA. Similarly, the reports submitted in regulatory applications have been criticised. However, extensive tables of data will accompany the regulatory application so that the regulators can run an independent analysis. In contrast, limited data are published in journals. The editor and the reviewer, when provided with the scientific paper to be published, are seldom provided with adequate data to allow a detailed critique. For the manufacturer, the findings from clinical trials form the basis of what is said about the efficacy, safety and quality of a new medicine when applying for a marketing licence and when persuading doctors to use the medicine. Whether the report is of a small academic investigation or part of the research for a future commercial product, its preparation justifies care and attention.

ICH GCP requires that all clinical trials involving human subjects should be reported, even if only one study subject is involved. This is another protective wall, along with ethical approval and informed consent, against unapproved and sloppy experimentation on humans.

Final Report

ICH Guideline E3 describes how the clinical trial report should be prepared. The format should allow someone to repeat the trial, using an identical design and to re-analyse it or examine it more closely. The writing of the report ought to rest with those who contributed most to it in terms of design, conduct and analysis. Several authors may contribute to the writing of the report, covering the medical aspects, the statistics and interpretation. A medical writer may be involved in editing the contributions so as to try to achieve uniformity of style and content. The pharmaceutical physician, either as the sponsor's medical input or as the investigator, should take particular interest in certain sections where his/her expertise will ensure that the correct medical terminology is used and that the interpretation is acceptable. The main findings of the study should be discussed in relation to the validity of the methods, the natural history of the disease and the subject population. The clinical relevance will need to be reviewed, and comparison of the study drug or treatment made with current practice. Limitations of the study, such as inconsistencies between measured parameters, protocol violations and target population, should be assessed.

Most clinical trials have problems, sometimes detected by inspection and audit. These can usually be resolved and, if so, the regulatory submission must include a full explanation of how they were dealt with. Therefore, an audit trail with all the data should be available, accompanied by a statement by QA confirming that the procedures have been audited.

A target date for completion should always be set to ensure that any further developments are not held up by the lack of a report. The report itself may form part of 20 or more reports prepared and assembled into a regulatory dossier. They should be uniform in format. Thus, the reader can easily read each of them and be equally comfortable when looking at an overall summary; for instance, the tables should be assembled in an identical format. Graphs should be consistent in format, for example bar charts running vertically or horizontally but not both. The aim is to assist the reader to assimilate evidence readily and to compare it between trials. The whole dossier should be one of accuracy, consistency and meticulous cross-referencing.

Regulatory Submissions

The assembling of a regulatory submission requires even more planning. The final written reports of a series of clinical trials are the "*building blocks*". However, the associated data must be uniform throughout and formatted in a manner that is consistent with the requirements of the regulatory agency that will review the submission. Once again, the effort to reach these objectives must be made in the early planning stages.

The processes are changing for regulatory submissions. Three major drives are taking place or are about to take place:

1. Electronic submissions or CANDAs are being made instead of paper submission, particularly in the US
2. The development of electronic standards for the transfer of regulatory information
3. The publication of the organisation of the Common Technical Document.

These changes mean that, very soon, submissions will be made globally using computer technology and with an identical dossier format. The advantages will be that the regulatory agencies will be able to interrogate the data, thereby avoiding delays in requesting responses from sponsors; the reviewers will have easy access to the whole submission, without the involvement of large amounts of paper; and there will be better consistency and quality in the reports because the format of the dossier will be clearly defined.

Expert Report

When the new ICH Common Technical Document is fully adopted, the pharmaceutical physician may be called upon to write an expert report or a clinical overview. It is essential that whoever writes the report or overview should have a good understanding of the trial. Inaccuracies are too frequent. The report is a comprehensive and critical review of the data submitted in the license application and should not be more than 25 pages long. The object of the report is to facilitate the review by the assessor and it should address the properties of safety and efficacy of the study drug, with cross-reference to the clinical study report. The report will need to support the proposed labelling. It has several sections including: a problem statement (i.e. product development rationale), clinical pharmacology, clinical trials, conclusions and a reference list. In general, summaries of this nature should be in a linguistic style that is appropriate to a non-specialist, in clear simple English with repetition studiously avoided.

Publications

The dissemination of information to the scientific community is essential for the progress of research. Publications in scientific journals provide a key source of information. In the case of medical research, patients' lives may be at stake. There are other reasons for publication. Publication will provide prestige to the investigator, to the sponsor and to the institutions involved in the research. In addition, in some circumstances the published paper will be quoted in reference dictionaries and pharmacopoeia, in advertisements and other promotions. The pharmaceutical physician should take every opportunity to publish high-quality scientific papers, even if the findings are not sensational but provide useful additional information. Publications must follow the journal style and therefore some rewriting of the final trial report will be required. The main problem is the provision of fewer data, usually in a summarised form, in a published paper. These amendments might be made by non-company authors or by editorial staff. The checking of these changes is crucial, as those making the changes have less knowledge of the database and may be prone to making mistakes. Proofreading must be thorough.

Authorship of Publications

The basic principle accepted by biomedical editors is for authors to be responsible for those sections of the work performed by them. It follows that company staff should be authors. Indeed, it is important for readers to know their involvement. However, from time to time some company executives argue that their involvement might be construed as biasing the trial and therefore that they should be excluded. This attitude is either timorous or reveals an element of complicity, or both. The professional role and standing of company staff and their personal development requires better support from senior executives. Some journals requests that authors specify the individual contributions of authors to a paper, for example original concept, statistical analysis, and writer. They also insist on statements about sources of funding and competing interests. These moves are welcome because they help to ascribe ownership and responsibility, and give a chance for more equal representation from commercial, academic and regulatory sources.

Quality Management

The final principle of ICH GCP states that "systems with procedures that assure the quality of every aspect of the trial should be implemented". The word "quality" is often misunderstood, although freely used when referring to processes and documentation in clinical trials. It means that a degree or standard of excellence has been reached; however, the standard set is frequently inadequate when the health of study subjects is at stake. Fortunately, some regulatory authorities such as the FDA requires evidence in the reliability and completeness of the data to support a quality claim. They conduct inspections of the investigator site and critically interrogate the clinical data collected. Regulatory frameworks such as ICH GCP have been established for all research destined to support the licensing of new medicines.

Unfortunately, the GCP guidelines are not always applied to other biomedical research and rarely to independent studies on marketed products initiated by clinicians without support from the manufacturer. There is still a double standard in therapeutic research and therefore in published papers arising from them. Editors and reviewers do not see the full documentation of non-sponsored biomedical research, whereas the regulatory authorities and their expert advisers will expect to see all data in the support of new medicines. The extent of the differences in standards is recognised when a potential investigating site is visited and one realises that there are no SOPs, that documentation of laboratory procedures is suboptimal and that staff are not properly trained. These facets are mentioned because the training that clinicians, scientists and technicians receive from company-based staff before and during a sponsored clinical trial adds considerably to the quality standards. In Europe, the new EU Clinical Trial Directive will change this situation. Non-commercial and commercial clinical trials will be required to meet the requirements of the Directive, including conducting studies to the GCP standard. In some pharmaceutical companies and institutions, the principles of Total Quality Management (TQM) or philosophies associated with European Foundation for Quality Management (EFQM) have been adopted. Schemes designed to encourage the involvement of factory workers in quality management do not always lend themselves successfully to clinical trial management. A more precise and, in many cases, a more vigorous approach is the series of quality management standards and guidelines called ISO 9000. Sweeney has provided details of how the original versions of ISO 9000 standards could be applied to clinical trials. However, all these quality systems can provide only a limited foundation. Independent reviewers, auditors from QA groups and inspectors from regulatory agencies must reinforce the quality systems.

Quality Control (QC) and Quality Assurance (QA)

Many scientists confuse the terms QC and QA. In terms of clinical trials, there is a very real difference. QC is the operational techniques and activities undertaken by all participants to verify that the quality requirements of the clinical trial have been fulfilled whereas QA verifies that the QC has satisfied these requirements. In other words, QC is where the data recorded is checked with source documents and that measurements and procedures followed are those described in SOPs and the protocol. QA is where independent individuals establish that QC is in place and report any deficiencies without bias.

Quality control (QC)

QC should be present at all phases of a clinical trial whether in the preparation, during or in the analysis of the clinical data and writing of the clinical trial report. The clinician still has hesitation in using QC in clinical research. This may be due to a fear of finding mistakes in processes that reflect on the professionalism as a clinician, a lack of time or in some cases, the clinician's arrogance that nothing could be wrong. This hesitation over using QC resulted in the drug industry recruiting non-medical scientists to independently monitor the activities occurring at the site.

At the investigator site, the investigator and his/her staff will have essential tasks and responsibilities, which if not scrupulously followed might alter the outcome of the trial. The site needs to have the right subject, with the right disease, who is receiving the right treatment in the right dose at the right time. The next requirements are the right observations made correctly, recorded accurately and checked as being complete. The objective measurements (such as blood pressure, peak expiratory flow, gastric emptying times, skin thickness, reaction times) can be defined, sometimes calibrated and the reproducibility of repeated measurements validated. Any variability should be related to physiological or other factors (for instance, diurnal changes, food intake, exercise, anxiety). Subjective endpoints have to some extent been structured and validated (for instance, anxiety or depression rating scales) but the training of staff in their consistent use in multicentre trials is often overlooked. All these observations will be recorded in CRFs and in many cases in the medical records of the subject.

Role of the clinical trial nurse or co-ordinator

Many investigator sites employ part- or full-time nurses to support the clinical trials. Nurses should never be considered to be an extravagance, because without them, the onus of administration and QC is solely on the investigator. The clinical trial nurse can help the investigator in many ways, but two of the most important are ensuring that the CRF reflects what is present in the source documents, such as essential events of the medical history of the subject, and close liaison with the sponsor's monitor.

Quality assurance (QA)

QA is no longer an activity conducted by rich pharmaceutical companies to prepare for possible regulatory inspections. All clinical trials should be subjected to QA, either by an in-house department or by external consultants. QA is defined as "all those planned and systematic actions that are established to ensure that the trial is performed and the data generated, documented (recorded), and reported in compliance with GCP and the applicable regulatory requirements(s)". Those persons undertaking QA should have sufficient independence of the clinical trial and its management to report any deficiencies without bias. QA will conduct audits to establish whether QC has taken place, whether SOPs are being followed and that the quality systems in place will provide accurate and correct clinical data to GCP standards. The word "audit" is often used for various QA and QC functions. However, some QA experts prefer not to use the word "audit" when operations are carried out by QC individuals because of the danger that the QC process is confused with that of QA. If a regulatory authority conducts an audit, it is usually called an "inspection".

QA has many other functions. As mentioned, QA should be part of the review board for new protocols and the associated documents, but in addition, individuals from the QA department will conduct audits of investigator site. The clinical data that have so laboriously been obtained may be of a high quality but the manner in which they are processed and analysed can reduce the quality and create numerous problems. The QA auditors should audit the processes of the data management, statistics and safety reporting groups on a regular basis. The clinical study report should also be audited. One would hope that vigorous QC processes are in place, but these processes can vary depending on the availability of suitable QC individuals and the frequent pressure to meet timelines.

Increasingly, the QA department conducts audits of systems and processes in the general organisation and management of the clinical department, any contracted research organisation and vendor. The regulatory agencies will expect all functions in the clinical trial that are subcontracted to meet the requirements of GCP. For example, the central laboratory, the software house that provides the programming for the electronic diary used in a particular study and the contract archives used to store documentation from a clinical trial need to be audited. Often the QA department will provide a supporting function in the preparation and revision of SOPs and in the training of staff involved in clinical trials.

Fraud/Misconduct

The FDA defines fraud as the deliberate reporting of false or misleading data or the withholding of reportable data. Although the Agency has used the word "fraud", in the US the word usually implies injury or damage to victims and therefore the word "misconduct" is preferred. Fraud in clinical research may be a rare phenomenon but no one really knows how many cases are undetected or not reported. In the UK, a pharmaceutical company reporting an investigator for fraud may experience a backlash from the local professional and lay community before the full facts become known. The motives of a fraudulent investigator may be financial gain or professional promotion, trying to produce results either too quickly or too precisely. In some cases, work overload or mental illness provide a backdrop to the crime.

The fraudulent investigator may add data where the original are missing, possibly not wanting to admit that they forgot to obtain or record them or that they lost them (for instance, broken blood sample tube). Serious cases involve falsification of subject data where study subjects do not exist or were not actually recruited. Ethical approval and consent documentation are "created" at the site.

With regular monitoring, an active QA unit and an increasing role for inspectors from the regulatory agencies, fraud should be contained. Statisticians should routinely scrutinise demographic differences in the subjects recruited at one centre compared with other centres, clustering of laboratory data, and variations in data to establish both the scientific significance of the results but also whether the data of a particular site need investigation for fraud.

As soon as fraud is suspected, a series of steps needs to be followed which have been thought out and written down as an SOP before any clinical research commenced. Where possible, additional evidence should be obtained, usually by the use of a competent QA auditor. In the meantime, only the minimum key individuals should be made aware of the problem until sufficient evidence has been obtained to establish the truth. The appropriate authorities such as the national drug industry organisation and the regulatory authorities should be informed if fraud has taken place. Sometimes, other sponsors will have reported additional evidence that fraud is taking place at a particular site. The site will need to be closed if study subjects are still being recruited and a full explanation provided to the authorities. Any clinical data collected will need to be reviewed and a decision made as to whether any of the data can be included in an analysis. To a pharmaceutical physician, fraud is never an easy situation. It usually involves a professional colleague and there is always the worry that the established facts have been misinterpreted. However, a fraudulent individual cannot be tolerated in modern clinical research.

Fraud is not limited to the investigator and his/her staff. Staff of pharmaceutical companies and institutions may alter CRFs, modify data sets, alter tables, suppress reported side-effects or bias written reports. The detection of such activities, inside or outside an institution, by investigators or company staff relies on others in the same team realising that something is suspicious. Double checking of data by colleagues and authentication of those data is the best deterrent to misconduct.

The therapeutic benefits and risks of a medicine, and therefore the choice of treatment for an individual patient, stem from evidence from a series of clinical trials. Taken together, these trials should reflect all likely therapeutic situations. From time to time a particular problem arises that generates a new hypothesis. In order to obtain an answer to the specific question we sometimes restrict the population sample to study subjects who do not possess a number of variables that may confound the outcome. In this manner, we move away from the realities of everyday clinical practice to an idealised, but artificial, environment. This is justifiable if the restriction is logical and if, with it, the hypothesis testing can be successfully completed. Otherwise the issue may never be settled. However, from time to time such restrictions on the population are perpetuated. The reasons may not be stated and even not recognised by many involved. This perpetuation of restriction may be an unthinking and even unwitting design feature, extended from the type of specific investigation to which we have just referred. On the other hand, the restriction may be deliberate in order to secure an early and clearcut therapeutic outcome. Such distortion of therapeutic situations and practice can be misleading. Specific groups of study subjects may not be adequately studied, even though they will represent part of the target population once the medicine is approved for general use.

The development of new medicinal products for narrower indications in serious, and usually poorly understood, diseases such as multiple sclerosis and motor neurone disease has resulted in a closer approximation of study subjects selected for the controlled clinical trial to the patients encountered in clinical practice. Many of these products are biologically derived, and while efficacy in the two situations may be similar, longer and larger trials will be needed to fully appreciate adverse event profiles.

The impact of pharmacogenetics and pharmacoeconomics on clinical trial design, regulatory action and clinical usage is only just being appreciated. Technological advances that will make genetic approaches, in their broadest terms, possible are coming at a time when there is high pressure to contain the cost of drug treatment. The move by governments to widen the prescribing of medicines for patients to healthcare professionals other than doctors, and indeed to increase direct sales of medicines to patients is part of a cost containment drive. One can envisage a market in which the following access to medicines may be present:

1. Direct sales to patients or via pharmacists and other healthcare professionals
2. Growth of the generic market as cheaper alternatives
3. Continued but decreasing number of small molecules, which, in order to gain a place in clinical usage, will have to satisfy increasingly stringent cost-effectiveness criteria
4. Development of high technology products for select groups.

Regulatory authorities will have to respond to such a challenge by defining what kind of clinical trials will be pivotal to gain marketing authorisation. For example, for a new medicinal product indicated for a genotypically (or phenotypically) defined subgroup of patients with essential hypertension, how much study subject exposure for safety evaluation will be required? If the hypothesis of "specific drug for specific disease/study subject" is valid in this example, how ethical will it be to conduct a placebo-controlled trial and how relevant is it to conduct a comparison with a non-specific active control?

The next few years will witness a greater partnership between industry, regulatory authorities and universities. Attempts to harmonise the conduct of clinical trials between these three agencies is a positive move. The perception that the impact of GCP and the new EU Directive will lead to bureaucracy and the stifling of investigator-instigated and non-commercial research is a pessimistic view. An improvement in the quality of the data and greater respect for the study subject should provide ample benefit over any disadvantages, especially if the regulators are receptive to the ever-changing climate of research. The regulatory authorities will continue to issue guidelines for the registration of drugs, but sponsors must be prepared to take the decision on their interpretation after due consultation. There is no evidence that the investment in manpower and other resources necessary to execute clinical programmes will decrease, and the use of specialist contract organisations in all areas – trial monitoring, data handling, report writing, and consultancy – is likely to continue. As companies strive harder for shorter, surer paths to regulatory approval, the well-conceived, well-executed and correctly interpreted clinical trial will continue to be pivotal.

6

HEALTH CARE SYSTEMS

It is quite fascinating how the organization, structure, and financing of health care services can be so very diverse in different countries around the world. One might think that leaders and policymakers would be aware of each other's national health systems and, by emulating the best features, that they would tend to move toward harmonization and greater similarity. Actually, this assumptions is false. National health care systems vary widely and are more related to variables in each country. In fact, the health system in a given country is a mirror of how that society functions at large. Health care delivery systems must be compatible with the: (1) economic system: socialist, capitalist, or mixed; (2) political system: major or minor role of degree of government centralization; (3) wealth of the country: use of primary care facilities, access to specialists and tertiary care facilities; (4) traditions and conventions as seen in their history—fundamental, visible things are difficult to change; (5) geography: whether the majority of the population is located in a few metropolitan areas, with the remainder scattered in rural areas, or whether the population is spread over hundreds of islands; (6) infrastructure: roads, communication systems, and air service; and (7) extent of and belief in high technology. There are other factors as well: the system from a previous colonial power, extent of literacy and education, and relationships with outside countries, to name a few.

The remainder of this article examines the health care delivery systems in six very different countries. Even though Canada and the United States are similar countries with a shared border and language and with open communication, their health care delivery systems could not be any more different. Each side of the border is aware of what happens on the other side, however, a series of complex and powerful forces keep them moving in their own directions. We look at six countries very briefly in this article to highlight the incredibly diverse approaches to health service organization and financing. In essence, most health systems fit into one of the following models:

1. State ownership and control—The best examples are the British National Health Service and the Swedish system in which clinics, hospitals, and most service providers are owned and operated by the government.
2. State health insurance program—Here, the government is the sole or major payer. However, some of the facilities and resources are in non-government hands. This is the case in much of Europe.
3. Mixed systems—This is seen in much of Asia and Central America and usually where there is a small wealthy class and a massive lower class. The lower class receives care from public facilities, and the small upper class uses private- sector, fee-for-service, and self-paid care.

   Other scenarios fit into this category as well. The United States has several independent health care systems including the military, veterans, Medicaid (a federal program for the medically indigent), Medicare (a federal insurance program for those 65 years of age and older), private-sector for-profit, and not-for-profit clinics, hospital chains, managed-care organizations, religious, prison health, and university teaching facilities.

4. Exclusively private sector—This category is shrinking as nations realize that health maintenance and disease prevention/wellness are important to their national goals of strength and productivity. Switzerland would still fit into this category, where most health care resources are in private hands.

Specimen National Systems

Canada

Organization

Canada uses a national health service, which provides medical services and hospital care to its entire population. The individual provincial governments operate health plans that conform to national legislation but can differ in various aspects. This "Medicare" program guarantees comprehensiveness, universal access, portability, and public administration. Health Canada is the national, federal health agency; however, the operation of health service provision is delegated to the provincial governments, which control virtually 100% of Canada's hospitals. There is a gatekeeper primary health care system, with GPs (general practitioners) or primary care family doctors serving as the entry point. Access to specialists, diagnostic testing, hospitals, and others is through the GP. Individual citizens have the freedom to choose their own doctors, 95% of whom are self-employed in private practice. The provincial government pays these doctors on a fee-for-service basis.

The individual provincial governments offer different supplemental benefits not covered by the national Medicare program, such as drugs, dental care, and vision care to the poor, elderly, and other specific groups. Supplemental benefits for the typical, employed, and non-elderly person come from the purchase of supplemental health insurance from private sources.

Pharmaceuticals

Canada created the Patented Medicine Prices Review Board (PMPRB) in 1987 to guarantee that pharmaceutical products would not have excessive prices in Canada. The board reviews prescribed and over-the-counter (OTC) prices and publishes annual guidelines for manufacturers. Compliance with PMPRB guidelines is voluntary; however, since 1993, the board has the authority to reduce excessive prices and return the excess amount to the government, and to punish the manufacturer. The PMPRB compares prices in Canada with those in seven industrialized nations to ensure that Canadian prices are in line with those of comparable countries. There is some controversy that existing drug products are well-controlled regarding prices, but that such is not the case with newly introduced pharmaceuticals.

Further controls exist at the provincial level at which each province maintains a published formulary of drugs that are reimbursable along with the reimbursement level. Quebec, observers perceive, lists nearly all new drug products, whereas Ontario appears to be slow to list newly approved products. Each province has additional control mechanisms. Ontario requires the first generic drug to be at least 40% less costly than the branded originator product. Some components of the reference price system are seen in British Columbia and Newfoundland.

There is growing harmonization among the provinces; however, there is still no national, standardized, and interchangeable list of drugs for ambulatory care use. In hospitals, drugs that are administered are paid for by Medicare. Each province has interesting and different features in its drug benefit plan. The Prince Edward Island plan pays for seniors; welfare recipients; nursing home patients; and those with rheumatic fever, diabetes, tuberculosis, multiple sclerosis, AIDS, and several other conditions. New Brunswick has an annual copayment cap for seniors and for organ transplant recipients and for selected other patient categories. A copayment is set at approximately $9 (Canadian) but is waived for some groups in Quebec, along with an annual copay ceiling of $750.

Other interesting features of the Canadian system include its 1998 mutual recognition agreement with the EU, prohibition of prescription drug advertising to consumers, a 20-year patent exclusivity period, and the establishment of the PMPRB to ensure fair pricing of medications.

Republic of South Africa

Organization

The Republic of South Africa (RSA) has a most diverse health care environment, with world-class practice and facilities in wealthy urban areas and some of the most primitive care in poor remote villages, with a vast array between these extremes. Primary care is now the focus of the ANC government in an effort to correct years of neglect and undemocratic practices under the earlier apartheid-oriented regimes. Public health services are being brought to the Black townships as rapidly as resources permit.

However, there are virtually no funds for new drugs against HIV infection in patients, a problem most prevalent in the RSA. To maximize the value of its drugs budget, the RSA has enacted legislation to create an Essential Drugs List for the public sector, along with generic substitution authority, the removal of some pharmacists' unique professional privileges, and legislation permitting the parallel importation of pharmaceutical products already registered in the RSA. Obviously, this conserves resources, stretching them for more patients, but this angers the RSA and multinational pharma firms.

South Africa is still the wealthiest country in Africa, with a (1997) GDP at approximately $130 billion. It must be noted, though, that aggregate numbers hide massive racial differences. It is improving, but the standard of living for Blacks is yet only slightly better than it is in neighboring countries, whereas whites enjoy a standard of living similar to that found in North America or Western Europe. An unemployment rate of over 30% (mostly among Blacks) exacerbates the fiscal situation.

Routine immunizations for children, conforming to the World Health Organization (WHO) recommended schedule is the governmental policy, but it is not yet accomplished in all regions. Infectious diseases including HIV remain a serious challenge. Planning and budgeting for resource allocation are difficult because accurate census figures do not exist. Total health expenditures appear to be in the area of $300 per person per year, and it is estimated that the private sector accounts for greater than 50% of total expenditures.

Public-sector expenditures emphasize primary care, lately, at the expense of tertiary care facilities. Private-sector spending is primarily through private "*medical schemes*." These are non-profit organizations supported by employer associations and employees. There are slightly fewer than 200 of these schemes, providing insurance and care payment for nearly 3 million workers and their 5 million dependents (of a total estimated RSA population of 40 million). The largest area of medical scheme expenditure is for medicines, which causes the pressures on pharmaceutical pricing addressed below. After drugs, the next largest expenditures are for private hospitals, medical specialists, general practitioners, and dentists.

The RSA Department of Health (DOH) has totally restructured the previous apartheid system of racial and provincial health systems into a coordinated national health program operated through health regions and local health districts. Still, there are major differences in knowledge, education, expectations, and wealth within different subpopulations.

Pharmaceuticals

Until recently, manufacturers were free to establish their desired price for a drug. Wholesalers and retailers added what they chose to reach the retail selling price for medications. In 1997, a proposed scheme of prices extending to the retailer was agreed on, but resistance was met from the Pharmaceutical

Manufacturers Association(PMA). In the legislation, a pricing board composed of members selected by the Minister of Health would establish prices for each product and a maximum selling price. Public-sector primary care drugs are reimbursed 100% by the government. Hospital care outpatient drugs can have copayments. The Essential Drugs List would be the core of what is to be available at public facilities, but there appears to be a long way to go before most of these agents will be regularly available on a consistent basis at primary care centers or at public hospitals.

The parallel importation of RSA-registered drugs available at lower prices abroad is the basis for PMA litigation against the Drug Legislation of 1997. In addition to the price-setting committee, DOH efforts to encourage the use of generic drugs has proven to be a source of conflict. Other features of the new legislation bar dispensing samples or making bonus payments to dispensers of medicines; the creation of a Code of Ethics for pharmaceutical marketing; and a series of safety regulations, dealing primarily with limiting practice to fully qualified and licensed professionals.

There is a fast lane for new drug approvals if the product is already in at least one of the following jurisdictions: the United Kingdom, Canada, United States, Sweden, or Australia. Approxmately 85% (by value) of pharmaceuticals go through the nearly 3,000 community pharmacies. Yet, approxmately 80% of the population rely on the public sector for drugs, received through clinics, hospitals, primary care posts, or military facilities. Although there is a 20-year patent period of exclusivity/protection, the parallel imports option effectively defeats this protection. It will be interesting to see how the access to drugs, price controls, and quality improvement forces will interact and what the actual situation will be in South Africa in the coming years, especially as the country complies with intellectual property and World Trade Organization policies and rules.

Japan

Organization

After North America and before Western Europe, Japan is the second largest pharmaceutical market in the world. Its population of 126 million spends $70 billion on pharmaceuticals each year. On average, each Japanese resident spends $2000 each year on health care with $550 of that on pharmaceuticals. Perhaps the primary single features of the Japanese market are the above-average proportion of elderly in the population and the higher than usual consumption of drugs. It has been estimated that by the year 2050, nearly 30% of the population will be older than 65 years of age. The high consumption rate is attributed to drugs being injected and/or sold by the physician, a practice used, in part, to increase the total price of an office visit. The primary funding source for health services in Japan is the Social Insurance System (SIS), made up of employee programs that pay for nearly 55% of care. The Medical Service for the Aged program covers another 35% of care. Private expenditures and a very small portion for public health promotion and disease prevention make up the difference. The Ministry of Health and Welfare (MHW) maintains overall responsibility for health care services and functions via a number of bureaus. Numerous sources comment that regulations are difficult to understand and interpret, often overlapping, and that this serves as a barrier to foreign firms desiring to enter a market. Physicians, for example, are authorized to own and operate hospitals, effectively excluding corporate owners or physicians not licensed in Japan. Universal health insurance was established in 1961. Nearly the entire population is covered through the employer plans or through programs for the unemployed, retired, or self-employed. Employees pay 10% of the cost of treatments, up to an annual ceiling, and also pay a portion of their premiums, with their employers.

Pharmaceuticals

The MHW sets prices for reimbursable drugs (those approved for the Social Insurance System). Physicians, clinics, and private hospitals are reimbursed at a price slightly higher than their actual acquisition cost. The government has scheduled annual reductions in the reimbursement prices to reduce this source of additional income to physicians. Patients make copayments of 20%, although for children and low-income elderly the copayment is waived, and recently a plan to eliminate copayments for persons 70 years of age and older was introduced.

The MHW reductions of 5–10% of the prices of existing drug products appear to have had the opposite of the intended impact. Doctors are prescribing more of the newest, high-priced pharmaceuticals that have not had their margins reduced yet, thereby earning a bigger amount from the wider difference between their actual cost and the listed reimbursement amount.

With regard to generic drugs, astute observers believe that the Japanese government wants its R&D-intensive firms to be successful. A regulation requires generics to be priced at not less than 40% of the innovator brand price. It is reasonable to assume that the margins for physicians are lower with generic drugs, and that these margins will continue into the future, as will the reference price scheme. There is a Japanese pharmacopeia that sets official standards and diverse government agencies that perform tasks undertaken by an FDA. It is rumored that the Japanese will establish a Western-style FDA in the near future.

One of the most disliked regulations in the view of foreign and multinational pharmaceutical companies is the requirement for duplicative clinical trials with humans in Japan, because those carried out elsewhere are not recognized. Also of interest is the fact that Japan, like Korea and Taiwan, has no separation between prescriber and dispenser of drugs. Called "Bungyo," it is a major source of revenue for doctors and clinics. Fewer than 20% of prescriptions ever reach a pharmacy for dispensing.

Good post-marketing surveillance practices (GPMSP) rules have been in place since 1993. Postmarketing experience reports are to be sent to a government agency. Both GPMSP and periodic safety reporting requirements are in place that require a review of the product each year while it is in its re-examination period, immediately after marketing approval. Unlike in the United States, where a new drug application is approved for an indefinite period, in Japan, there is a periodic full reassessment. Such re-evaluations are conducted every 5 years once the initial re-examination period for a drug product has ended.

Drug products are distributed primarily via the 2000 wholesalers, and in addition, there exists a small second channel with drugs going directly to hospitals, GPs, and pharmacies. There are approximately 66,000 pharmacies, most of which are family-owned independents. There are chains as well. However, a growing market for OTCs is found in convenience stores.

Physicians administer and sell drugs to patients as a highly profitable sideline. The incentive is for the physician to use as much of the most costly drug products as possible. There is only a small OTC market, because physicians try to prescribe and dispense as much as is possible. Other than some concern about a drug lag, the pharmaceutical environment in Japan is robust. Periodically, there are calls to separate prescribing and dispensing; however, this is not likely in the near future given the powerful forces backing the status quo.

United Kingdom

Organization

With a population of more than 60 million and GDP per capita of more than US $22,000, the United Kingdom is one of the richest nations in the world. It is one of the G7 countries, a member of the European Union, and a member of the Organization for Economic Co-operation and Development (OECD). In 1996, total health care expenditure in the United Kingdom was approximately 7.0% of the GDP. Public expenditure by the National Health Service (NHS) accounts for most of the health care costs. The NHS was set up after World War II, with the aim of unifying health care services by voluntary and local hospitals. The NHS offers free health services to all U.K. residents, funded through general taxation.

Two of the major characteristics of the U.K. health care system include health authorities responsible for hospital services and GP fundholders responsible for primary care. In 1996, 100 health authorities became operational in England, responsible for the provision of NHS hospital and community health services covering geographic boundaries with populations ranging from 125 thousand to over 1 million. There are four levels of hospital services. At the community level, community hospitals offer basic medical care for the treatment of acute cases and patients requiring convalescent and long-term/terminal care. General practitioners are the key staff here. At the district level, district general hospitals operate the key acute units, serving an average population of a quarter-million. At the regional level, major specialty services such as neurosurgery, open-heart surgery, and radiotherapy are provided. At the national level, highly specialized hospitals provide complex services for parts or for the entire country.

GPs are the gatekeepers and fundholders of the health care system. The principle of fundholding is that GPs manage their own budgets. They can obtain a defined range of services from hospitals and manage patients at the GP level whenever possible to reduce costs. In the late 1990s, GPs fundholders were organized into Primary Care Groups (PCGs). These networks of GPs cover wide geographic areas with an average population of 100,000. In 1999, there were 481 PCGs in England and Wales, and all have unified budgets (e.g., drugs, hospital care services). With a population of a small to medium-sized HMO in the United States, these PCGs have a very broad influence on patient health care and the selection of drugs through formularies.

Pharmaceuticals

The regulatory authority in the United Kingdom is the Medicines Control Agency (MCA) under the Department of Health. The agency's responsibilities include drug licensing, clinical trials licensing, pharmacovigilance and drug safety, communication and provision of information on medicines, inspection of facilities and enforcement of regulations, and the British Pharmacopoeia. The United Kingdom is a reference member state for the European Union mutual recognition procedure. The European Union's pharmaceutical registration system came into effect for all member countries in 1995. The aim of the EU system is to harmonize pharmaceutical regulations throughout the EU. The centralized registration procedure is handled by the European Medicines Evaluation Agency (EMEA). Authorization through the central registration procedure is immediately valid in all EU member countries. The decentralized procedure relies on the principle of mutual recognition. After registration has been obtained in a member country under the centralized procedure, application may be made for registration in one or more other member countries via the decentralized procedure.

The majority of pharmaceuticals are distributed through wholesalers to retail pharmacies, with large pharmacy chains now dominating the market. There are approximately 11,000 community pharmacies in the United Kingdom. In recent years, pharmacy services are increasingly available in supermarkets at the expense of local independent pharmacies.

Total expenditure on pharmaceuticals in the United Kingdom amounted to approximately 8650 million pounds in 1999, accounting for approximately 17% of the total health expenditure. The NHS covers prescription drugs. However, the government does not reimburse for over-the-counter (OTC) products. The Department of Health indirectly controls pharmaceutical prices. Because the price control scheme is related to profit control, rather than to the prices of individual products, pharmaceuticals are relatively free-priced in the United Kingdom. The government operates a negative list for products that are not reimbursable. The cost of most licensed prescription products is fully reimbursed. However, cost constraints and prescribing budgets mean that GPs will often prescribe a generic when one is available. As a result, new prescription drugs usually have a slower penetration rate in the United

Kingdom than in the United States. The recently introduced National Insti-tute for Clinical Excellence (NICE) will add more barriers to the introduction of new pharmaceutical products in the United Kingdom.

National institute for clinical excellence

Funded by the government, the National Institute for Clinical Excellence (NICE) was set up as a Special Health Authority in the United Kingdom in 1999 and, as such, it is a part of the National Health Service (NHS). It was set up to "provide the NHS (patients, health professionals, and the public) with authoritative, robust and reliable guidance on current best practice." Its key functions are "to appraise the clinical benefits and the costs of those (health care) interventions and to make recommendations." Guidance is issued from each appraisal based on the clinical benefits, cost-effectiveness, and total economic impact on the National Health Service. The government does not have to adhere to the recommendations by the NICE in its guidance and financial payment to health care providers. However, many believe that a negative recommendation from the NICE will have a detrimental impact on the pricing, reimbursement, and sales of the appraised product not only in the United Kingdom but also throughout Europe, Australia, and Canada.

The guidance covers both individual health technologies (including medicines, medical devices, diagnostic techniques, procedures, and health promotion) and the clinical management of specific conditions. The Institute may recommend a technology for general use, for specific indications, or for defined subgroups of patients. Based on the appraisal, a therapeutic intervention (e.g., drug) will be classified into one of three categories: category A, routine use in the NHS; category B, further trials needed; and category C, not recommended for routine use in the NHS. The NICE has a board reflecting a range of expertise including the clinical professions, patients and user groups, NHS managers, and research bodies. The Board ensures that the NICE conducts its business on behalf of the NHS in the most effective manner. Details of the appraisal process and membership of the Appraisals Committee are available on the NICE Web site. Because the NICE was new at the time of completion of this article, its impact on the pharmaceutical industry is still not clear.

Germany

Organization

With a population of approximately 82 million in 1998 and a GDP per capita of more than $26,000, Germany is one of the world's largest economies and health care markets. The population enjoys a generally good standard of health with a high degree of public awareness about health-related issues. Life expectancy in Germany is among the highest in the world. In 1997, the life expectancy for males was 74 years and for females 80. Approximately 15.8% of the population were over 65 years in 1997, and it has been projected that by 2020, the number of German inhabitants aged over 60 years will be 28.2%.

In 1997, health expenditures in Germany totaled $298 billion, equal to 14.2% of the GDP. The health care system in Germany is decentralized, and health care expenditures are covered by a variety of sources/payers. The statutory insurance system (GKV) represents the biggest proportion of the total care coverage (for almost 50%). Employers, government budget, private households, private insurance, retirement insurance, and accident insurance cover the remaining 50% of the health care expenditures. The largest spending sector is hospital expenditure, representing 34.3% of the total GKV health care expenditures.

The federal government has little executive responsibility for the provision of health care in Germany. Its primary responsibility is to provide a regulatory framework within which the individual Lander have to operate. The health ministries of the individual Lander are responsible for implementing the federal legislation, enacting their own legislation, supervising subordinate authorities and the medical profession, hospital planning, and regional administration. Hospitals in Germany can be classified into three major categories based on ownership: public, non-profit, and private. In 1997, the public sector operated approximately 40% of general hospitals, and non-profit organizations operated another 40%. However, the number of privately owned facilities has been increasing steadily over the past decade.

The number of practicing doctors has risen steadily for the past 10 years. More than 70% of the practicing doctors are specialists, with general medicine as the largest specialty. Fewer than 30% of doctors practice without any specialty.

Pharmaceuticals

Germany is a reference member of the EU pharmaceutical registration system. The European Medicines Evaluation Agency (EMEA) handles the centralized registration and the decentralized registration procedures in individual countries. After marketing authorization of a product with a new active substance has been granted in one country, the mutual recognition procedure is compulsory in other member countries. The mutual recognition procedure is also compulsory for line extensions and generic products. Marketing authorization approvals in Germany are valid for 5 years and renewable thereafter in 5 year periods.

Germany is the home of some major multinational pharmaceutical companies such as Aventis, BASF, Bayer, Boehringer Ingelheim, Merck KGaA, and Schering AG. VFA is the research-based manufacturers' association, whereas the Bundesverband de Pharmazeutischen Industrie (BPI) represents small and medium-sized companies. Because North America is the largest pharmaceutical market in the world, many of the VFA pharmaceutical companies locate their key operations in the United States. Exports to Western European countries represent a major source of income for many of the German pharmaceutical companies.

The pharmaceutical market in Germany is one of the largest in the world. Based on drug use per capita, Germany is second only to Japan in the consumption of pharmaceuticals. The principal distribution channels for pharmaceuticals in Germany are public retail pharmacies and hospital pharmacies. In 1998, there were 47,322 pharmacists in Germany, equal to 0.6 pharmacists per thousand population. Public (retail) pharmacies employed 96% of all pharmacists in 1998 and they obtained their supplies primarily from whole-salers. Prescribed drugs, including both branded and generic products, can only be dispensed in a pharmacy with a doctor's prescription. The generics market in Germany is one of largest and fastest-growing in Western Europe, representing approximately one-third of the European generics markets. OTC products can be divided into three overlapping categories: prescription OTC medicines, non-prescription OTC medicines, and freely available OTC products that can be sold freely through all retail outlets such as health food stores, supermarkets, and other retail outlets.

Mexico

Organization

Mexico is a federal republic of 31 states and a federal district. The population was officially estimated to be 97.7 million in 1997. GDP per capita was estimated at approximately US $4400 in 1998. As a developing nation, communicable diseases are still one of the major causes of mortality, although chronic and degenerative diseases have become the leading cause of death during the past decade. One of the major challenges for the government is to address the inadequacies of the Mexican health care system. Approximately 10 million people have virtually no access to regular basic health care services, and another 20 million people have less than adequate access. In 1996, the total health care expenditure in Mexico was equivalent to approximately 4.6% of GDP. Spending by the public sector accounted for approximately 60% in 1996. There are three sectors in the Mexican health care system: public, social security, and private. The public sector is primarily directed and operated by the Secretariat of Health. The public sector of health services is under the Secretariat of Health and is coordinated by over 200 health districts. The Federal District Department provides health care services to some 3.2 million people in Mexico City. The Mexican Social Security Institute (IMSS) Solidarity program covers another 10 million people in rural areas.

The social security system covers health services for government employees, managed by the Social Insurance Institute of State Employees (ISSSTE), and for private-sector workers, managed by the Mexican Social Security Institute (IMSS). The two agencies operate their own networks of hospitals and clinics and provide similar benefits. Some other smaller social security agencies exist, providing medical services for special groups such as the army, navy, and state oil company personnel. The private (commercial) sector includes private hospitals, doctor's offices, and practitioners of traditional medicine. Charity organizations such as the Red Cross also play a role in the Mexican health care system.

Pharmaceuticals

The regulatory authority in Mexico is the Dirección General de Control de Insumos para la Salud (DIGE-CIS). The Health Secretariat issues pharmaceutical registration. Safety and efficacy must be proven by phase III clinical trials in Mexico to register drugs that are new to the Mexican market. All major pharmacopeia are acceptable in Mexico. Most domestic producers in Mexico are wholly owned or licensed subsidiaries of multinational pharmaceutical firms. Exports have been growing fast, with other Latin American countries as the major destination markets. However, the United States is the major supplier of pharmaceutical imports in Mexico.

Pharmaceuticals in Mexico are subject to government price control. The private sector accounts for approximately 85% of the pharmaceutical market. Prescription drugs account for the majority of the pharmaceutical market, with antibiotics as one of the largest classes. Because the use of generics is still a relatively new phenomenon, most of the prescribed pharmaceuticals are branded products. OTC products represent approximately one-fifth of the total pharmaceuticals market. As presented, these six representative countries use vastly different organizations, financing mechanisms, goals, and provision structures. In fact, few systems around the world are identical because the systems represent the values and priorities and political as well as economic leanings and traditions of that country. If there were one perfect system, we would be seeing migration toward that model. However, because this is not the case, it is reasonable to assume that most of the various systems encountered around the world are at least satisfactory in their foundations and macrolevel characteristics, even if some of the operating details are not always popular.

The world is full of interesting additional approaches that a serious student of this subject might wish to explore further. Some of these include the "need clause" used in Norway, where, for example, their FDA had the authority to refuse to accept and review a new drug because Norway already had six benzodiazepines on the market. The FDA deemed that sufficient unless the sponsoring company knew of a new indication or other therapeutic breakthrough from its use. The Swedes bought all of the then-existing community pharmacies in the country in 1970 to rationalize distribution, and service level and to create a monopsonistic body for negotiating with manufacturers in price-setting. The French and others place new drugs into one of several reimbursement categories. Clearly, life-saving drugs are put in the 100% reimbursement (to the patient) category. Most others strive for the 70% reimbursement category; however, if the manufacturer cannot agree on a price satisfactory to the Social Security agency, the product will be placed in a lower reimbursement category, effectively hampering its market success. This is a powerful bargaining chip for the government to contain drug prices.

It will be interesting to watch the future in this area to see how medications previously requiring a doctor's prescription that move to OTC status are handled, and how nutraceuticals, herbals, homeopathic, and naturopathic drugs, without the benefit of rigorous, randomized clinical trial or outcome data are handled as well. Similarly, we can be certain that there will be excitement galore when the nations in Central America and the Middle East decide to control pharmaceuticals and to end the practice of lay-person purchases of virtually any product without the benefit of a physician's order. Separation of pharmacy and physician functions will occur in the Far East in the not too distant future, causing even more excitement or grief. If logic dictates, we should expect to see in the future a trend to offer incentives for prescribers who use the most cost-beneficial products (bonuses) and disincentives for patients (reimbursement level co-payment differences) and physicians when less than optimal choices are made. Irrespective of whatever does actually occur, it will be most interesting to observe.

7 Immunological Products

The concept of vaccination was introduced in the late 18th century by Edward Jenner when he used cowpox virus as a vaccine to protect humans against smallpox virus infections. This led to the development of vaccines over the next 2 centuries to provide protection against various bacterial and viral pathogens. Undoubtedly, the effective vaccination against infectious diseases is the best method of reducing suffering of human and animals caused by viral, bacterial, and parasitic infections. Over the last 200 years, the technology of vaccine development and production has not changed significantly. This usually involves the use of either a killed pathogen combined with an adjuvant or a live-pathogen with reduced virulence. Apart from the tremendous success of killed and attenuated virus vaccines over the years, many of such vaccines do not provide satisfactory protection, and there are a number of other disadvantages associated with these vaccines. Additionally, there are important pathogens against which attempts to develop effective vaccines using traditional approaches were unsuccessful. Various protective viral antigens (envelope and/or capsid proteins or glycoproteins and other viral proteins) and bacterial antigens (surface, internal, or fimbria proteins; bacterial polysaccharides; bacterial toxins; and other proteins involved in bacterial metabolism) have been identified as potential vaccine candidates. These protective antigens are used by various means to develop effective vaccines. The field of vaccine technology is not limited to infectious diseases but has shown potential in other areas, such as cancer treatment, reproduction, and modulation of animal productivity.

Conventional Vaccines

Inactivated vacci

Inactivated (killed) pathog nic rganisms can be used in vaccines. This is the simplest way to produce vaccines, provided the organisms can be cultured easily. Therefore, this method is often first tested to develop a potential- vaccine. As with any other technique of vaccine production, this procedure is only good for some organisms. There are a number of methods of inactivating pathogenic organisms; the most common are treatment with chemicals (formalin, formaldehyde, or propiolactate), heat, or γ-irradiation. In some instances, the procedure of inactivation may enhance antigenicity of some antigens important in protection. Inactivated vaccines usually result in good humoral immune response after multiple inoculations. Because inactivated vaccines in general fail to elicit effective mucosal and cell-mediated immune responses, they may provide limited protection against mucosal and intracellular pathogens. Failure to inactivate the pathogenic organisms completely could result in disease instead of protection. During the 1950s, some lots of poliovirus vaccine were not inactivated completely. Now, the methods used to detect residual infectivity are more stringent, therefore, inactivated vaccines are considered safe with extremely low or no chance of infection.

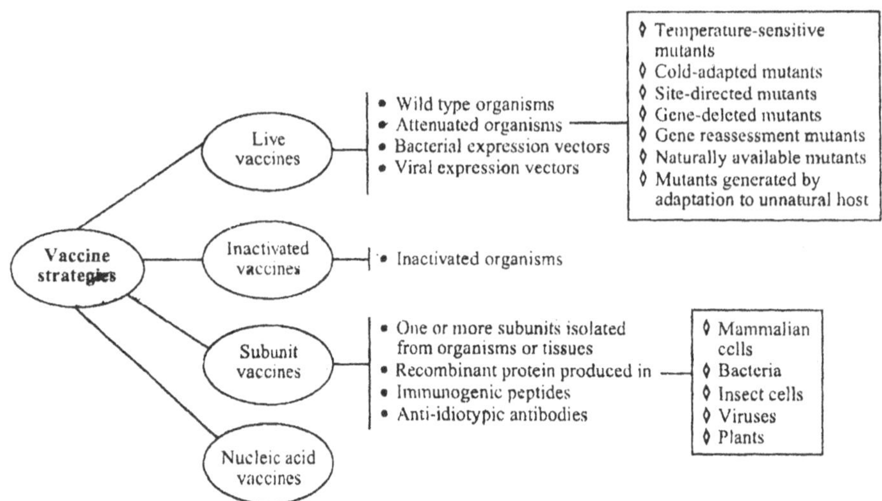

Fig. 7.1. Overview of vaccine strategies.

There have been instances in which inactivated vaccines led to atypical disease or enhanced disease severity. For example, in the 1960s, formalin-inactivated respiratory syncytial virus (RSV) vaccine actually enhanced the disease symptoms when vaccinated children were naturally exposed to RSV. It was later discovered that a change in the antigenicity of RSV F and G glycoproteins resulted not only in alteration in humoral immune response but also in the Th1 and Th2 components of the CD4+ T-cell response to RSV.

Live attenuated vaccines

Mostly attenuated organisms are being used as live virus vaccines; however, in some instances, even virulent organisms could be used, provided they are not administered via the natural route of infection. For example, human adenovirus types 4 and 7 may cause acute respiratory infections in humans when administered via the oronasal route but provide protection when given orally in enteric-coated capsules.

There are different ways to attenuate pathogens for vaccine production. Attenuation of organisms can be achieved by growing them under abnormal conditions, which include cultivation in unnatural hosts or cell lines. Some organisms are attenuated when they replicate at different pH levels and/or temperatures. In cells infected with multiple viruses with a segmented genome (e.g., influenza virus, reovirus), genome segments are randomly recombined in the progeny. This process of recombination is known as reassortment and is also useful in generating attenuated viruses. A natural pathogen of one host may be attenuated for another host, e.g., vaccinia virus worked as an attenuated vaccine for small poxvirus eradication program during the 1960s and 1970s, and turkey herpesvirus works as an attenuated vaccine for Marek' s disease virus (a chicken herpesvirus). In an inoculated host, the attenuated organism replicates without causing disease symptoms, thereby leading to induction of immune response somewhat similar to the natural infection with the disease-causing organism. The Bacille Camet–Guerin **(BCG)** strain of *Mycobacterium tuberculosis* was attenuated after more than 200 passages on media containing increasing amounts of bile. The Sabin polio- virus vaccine was attenuated by a number of passages in monkeys and in monkey kidney epithelial cells. Measles virus was initially adapted to monkey kidney cells and subsequently attenuated in duck embryo and human tissue culture cell lines.

Temperature-sensitive (*ts*) mutants have proven to be the most useful type of mutants for a number of viruses and bacteria because of their conditional-lethal phenotype. The (*ts*) mutants are produced by alteration in the nucleotide sequence of a gene so that the resulting protein product of the gene is unable to assume or maintain its functional configuration at the non-permissive (37–39°C) temperature. The protein, however, is able to assume a functional configuration at the permissive temperature (32–34°C), e.g., herpes- viruses, adenoviruses, and influenza viruses. Thus, these mutants can replicate in mucosal sites with a lower temperature, e.g., the nasal cavity, but are unable to cause systemic infections and disease.

A number of advantages associated with live vaccines are that: (1) they are cheap to produce because the inoculum dose is relatively less; (2) they require fewer inoculations; (3) they do not require adjuvants; (4) they elicit both humoral and cell-mediated immune responses; and (5) they can be inoculated by the natural route of infection. Some of the disadvantages associated with live vaccines are that: (1) they are usually less stable than inactivated vaccines and may require refrigeration for storage; (2) some of these vaccines under certain situations may revert to virulent form in the host and thereby lead to clinical disease; (3) they may not be recommended for immunosuppressed, immature, older, or pregnant hosts; (4) they may have a low level of residual virulence; and (5) they may be contaminated with other adventitious organisms.

Recombinant Vaccines

Recombinant vector vaccines

Viral vectors

For the development of an effective vaccine strategy for protection against mucosal pathogens such as respiratory and enteric viruses, a vaccine- delivery system that can induce a protective mucosal immunity in the form of secretory IgA antibody, in addition to a systemic immune response, is extremely important. The route of vaccine delivery also plays an important role in determining the type of resultant immunity induced. A number of viruses, such as adenoviruses, poxviruses, herpesviruses, picornaviruses, togaviruses, orthomyxoviruses, paramyxoviruses, and others, have demonstrated considerable potential as vectors for antigen delivery at mucosal surfaces. Immunogenic foreign epitopes can be expressed on the virus surface by modifying the viral capsid or envelope protein. A wide variety of foreign viral antigens has been expressed in viral vectors, and vaccination-challenge studies in experimental animals have demonstrated moderate to complete protection. Immunization with such vectors leads to the foreign viral antigen expression similar to that of natural infection without causing disease. Antigenic peptides are expressed along with major histocompatibility (MHC) class I and class II antigens and, thus, result in both humoral and cytotoxic T-cell responses. Both adenovirus-and poxvirus-based vectors have a number of common advantages including that (1) vector construction is easy; (2) relatively high levels of foreign protein expression are easily attained; (3) relative thermostability; (4) they have a large capacity for foreign DNA insertion; (5) vector derivatives are nonpathogenic; and (6) they have a wide host range. More than one foreign antigen can be expressed in the same vector to provide protection against a number of diseases by inoculation with a single vector.

Vaccinia virus expressing rabies glycoprotein has been licensed for use to control rabies in the wildlife population, especially raccoons, foxes, skunks, and coyotes. Baits containing a live vaccinia-rabies glycoprotein recombinant virus vaccine are distributed in the rabies endemic area with the intention that rabies-susceptible wild animals that eat these baits will become immunized against rabies virus, and this approach has demonstrated satisfactory results. Vaccinia virus expressing the F and H gene of rinderpest virus has shown potential for its use to control rinderpest in developing countries.

To increase the safety of viral vectors for immunocompromised hosts and to control their indiscriminate spread, replication defective viral vectors have been developed. These vectors can be grown to high titers in vitro, but they are defective for in vivo replication.

Replication-defective vectors undergo an abortive infection in an inoculated host that leads to foreign antigen expression similar to replication-competent vectors. Replication-defective adenovirus vectors are generated by deleting the early region 1 (E1) genes. E1-deleted vectors can be grown in an E1-complementing cell line, and animals immunized with such vectors elicit a protective immune response. Avian poxviruses grow normally in avian cells but would result in an abortive infection in mammalian hosts. Dogs and cats immunized with an avipox-rabies glycoprotein recombinant are protected against rabies virus infection.

Bacterial vectors

Similar to viral expression vectors, attenuated bacteria can be developed as vectors for foreign gene expression and delivery for the purpose of multivalent vaccines. Immungenic foreign epitopes can be expressed on bacteria surfaces by modifying cell surface proteins, fimbria, or flagella. It has been demonstrated that *M. bovis* BCG strain induces both strong humoral and cell-mediated immunity, therefore, it has been developed as a delivery vector with the assumption that foreign proteins expressed by *M. bovis* in inoculated individuals will also raise a strong protective immune response. Because *Salmonella* and *Vibrio* colonize in the intestinal tract, attenuated strains of these bacteria were developed as vectors for mucosal delivery.

Various bacterial vectors have been used to express a number of bacterial (*B. pertussis*, *S. pneumoniae*, *Y. pestis*, and *L. monocytogenes*), viral (herpesvirus, influenza virus, human immunodeficiency virus, simian immunodeficiency virus, and hepatitis B virus), and parasitic (*S. mansoni*, and *L. major*) antigens. Significant improvements in attenuation of bacteria, and the stability, localization, and expression levels of heterologous antigens are required to market the bacterial vector-based vaccines for use in humans or animals.

To enhance foreign gene expression, "*balanced lethal*," plasmid-based expression vehicles have been developed. A foreign antigen may form inclusion bodies or localize in intracellular compartment of the vector thereby affecting the type, levels, and duration of immune response elicited against the antigen. The *Escherichia coli* α-hemolysin secretion system (HSS) that includes HlyB, HlyD, and TolC is involved in exporting the HlyA-fused foreign antigens to extra- cellular compartment. Using the HSS system for attenuated *Shigella dysenteriae* the expression and secretion of Shiga toxin-B subunit were obtained.

Gene-deleted vaccines

Many attenuated vaccines are derived after introduction of random mutations in the genomes of various pathogens. In situations in which these random mutations may be point mutations, attenuated organisms may regain virulence owing to back mutations. Because of our increased understanding of virulence of various pathogens at the molecular level, one or more genes responsible for virulence has been identified in many pathogens. The genes associated with virulence may be genes involved with nucleic acid replication and other non-structural and structural components of the organism. This has made it possible to delete one or more of these genes involved in virulence—another strategy to produce safer attenuated vaccines.

Pseudorabies virus has been attenuated by deleting genes associated with viral virulence. These genes include the thymidine kinase gene (non-structural protein) involved in viral DNA replication and the gC, gG, and gE genes (non-essential glycoproteins) involved in virus assembly. A gene-deleted vaccine of pseudorabies virus has proved highly effective in controlling this viral infection under field conditions. It has been demonstrated that *Salmonella typhimurium* aroA, aroB, and aroC deletion mutants fail to grow in its host because of the absence of aromatic amino acid production. These genes have been targeted to reduce the virulence of the bacterium. *S. typhimurium* gene-deleted mutants are capable of replication at least for a short period in its host, thus raising a protective immune response. Vaccination with gene-deleted vaccines also allows eradication of wild-type pathogens from the population. Because antibodies against the deleted gene product will only be developed in infected animals, it is feasible to differentiate between vaccinated and naturally infected animals. The process of gene deletion not only attenuates the pathogen but also offers a unique opportunity to insert foreign genes for developing viral or bacterial-vectored vaccines.

Subunit vaccines

A subunit vaccine consists of one or more immunogenic epitopes, proteins, or other components of a pathogenic organism. Immunogenic epitopes can be chemically synthesized and are known as peptide vaccines, e.g., peptide vaccine candidates for foot- and-mouth disease virus. The pathogen could be disrupted, and one or more immunogenic proteins such as bacterial cell wall proteins; flagella or pili; and viral envelope, capsid, or nucleoproteins can be purified. The isolation of such components in purified form is sometimes cumbersome and expensive. However, bacterial exotoxins can be easily purified, inactivated, and used as toxoid vaccines.

A number of expression systems including bacteria, yeasts, mammalian cells, insect cells, and plants are now available for foreign protein expression. High amounts of a foreign protein can be produced in a bacterial- expression system at a low cost. Because scale-up and downstream processing have been well worked out for bacterial-expression systems, they are usually first tested for subunit vaccine production. Many of the immunogenic proteins, especially of viral origin, require secondary modifications that are important for their antigenicity. A bacterial-expression system may produce proteins of altered immunogenicity because the bacterial system lacks many posttranslational processes. However, some viral glycoproteins expressed in bacteria induce protective immunity, e.g., the gp 70 gene of feline leukemia virus. A yeast-expressed hepatitis B virus surface antigen (HbsAg)-based subunit vaccine is currently in use for humans and has demonstrated excellent protection against hepatitis B virus infection. This vaccine is an excellent example of the potential of recombinant subunit vaccines for providing protection against many viral and bacterial infections.

Because mammalian cells are known to process viral glycoproteins to their functional form by secondary modifications, they are considered one of the means to produce viral antigens for subunit vaccine production. However, the expression of such proteins in mammalian cells is usually too low. It was demonstrated that the stable expression of the transmembrane anchor-deleted form of many viral glycoproteins in mammalian cells results in the secretion of truncated products in the medium in large quantities that could be used as a subunit vaccine without further purification. However, the removal of transmembrane anchor may potentially alter antigenicity of the secreted protein. A number of viral glycoproteins that were expressed either in mammalian or in insect cells and secreted in form of proteins were suitable for providing protective immune response include F and G genes of respiratory syncytial virus, the HN and F genes of parainfluenza virus, and the gD gene of bovine herpesvirus type 1.

Immunogenic antigen production in plants

In the past decade, significant progress has been made in the stable integration and expression of a wide variety of genes in plant cells, resulting in the creation of novel plants for agricultural and industrial use. The inserted genes confer resistance to insect pathogen and herbicides; enhanced tolerance to drought, salt, and frost; and improved agricultural production. Undoubtedly, improvements in plant attributes by genetic engineering will have a great impact on agriculture production. However, it has been estimated that the major economic (over 90%) gain of plant biotechnology will result from the use of plants as bioreactors to produce high- valued products such as vaccines, industrial enzymes, and other pharmaceuticals.

Production of subunit vaccines in mammalian cells is usually expensive because of the low level of foreign gene expression and high processing cost. High levels of foreign gene expression can be obtained in bacteria and yeast, but many animal viral or mammalian proteins expressed in these systems fail to undergo proper secondary modifications such as glycosylation, phosphorylation, sulfation, etc. Therefore, these recombinant proteins may have altered antigenicity. Because most mechanisms regulating secondary modifications of proteins are present in plants, transgenic plants offer an attractive alternative to produce functional viral, bacterial, or parasitic proteins in large quantities at a very low cost for subunit vaccine production. Similarly, the production of functional multimeric antibody molecules in plants has made it possible to manufacture antibodies in bulk amounts for passive immunization.

Two major strategies have been devised to produce foreign proteins in plants. These are: (1) the stable integration of chimeric gene into the plant genome under a suitable constitutive or inducible plant promoters, and (2) manipulation of plant pathogenic viruses. Foreign protein expression in plants usually range from 0.01 to 1% of the total plant protein.

The hepatitis B virus (HBV) surface antigen HBsAg produced in transgenic tobacco elicits an immune response when injected in mice. Mice fed transgenic potato tuber expressing B subunit of heat-labile enterotoxin (LT-B) of enterotoxigenic E. coli developed antibodies to LT-B, particularly IgA antibodies. Dalsgaard et al. demonstrated that immunization of mink with the VP2 capsid protein of mink enteritis virus, expressed in cowpea after infection with modified cowpea mosaic virus, elicited a protective immune response. Protection against challenge with virulent foot- and-mouth disease virus (FMDV) in mice inoculated with the structural protein VP1 of FMDV produced in transgenic *Arabidopsis* has been shown. It has been hypothesized that transgenic plants could serve as "*edible vaccine*," thereby providing a very inexpensive mean of oral immunization.

Anti-idiotypic vaccines

Another approach to provide protective immune response is the use of anti-idiotype antibodies as vaccines. Antibodies have unique sequences in the variable (V) region in their binding site known as "*idiotypic determinants*". Some of the idiotypic determinants make up the antigen-binding site (paratope) of the antibody. The part of the antibody that binds to the antigen is called a paratope. Antibodies to a specific paratope of an idiotype mimic the epitope of immunizing antigen and are known as anti-idiotypic antibodies. Thus, anti-idiotype antibodies are mirror images of antigens and can be used instead of immunogens to elicit a protective immune response. Monoclonal antiidiotypic antibodies could serve as a source of antigen. Anti-idiotype vaccines are useful in cases in which actual antigen is poorly immunogenic or similar to host antigens. Some of the pathogens against which anti-idiotype vaccines have been tested include *Listeria monocytogenes*, *Streptococcus pneumoniae*, hepatitis B virus, Semliki forest virus, and Sendai virus. This type of vaccine is still in the developmental stage.

DNA Vaccines

Immunization of mammalian hosts with a plasmid DNA containing a gene under control of a heterologous promoter has introduced a new approach in the area of recombinant vaccine design. The introduced DNA is taken up by cells, and the gene of interest is expressed. The cells expressing the foreign antigen are recognized by the host immune system, leading to humoral and cell-mediated immune responses. DNA vaccines can also be called polynucleotide vaccines or nucleic acid (NA) vaccines. Such vaccines appear to have the primary advantages of both attenuated and inactivated vaccines but without their known limitations. NA vaccines elicit an immune response similar to that obtained with live attenuated vaccines. They also provide safety similar to that of inactivated vaccines, however, without the obvious side effects of adjuvants or animal-derived proteins.

The concept of NA vaccine evolved from initial studies in experimental animals in which the inoculation with naked plasmid DNA resulted in a protective immune response. After inoculation into a muscle, the efficiency of cellular uptake of the naked DNA is poor, and a large portion of the DNA is degraded before it reaches the nucleus for transcription. To increase the efficiency of DNA uptake by host cells and to reduce DNA degradation within the cell, a number of delivery systems, such as bombardment with gold microparticles coated with NA, incorporation of NA into liposomes and other polycationic lipids, biological erodable polymers, and others, have been developed. Recently, it has been demonstrated that alginate microspheres can be used for the encapsulation, delivery, and expression of plasmid DNA. Inoculation of mice with microspheres containing both plasmid DNA and bovine adenovirus type 3 (BAd3) resulted in a significant increase in transgene expression compared with those inoculated with microspheres containing only the plasmid DNA. As with other delivery systems, alginate microspheres led to a stronger mucosal or systemic immune response, depending on route of inoculation. Because alginate microspheres are most likely taken up by macrophages and dendritic cells, it may have a positive effect on the type of immune response elicited.

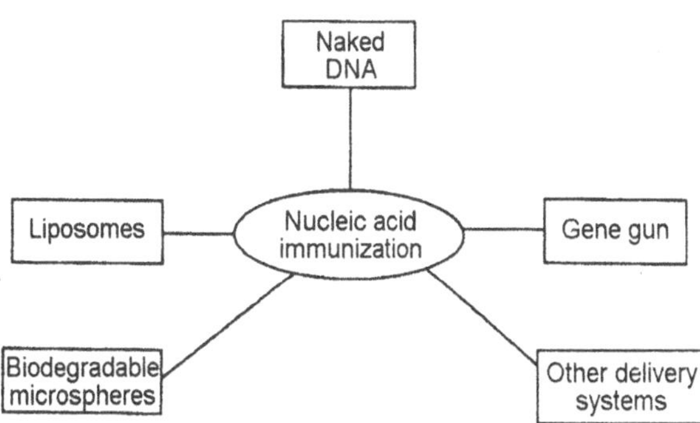

Fig. 7.2. Methods of nucleic acid delivery.

A number of factors that have an impact on the level and type of immune response produced by an NA vaccine include the type of immunogen, the dosage and number of inoculations, the heterologous regulatory sequences, the delivery system, the route of inoculation, and the presence or absence of immunomodulatory molecules. A variety of immunogenic antigens including HIV-1, SIV, HTLV-1, influenza virus, hepatitis B virus, hepatitis C virus, herpesvirus, M. tuberculosis, *Leishmania*, malaria, and many more have been expressed by NA vaccines and have demonstrated encouraging results.

Adjuvants

Adjuvants are compounds that, when administered in combination with antigens, enhance the immune response to those antigens. This enhanced immunogenicity can be measured as an increase of antigen-specific antibody levels in serum and/or mucosal secretions, a response against an increased number of epitopes, an increase of cell-mediated immune responses, or a combination thereof. Adjuvants are particularly important for the induction of protective immune responses against weak immunogens such as subunit vaccines. The mechanisms by which adjuvants enhance the immunogenicity of antigens are not completely understood, but they include immunostimulation, altered processing of antigens, and sustained release of antigens (depot effect). A different type of immune response is obtained by administration of antigens via the oral route, and this has different delivery requirements.

Many compounds can act as adjuvants. Their classification is made difficult by the variety in chemical composition and the overlapping, often poorly understood, mechanisms of action. Only aluminum adjuvants are approved by the FDA for use in human vaccines. Quil A is a saponin that is commonly used as an adjuvant in veterinary vaccines and is also a component of immune-stimulating complexes (ISCOM).

Immunostimulation

The immune system can be divided into the adaptive immune system, comprising of B and T lymphocytes, and the innate immune system, which includes neutrophils, macrophages, dendritic cells, and soluble factors such as the complement system. The innate immune system plays a critical role in the activation of the adaptive immune system. Dendritic cells are antigen- presenting cells that integrate the signals from the innate immune system and activate T-cells and possibly B-cells. T-cells have antigen-specific receptors that recognize peptides displayed by MHC I molecules ($CD8^+$ cytotoxic T-cells) and MHC II molecules ($CD4^+$ T helper cells). Engagement of the antigen- specific T-cell receptor is not sufficient, and T-cells also need to receive costimulatory signals delivered via CD28 and CD40-ligand. Dendritic cells express both MHC I and MHC II and, on activation, increase the expression of the costimulatory molecules CD80 and CD86 (ligands for CD28) and CD40. The signals that activate dendritic cells include microbial molecules. The innate immune system is equipped with receptors (called pattern-recognition receptors) that can recognize molecules that are expressed by pathogens, but not by mammalian cells, and alert the innate immune system on infection. These molecules, pathogen- associated molecular patterns, include lipopolysaccharides (LPS), mannose, and bacterial DNA with unmethylated CpG motifs. In addition, dendritic cells are stimulated by host cell components that are expressed and/ or released by cells when they undergo stress and pathologic cell death (necrosis). The identity of these components, called danger signals, is uncertain but may include heat shock proteins. The microbial molecules and danger signals can directly activate dendritic cells, or they can activate other components of the innate immune system resulting in the secretion of cytokines and other mediators that activate dendritic cells. The activated dendritic cells, in turn, activate T- and B-cells.

Immune responses can be divided into type 1 and type 2, based on the pattern of cytokine secretion and functional outcome of the immune response. Type 1 immune responses are characterized by secretion of IFN-gamma, production of IgG2a in mice, and activation of macrophages, NK cells, and cytotoxic T-cells. Type 2 responses are characterized by secretion of IL-4, IL-5, and IL-13 and by IgG1 and IgE production. The responses are reciprocally regulated. How the polarization of the immune response toward type 1 or type 2 is determined is not exactly understood. IL-12 is an important factor that drives the type 1 response, and IL-4 is implicated in the type 2 response. Microbial products such as LPS and bacterial DNA stimulate the secretion of IL-12 by dendritic cells and preferentially induce type 1 immune responses.

It is likely that the primary mechanism by which adjuvants stimulate the immune response is by direct or indirect signaling through pattern-recognition and danger signal receptors. Very strong adjuvants are often composed of or include microbial components such as LPS and mycobacteria or derivatives thereof. These type of adjuvants bind to pattern-recognition receptors to stimulate IL-12 production and a type 1 immune response. Coadministration of cytokines can directly activate and influence dendritic cells and the outcome of the immune response. This was clearly demonstrated with an experimental Leishmania vaccine using IL-12 as an adjuvant. Immunization of genetically susceptible BALB/c mice with a Leishmania antigen did not result in protection, but when IL-12 was injected with the antigen, the mice became markedly resistant to infection. The effect of IL-12 correlated with increased IFN-γ and decreased IL-4 secretion by antigen-specific T-cells in vitro.

Altered Processing of Antigens

Most T-cells that carry the α-β-T-cell receptor do not recognize and react with intact proteins. Instead, the T-cells recognize small peptides that are derived from proteins and that are linked to MHC I and MHC II molecules. The MHC I-linked peptides are generated in the cytoplasm (endogenous pathway) and recognized by $CD8^+$ T-cells. Proteins in the cytoplasm are degraded by a complex of proteolytic enzymes, the proteasome, and the peptides are transported into the rough endoplasmic reticulum where they associate with MHC I molecules. Peptide binding stabilizes the MHC I molecules, and the complexes are transported to the cell surface. In contrast, proteins that enter cells by endocytosis are partially degraded into peptides in endosomal vesicles. The peptides bind MHC II molecules that have been transported from the endoplasmic reticulum to the endosomes. The MHC II-peptide complexes are then displayed on the cell surface and are available for recognition by $CD4^+$ T-cells. Vaccines that contain single proteins or inactivated pathogens can readily activate $CD4^+$ T-cells because the antigens are endocytosed and processed by MHC II-positive antigen-presenting cells. Activation of the $CD4^+$ T-cells can result in a type 1 or a type 2 immune response, depending on the type of adjuvant included. However, such vaccines usually do not activate $CD8^+$ cytotoxic T-cells because activation of $CD8^+$ T-cells requires processing of antigen via the endogenous pathway. Certain adjuvant formulations such as liposomes, the saponin QS-21, and poly-(lactic-co-glycolic acid) (PLGA) are able to induce cytotoxic T-cell responses to protein antigens. These adjuvants appear to target some of the injected antigens into the cytosol of antigen-presenting cells for processing via the endogenous pathway. The mechanism by which this occurs is not known.

Sustained release of antigens

The slow and continued release of antigens has been postulated to induce a strong immune response through continued activation of the immune system. This may contribute to the adjuvant effect of aluminum-based adjuvants and mineral oils. Newer technologies may allow for the design of vaccines that release antigens from a depot at certain time intervals after a single injection. One example is the use of poly PLGA micro- spheres for encapsulation of antigens. By varying the polymer composition and size of the microspheres, the release of antigen can be varied. Pulsatile release of antigen can be attained by combining multiple variations of PLGA microspheres in a single dose of the vaccine. Relatively little is known about the desired pattern of antigen release to obtain a maximal response. It was recently suggested that continued release of antigen is not desirable for the induction of strong memory cell responses. Mathematical models may help design appropriate strategies for the release of antigens from depots after a single injection.

Aluminum

Aluminum adjuvants in human vaccines are either aluminum hydroxyphosphate (commonly referred to as aluminum phosphate) or aluminum oxyhydroxide (aluminum hydroxide). Aluminum-based vaccines are prepared by adsorption of antigen to commercial aluminum hydroxide or aluminum phosphate gels or by mixing antigen with alum (potassium aluminum sulfate), resulting in precipitation. The alum-precipitated adjuvants resemble aluminum phosphate in their chemical and physical properties. The surface charge and morphology of the aluminum adjuvants affect their adsorptive capacity. The rate and degree of adsorption are further dependent on the pH, ionic strength of the antigen solution, and isoelectric point of the antigen.

Aluminum adjuvants are universally used in diptheria–tetanus–pertussis (DTP) vaccines and in most hepatitis B vaccines and have an excellent safety record. They are not ideal adjuvants, however, because the enhancement of the immune response is relatively weak, they are not effective with all antigens, and, most important, they only enhance the humoral (type 2) immune response and have little effect on the cell-mediated (type 1) immune response.

The mechanism by which aluminum enhances the immune response is not clear. Early studies suggested that aluminum adjuvants slowly release the adsorbed antigen over time (depot effect). However, recent experiments demonstrated that antigens are rapidly desorbed after injection in animals. Moreover, aluminum phosphate enhanced the immune response to DNA-encoded antigen after DNA immunization, clearly indicating that adsorption may not be critical to the adjuvant effect of aluminum compounds. These data indicate that aluminum enhances the immune response via other mechanisms. A satisfactory explanation of the adjuvant effect of aluminum also needs to take into account its selective mode of enhancing the immune response, i.e., a predominant type 2 immune response. Aluminum adjuvants induced differentiation toward type 2 immune responses, even in the absence of IL-4 or IL-13. Aluminum stimulated a type 1 and type 2 immune response in genetically engineered mice with a defective IL-4 and IL-13 response, suggesting that aluminum-induced IL-4 and/or IL-13 secretion suppresse the type 1 response but are dispensable for a type 2 response in intact animals. The lack of a type 1 immune response is a drawback for the use of aluminum in vaccines for intracellular pathogens and tumors. A recent study demonstrated that aluminum adjuvant with adsorbed IL-12 induces a strong type 1 response, indicating that it is possible to overcome the aluminum- induced suppression of type 1 responses.

Saponins

The saponins of the bark of the *Quillaja saponaria* Molina tree have long been known to have immunostimulatory activity. A partially purified fraction, Quil A, has reduced toxicity and more potent adjuvant activity and is used in veterinary vaccines. Quil A can be further fractionated into fractions that have different degrees of toxicity. QS-21 is a less toxic component with strong adjuvant activity. Saponins probably act by direct stimulation of the immune system. They stimulate both the humoral (primarily IgG2a antibodies in the mouse) and cell-mediated immune responses. QS-21 causes protein antigens to be processed and presented via the MHC I pathway, resulting in cytotoxic T-cell responses. Cytokine analysis indicates that QS-21 stimulates type 1 cytokine production.

Immune-stimulating complexes (ISCOMs) are 30–40 nm particles consisting of Quil A, cholesterol, antigen, and phospolipids. They are used in a commercial vaccine for equine influenza. ISCOM-adjuvanted vaccines stimulate a strong humoral and cell-mediated immune response caused by the immunostimulatory actions of Quil A and targeting of the particles to macrophages. As with Quil A, ISCOMs target antigens for processing via the MHC I pathway, resulting in induction of cytotoxic T-cell responses.

Delivery of Vaccines

Parenteral vs. mucosal route

The success of vaccination depends primarily on the method of presenting the antigen to the host immune system. Antigens have usually been delivered by par- enteral (such as intravenous, intramuscular, intraperitoneal, intradermal, and subcutaneous) administration, but recent studies have shown that other routes of delivery such as intranasal, oral, and transdermal delivery have also been effective. In some cases, vaccination through mucosal routes resulted in better responses in IgA production. Because non-parenteral vaccine delivery presents many obvious advantages, numerous attempts have been made on the development of non-parenteral delivery of vaccines.

Parenteral route

Parenteral vaccination remains the immunization method of choice for most antigens because it provides more effective immune response than do any other routes of vaccination in most cases. Every years millions of people receive inactivated influenza vaccine by parenteral administration. Subcutaneous vaccination with inactivated influenza vaccine is known to induce simultaneous immune responses in the blood and upper respiratory tract of subjects. The immune response, i.e., the increase in the number of influenza virus-specific antibody-secreting cells in peripheral blood and tonsils, increased rapidly to reach a peak within 1 week after vaccination. Parenteral vaccination of a DNA vaccine encoding glycoprotein D of herpes simplex virus type 2 resulted in systemic cellular and humoral responses. The mucosal humoral responses generated by intramuscular and intradermal vaccination were comparable with those obtained by mucosal vaccination. The DNA vaccine was able to stimulate a response in the Peyer's patches, a major inductive site for mucosal responses. For many other antigens, however, the usefulness of parenteral vaccination is limited by the insufficient induction of mucosal immune responses.

Parenteral vaccination is difficult for those living in the developing countries where medical care is not well-established. Vaccination of a large number of subjects using hypodermic needles, which is a highly labor-intensive procedure requiring healthcare personnel, is not practical. The problem becomes even more significant for vaccination of millions of animals. For example, vaccination for routine control of Newcastle disease in chickens by intramuscular injection requiring individual handling of the birds is not practical. Recent advances in needleless injectable systems have made the parenteral vaccination easier, but it still requires individual handling. Examples of needleless injection systems are PowderJect, Medi-Jector, Biojector, Vitajet, Bio-Set, and Intraject. They all use high pressure released in a very short period to deliver drugs through the skin. A jet-immunization technique was used for intraoral administration of DNA in the cheek, resulting in high IgA mucosal responses. The intraoral jet-injection technique for DNA vaccine delivery has the advantages of being a simple and rapid way to administer the DNA in solution and to provoke specific mucosal IgA after administration in the mucosal-associated lymphoid tissue.

The results of parenteral vaccination depend on the route of administration. For plasmid DNA vaccines, the highest levels of antibodies were induced by intramuscular and intravenous injections, although significant titers were also obtained with sublingual and intradermal delivery. Delivery to the skin by the gene gun induced exclusively IgG1 antibodies (Th2-like) at 4 weeks and only very low IgG2a levels at later times. Other routes, such as intraperitoneal, intraperineal, subcutaneous, intranasal inhalation, intranasal instillation, intrarectal, intravaginal, ocular, and oral, did not result in significant immune responses.

Dual-chamber syringe

For delivery of two established vaccines (e.g., polyribosyl ribitol phosphate conjugated to tetanus toxoid and diphtheria–tetanus– whole cell pertussis and inactivated poliovirus vaccine) at the same time, a dual-chamber syringe delivery system can be used. The proximal chamber may contain a vaccine in the freeze-dried solid state, and the distal chamber contains a vaccine in the liquid formulation that allows reconstitution of the vaccine in the proximal chamber. The immune response by the dual- chamber delivery of vaccination was equivalent to that by the separate-injection method of vaccination. The dual-chamber syringe can be used for safe and effective delivery of two different vaccines that are not yet available as a single formulation for pediatric applications. The primary advantage of the dual-chamber syringe is that it reduces the cost of vaccine delivery and, at the same time, increases the vaccine acceptability and coverage rate of vaccines.

Mucosal route

Vaccination through mucosal routes provides new avenues of vaccination with a unique advantage of mucosal immunity, that may not be obtained, through parenteral vaccination. Mucosal immunization presents a realistic alternative to parenteral administration for inducing protective immune responses. Vaccination by mucosal route provides a number of advantages over parenteral vaccination. First, mucosal vaccination does not involve hypodermic needles, which are not user-friendly. Second, the total surface area of the mucosal surfaces in the gastrointestinal, respiratory, and urogenital tracts where many infectious pathogens come into contact with the host is huge. Thus, preventing infections at the mucosal surface provides an immunological first line of defense against diseases. This makes priming of the mucosal-associated lymphoid tissue (MALT) by vaccination most desirable. Parenteral vaccination alone is quite often insufficient in inducing mucosal immune responses, because stimulation of the MALT usually requires direct contact between the immunogen and the mucosal surface. The mucosal tissues are protected by interconnected local immune system, which is essentially separated from systemic immunity. In a common mucosal-defense system, an antigen interacting with localized lymphoid tissue can stimulate IgA precursor cells that may then migrate to other mucosal surfaces to elicit immune reaction in other mucosal tissues. It is known that the mucosal immune system produces 70% of the body's antibodies. Mucosal delivery of numerous antigens by a variety of routes (oral, nasal, tracheal, and rectal) has been shown to elicit immunity at mucosal surfaces mediated by secretory IgA. The presence of MALT indicates that mucosal vaccination at a certain site in the body can be achieved by mucosal immunization at the distal site of the body. Although the mucosal and systemic humoral immune

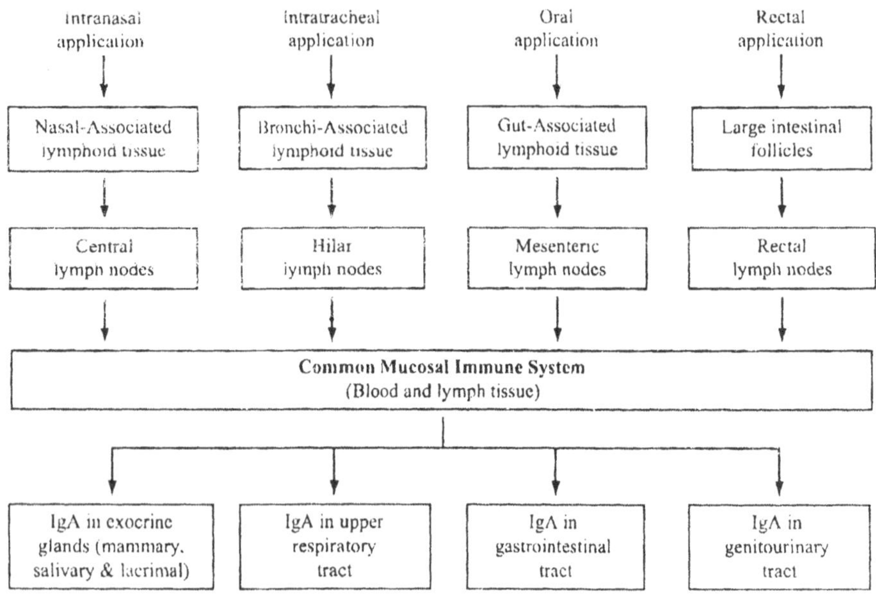

Fig. 7.3. Mucosal immunization and production of IgA antibodies in various mucosal surfaces via the common mucosal-simmunization system.

systems function essentially independent of each other, an antigen administered by one route can modify responsiveness to subsequent immunization by an alternate route.

Oral vaccination of the various mucosal routes, oral vaccination is the most preferable mode of vaccination because of its ease of use and low cost of manufacturing. Furthermore, the gastrointestinal (GI) tract provides the largest component of the mucosal immune system that has been well-characterized. Oral administration of vaccines has high acceptability, by avoidance of injection, to individuals of all ages. After oral vaccination, an antigen, which is typically loaded in microspheres, is taken up by M-cells in the Peyer's patch of the gut-associated lymphoid tissue. The antigen is then passed to the macrophages and B-cells (B). These cells in turn present the antigen to T helper lymphocytes. These cells migrate into the blood via the mesenteric lymph nodes (MLN) and the thoracic duct (TD). These cells subsequently localize in the effector sites, i.e., mucosal membranes of the GI tract, upper respiratory tract, genitourinary tract, and glandular tissue. At the effector sites, the migrating B-cells develop into plasma cells that produce IgA antibodies. Polymeric IgA is then released as secretory IgA (sIgA) through epithelial cells.

The maximal intestinal immunization can be achieved by intra-Peyer's patch immunization, and thus this method can be used to screen oral vaccine candidate antigens without the added complication of simultaneously testing oral-delivery systems. Immunization of subjects against *Helicobacter pylori* by intra-Peyer's patch resulted in an 84–91% reduction in *H. pylori* infection compared with unimmunized controls. The therapeutic efficacy of the recombinant *H. pylori* urease vaccine in mice was shown to be comparable with that achieved with the combined antibiotic/antacid treatment in humans. The oral vaccination is preferred to conventional treatment of ulcers because it is a very simple and quick procedure compared with long-term conventional treatment. In addition, vaccines use the defense mechanisms of the body to establish long-lasting immunity.

One of the limitations of oral vaccination is that it does not always induce sufficient immunity. There are a few good reasons for this. First, the GI tract is designed to digest proteins by acidic and enzymatic degradation for absorption. Because most antigens are proteins in nature, they may be degraded by enzymes in the GI tract as well as by acids in the stomach. This is why soluble antigens administered orally are not effective. Thus, prevention of the antigen degradation is the first step toward successful oral vaccination. Adding protease inhibitors before oral vaccination may induce complete immunity, but this approach is not practical. There are many different enzymes that may not be inhibited by a particular protease inhibitor, and, more important the action of protease inhibitors may not occur at the same time that the antigens are present in the GI tract. Second, the systemic uptake of antigens from the GI tract is very poor. Even after oral intake of gram quantities of antigen, only a nanogram range of antigenic material was found to pass the intestinal barrier. It is also possible that for certain antigens, oral vaccination may simply be less effective than parenteral vaccination in induction of systemic immunity. The protection resulting from oral vaccination is known to last for a relatively short period, ranging from a few months to 1 year. To obtain the desirable immunity equivalent to systemic immunization, oral vaccination requires much higher and more frequent oral doses. The use of highly effective adjuvants in oral vaccine formulation may result in strong and long-lasting immunity in mucosal tissues.

The issues of degradation of antigens in the GI tract and the poor systemic uptake of antigens from the GI tract have led to encapsulation of antigens in microparticles (also called microcapsules or microspheres). Antigens that are encapsulated in microparticles are protected from degradation, and the microparticulate nature allows better uptake by the M-cells in the Peyer' s patches. A large number of studies have shown that antigens orally delivered in microparticles resulted in good mucosal immunity. It is noted here that virus itself can be regarded as a particulate vaccine-delivery system. Many viruses are highly effective in inducing immunization after oral vaccination. Norwalk virus, which is a major cause of epidemic gastroenteritis, was immunogenic in healthy human adults even when administered without adjuvants. Influenza virus can also elicit immune response after oral administration. Successful oral vaccination relies on targeting of microparticles to the Peyer's patches. It is known that the surface chemistry of microparticles affects the targeting to and uptake by M-cells in the Peyer's patches. The exact relationships between the surface chemistry and the uptake by Peyer's patches, however, have not been fully understood. Development of better oral vaccines requires understanding of such relationships.

Intranasal vaccination route has received growing interest for non-invasive immunization. Intranasal immunization has been quite effective for various vaccine-delivery systems. Both solution and microsphere formulations tend to show good immune responses after intranasal administration. Immunization of mice with tetanus toxoid, in solution and microsphere-encapsulated formulations, resulted in high levels of specific IgG and IgA antibodies. Nasal vaccine delivery is known to be superior to oral delivery in inducing specific IgA and IgG antibody responses in the upper respiratory tract. Nasal immunization is also known to be preferable to the oral route for distant mucosal vaccination that might be used to prevent adhesion of pathogens to the urogenital tract. It is interesting to note that the volume of.the nasally instilled vaccine is important. The larger-volume (e.g., 50 μL) of microsphere suspension resulted in the higher percentage of particles entering the lungs than did the lower, volume (e.g., 10 μL) instillation. It is generally believed that microspheres that adhere to the nasal mucus elicit better immune response, and for this reason, many microspheres made of mucoadhesive polymers, such as chitosan, have been used extensively in the preparation of nasal vaccine formulations.

Transdermal vaccination or transcutaneous immunization, is attractive, because it does not require specially trained personnel necessary for needle injections. Topical application of antigens to intact skin has shown promising results for the administration of DNA-based vaccines. Noninvasive gene delivery by pipetting adenovirus- or liposome-complexed plasmid DNA onto the outer layer of skin was able to achieve localized trans- gene expression within a restricted subset of skin in mice. It also elicited an immune response against the protein encoded by the DNA. For improved results, transdermal electroporation was also tried to explore the feasibility of non- adjuvant, needle-free skin immunization. The trans- dermal electroporation route elicited higher responses to a myristylated peptide than did intradermal immunization. For diphtheria toxoid, however, the result was the opposite. It appears that transdermal electroporation is a promising technique for non-adjuvant skin immunization, especially with low-molecular-weight, weakly immunogenic antigens. Topical application of antigen and cholera toxin or bacterial exotoxin to the skin surface resulted in detectable antigen-specific IgG in plasma and mucosal secretions. It appears that transcutaneous immunization can induce potent, protective immune responses to both systemic and mucosal challenge.

Pulmonary vaccination is especially useful in mass vaccination campaigns. A conventional method of pulmonary delivery of drugs using metered-dose, propellant-driven, small-particle aerosols was used to deliver killed whole bacterium vaccines. The results showed good stimulation of mucosal immunity against respiratory infections in animals. Recent advances in powder inhaler devices have made it possible to deliver vaccines via the pulmonary route using dry powder inhalation technologies Dry powder vaccine in the size range from 1 to 5 μm in diameter is used for the maximum alveolar (deep lung) deposition.

Direct gene transfer into the respiratory system can be carried out for either therapeutic or immunization purposes. Cells in the lung can take up and express plasmid DNA whether it is administered in naked form or formulated with cationic liposomes. For a given dose of DNA, the results can be improved when the DNA is mixed with the minimum amount of lipid that can complex it completely. Such a complex formation can be considered a formation of microparticles that can enhance cellular uptake and subsequent immune responses.

Parenteral and mucosal combination vaccination

The combination of mucosal and systemic immunization routes (e.g., parenteral immunization followed by oral immunization or vice versa) generally induces mucosal immune responses that are superior to immunization by either route alone. Pigs showed some protection after intramuscular inoculation with formalin-inactivated *M. hyopneumoniae* vaccine in incomplete Freund' s adjuvant and a booster inoculation with the same vaccine in microspheres onto the mucosal surface of Peyer's patches by a surgical operation.

Antigen delivery systems

The primary goal of antigen-delivery systems is to maintain a stable dosage form during storage and, when administered to present antigens to elicit a vigorous immune response in vivo. It is necessary to develop vaccine formulations that would preserve the antigen and deliver it to a specific target organ over a desired period. Continuous release or multiple pulsatile release during the desired period would eliminate the inconvenience of multiple vaccine administration for obtaining satisfactory immune responses. The antigen-delivery system plays one of the most crucial roles in the outcome of the immunization. The way that antigens are delivered affects the immune response significantly. Currently, antigen-delivery systems are classified into two systems: live attenuated microorganisms and non-living microparticulate systems.

Live attenuated organisms

Live attenuated bacteria and viruses have been used not only as vaccines but also as a delivery system that elicits humoral, mucosal, and cellular immune responses against exogenous antigens. Since the success with live attenuated oral vaccines against tuberculosis and polio more than 3 decades ago, a number of live attenuated microorganisms have been used as antigen-delivery systems. Live vaccines are relatively easy and cheap to manufacture, because they do not require purification of antigens or formulation with adjuvants. Attenuated strains of microorganisms can be formed spontaneously or induced by heat, chemical, or UV mutagenesis. Another advantage of the attenuated live vaccines is that they can be administered by the natural route of infection. Recently, pathogenic microorganisms have been attenuated by genetic engineering, i.e., mutating specific genes or removing some toxic genes. Because much of the infection occurs through the mucosal surfaces, live attenuated vaccines are best suited for protection against pathogens that access the body through the mucosal surfaces. Live attenuated oral vaccines are expected to provide the most convenient and effective means of vaccinating against enteric disease. Orally administered attenuated *Salmonella* are known to interact with the MALT. Other examples of live attenuated microorganism vaccines are BCG (bacilli Calmette–Guerin), adenovirus, and poliovirus.

Some viruses and bacteria are inherently quite stable. For example, polio virus can be formulated as a frozen liquid. A live poliovirus vector expressing a foreign antigen generates both antibody and cytotoxic T-lymphocyte responses in mice. Most live bacteria and viruses, however, are usually stored as powders after freeze-drying or lyophilization. Preserving the live state through freeze-drying often requires the presence of a stabilizer, which is selected primarily through trial and error. The most widely used nonspecific stabilizers are sugars, amino acids, polyols, and neutral salts which are known to act as bound water substitutes for maintaining the conformational integrity of proteins. An example of lyophilized vaccine products is *S. typhi* bacteria lyophilized to a powder that is encapsulated into gelatin for oral administration.

One of the drawbacks of using live microorganisms is that attenuated pathogens may invoke the very disease they are designed to prevent if they are insufficiently attenuated. Even if they are sufficiently attenuated, they still may cause severe infections in immunocompromised individuals. In addition, they always have a potential to revert to full virulence if lesions causing attenuation are not fully characterized. If pathogens are over-attenuated, they fail to trigger an appropriate immune response. Thus, it is highly important to attain the right balance between minimal virulence and maximal immunogenicity. This balance can be achieved in a normal population but may not be the same in a population with even minor defects in immune competence. Another aspect to notice in using live vaccines is that the distribution of live vaccines requires a cold chain that may not be readily accessible in many developing countries, and this may offset advantages of using live-vectored vaccines.

Non-living microparticulate delivery systems

Non-living immunogens generally result in immune responses of lesser magnitude and of shorter duration than do those by living immunogens. Nonliving immunogens are usually made of microparticulate forms to protect antigens and to improve cellular uptake. Nonliving microparticulates that can be used as antigen-delivery systems include polymeric microparticles, liposomes, virus-like particles, neosomes, and cross-linked protein crystals. The definition of microparticles should be broad enough to include all other forms, such as protein aggregates. The size of microparticles used in the vaccine area is usually less than 50 μm. It is common, however, to call any particles less than a few hundred micrometers microparticles. For this reason, it is important to specify the average size of microparticles for particular applications, because the size of microparticles often affect the outcome.

Polymeric microparticles and liposomes have been used extensively as controlled-release dosage forms for many drugs including antigens. They have been quite useful in oral delivery of antigens because encapsulation in microparticles can protect antigens from acidic and enzymatic degradation in the GI tract, and thus serve as a stable vaccine vehicle with extended shelf life. Delivery of antigens by microparticulate-delivery systems has the potential benefits of reducing the number of inoculations, enhancing the immune response via both parenteral and oral vaccination routes, and reducing the total antigen dose required to achieve immune protection. Microparticulate vaccine-delivery systems show improved immune responses because of the protection of the loaded antigens from degradation and the slow release of the antigens. For this reason, microparticulate-delivery systems are often considered adjuvants. Polymer microparticles, a large number of polymers, such as poly(methyl methacrylate), poly(butyl cyanoacrylate), poly(lactide-co-glycolide), polyarcyl-starch, dextran, albumin, and alginic acid, have been used for making microparticles for vaccine delivery.

All the polymers that have been used for controlled drug delivery can be used for vaccine delivery. Preparation of microparticles from water-insoluble polymers [e.g., poly(methyl methacrylate), poly(butyl cyanoacrylate), and poly(lactide-co-glycolide)] requires use of organic solvents or high temperature, both of which may not be good for maintaining tertiary structures of antigens. Preparation from water-soluble polymers frequently requires cross-linking reaction to make the polymers remain insoluble. It is possible that cross- linking agents cross-link not only polymer chains but also antigen molecules. Absorption of water into hydrophilic polymers results in swelling of the network, i.e., formation of hydrogels, or aquagels. Preparation of microparticles from hydrophilic polymers is preferred because it does not require organic solvents or high temperature. Polymers that have been used in the immunization vary depending on the route of administration.

For parenteral vaccination, biodegradable polymeric microparticles made of poly(lactide-*co*-glycolide) are commonly used as vaccine carriers. Poly(lactide-*co*-glycolide) has been well-characterized and known to be highly biocompatible. The size of microparticles can be easily controlled, and microparticles of less than 100 μm in diameter can be easily administered by injection through standard-sized needles (22 gauge or smaller). Because of the slow degradation of the polymer, antigens are slowly released from the microparticles for long term in much the same way as do alum adjuvants, and this results in enhanced immune responses. Other polymers, such as chitosan, have been used for preparation of vaccine formulations. Because one of the important roles that microparticles play in immunization is the slow release of antigens, a number of approaches have been tried to achieve antigen release at desired rates. The surface of microparticles can be modified to alter the adsorption and desorption kinetics of antigens. Alternatively, the pore size can be varied to control the release of antigens from microparticles.

The size of microparticles is known to play a critical role in oral immunization. In addition to protecting antigens from acidic and enzymatic degradation in the GI tract, microparticulates are known to enhance uptake by M-cells in the Peyer's patches, and the effectiveness of the uptake depends on the size of microparticles. It is generally thought that microparticles smaller than 10 μm are preferentially absorbed by M-cells, and the smaller the size, the better the absorption. One study using microparticles of different sizes showed that the efficiency of uptake of 100-nm particles by the intestinal tissue was 15- to 250-fold higher than that of larger size microparticles. In addition to the small size, microparticles with more hydrophobic surface property are absorbed better than those with more hydrophilic surface property. There are, however, no definite studies confirming or supporting these assumptions. Once microparticles are placed in the GI tract, adsorption of numerous proteins and polysaccharides present in the GI tract would alter the surface chemistry drastically, and it is difficult to correlate a particular surface chemistry of the native microparticles with the absorption ability.

Virus-like particles (VLPs) consist of one or more viral-coat proteins. They are very immunogenic molecules that allow for covalent coupling of the epitopes of interest. Recently, parvovirus-like particles have been engineered to express foreign polypeptides in certain positions, resulting in the production of large quantities of highly immunogenic peptides, and to induce strong antibody, helper T-cell, and cytotoxic T-lymphocyte responses. Parenteral administration of recombinant VLPs of papillomavirus induced VLP-specific humoral and cellular immune responses. Immunization of VLPs without adjuvant via mucosal route is also known to elicit specific antibody at mucosal surfaces and also systemic VLP epitope-specific T-cell responses.

Liposomes are vesicles composed of naturally occurring or synthetic phopholipids. The bilayer structure can be single- or multicompartment. The size can also vary from smaller than 1 μm to larger than 10 μm. When negatively charged lipid molecules, which form liposomes, interact with divalent cations, a solid, multi-layered, crystallaine structure called cochleate is formed. Because liposomes and cochleates can protect antigens from the GI tract and deliver them to the Peyer's patches, they have been exploited as an effective delivery system for oral vaccination.

Liposomes, like other vaccine-delivery systems, can exert immunoadjuvant effects. The surface charge of liposomes is known to affect the immune responses. Positively charged liposomes containing soluble antigens were reported to function as a more potent inducer of antigen-specific, cytotoxic T-lymphocyte responses and delayed-type hypersensitivity responses than negatively charged and neutral liposomes containing the same concentrations of antigens. Studies showed that the positively charged liposomes delivered proteinaceous antigens efficiently into the cytoplasm of the macrophages/antigen-presenting cells where the antigens are processed to be presented by class I MHC molecules to induce the cell-mediated immune response. Liposomes containing highly immunogenic glycoproteins of the Sendai virus on their surface, which are called fusogenic liposomes, showed enhanced antigen- specific humoral immunity in mice. The levels of antiovalbumin antibody were markedly increased in serum from mice immunized with OVA encapsulated in fusogenic liposomes. It appears that the fusogenic liposomes function as an immunoadjuvant in inducing antigen-specific antibody production.

Virosomes are liposomes containing viral fusion proteins that allow efficient entering into cells fusion with endosome membranes. Viral fusion proteins become activated in the low pH environment in the endosome to release its contents into the cytosol. Hepatitis A and influenza vaccines constructed on virosomes elicited fewer local adverse reactions than did their classic counterparts and displayed enhanced immunogenicity. Virosome-formulated influenza vaccine has also been shown to be safe and immunogenic when administered by the intranasal route. Other studies have suggested that immunopotentiating reconstituted influenza virosomes can be a suitable delivery system for synthetic peptide vaccines. The virosomes have a great potential for the design of combined vaccines targeted against multiple antigens and multiple pathogens.

Micelles are aggregates of detergent molecules in aqueous solution. Detergents are water-soluble, surface- active agents composed of a hydrophilic head group and a hydrophobic or lipophilic tail group. They can also align at aqueous/non-aquous interfaces, reducing surface tension, increasing miscibility, and stabilizing emulsions. Polymeric micelles made of block copolymers, such as poly(ethylene oxide)-poly(propylene oxide)-poly(ethylene oxide), have been used as a delivery system for hydrophobic drugs. They can also encapsulate antigens for vaccination.

Niosomes are non-ionic surfactant vesicles. They have been used to develop a vaccine-delivery system by peroral and oral routes. Ovalbumin was encapsulated in various lyophilized niosome preparations consisting of sucrose esters, cholesterol, and dicetyl phosphate. Encapsulation of ovalbumin into niosomes consisting of 70% stearate sucrose ester and 30% palmitate sucrose ester (40% mono-, 60% di/triester) resulted in a significant increase in antibody titers in serum, saliva, and intestinal washings.

Cross-linked protein crystals have been used as antigens. The immunogenicity of cross-linked protein crystals of human serum albumin was 6- to 30-fold higher in antibody titer than that of the soluble protein over an almost 6-month study. It is likely that the cross-linked protein crystals release antigen in a slow- release manner, and in this sense, the cross-linked protein crystals function as a depot. The cross-linked protein crystals present high stability, purity, biodegradability, and ease of manufacturing, all of which are highly attractive features for vaccine formulation. Because the cross-linked protein crystals are microparticulates, they can also be used for vaccination through various routes.

Immunomodulation

Immunomodulation refers to treatments that alter immune responsiveness in a non-antigen-specific manner. Enhancement of the immune response is desired in the treatment of chronic infectious diseases and neoplastic diseases, whereas suppression is needed in cases of inappropriate or exaggerated immune response, including allergies and autoimmune diseases. There are numerous treatments that affect the activity of the immune system. The effect of currently available immunosuppressive drugs is very broad, giving these drugs undesirable side effects. The aim of the research in this area is to design treatments that selectively enhance or suppress immune responses. Some of the newer treatment options are those that target costimulatory molecules, and the use of CpG DNA, and cytokines.

Costimulation

Activation of T-cells requires two signals. The first signal is provided by recognition of MHC/ peptide complex by the T-cell receptor. This does not result in proliferation and differentiation of the T-cell unless the T-cell receives a second, costimulatory signal. Several costimulatory signals have been identified, but the major costimulatory signal appears to result from the binding of CD28 on T-cells to B7 molecules on antigen-presenting cells. There are at least two B7 molecules, B7-1 (CD80) and B7-2 (CD86). Activation of antigen-presenting cells results in increased expression of B7-2, followed by B7-1. A second T-cell ligand of the B7 molecules is cytotoxic T lymphocyte antigen-4 (CTLA-4 or CD152) that, other than its name implies, is rapidly expressed on both $CD4^+$ and $CD8^+$ T-cells after binding of the T-cell receptor to the MHC/ peptide complex on antigen-presenting cells. However, in contrast to the positive signal provided by CD28, CTLA-4 down-regulates T-cell responses. CTLA-4 has a higher affinity for the B7-molecules than does CD28 and may prevent the activation of T-cells when B7 expression by dendritic cells is low and terminate the immune response when its expression is strongly increased. A soluble chimeric protein, CTLA4Ig, blocks the binding of both CD28 and CTLA-4 to the B7 molecules and, thus, may prevent T-cell activation. Administration of this protein to patients with psoriasis vulgaris, an immune-mediated skin disease, in a phase I clinical trial resulted in significant improvement in approximately 50% of the patients. Selective inhibition of CTLA-4 with specific antibodies may boost the immune system. The combination of surgery and anti-CTLA-4 antibody therapy was highly effective in the prevention of metastatic recurrence in a mouse prostatic carcinoma model. Other CD28 and B7 homologs continue to be identified and appear to play a role in costimulation. These molecules may provide additional targets for immunomodulation and suggest that it may be possible to fine-tune the immune response through pharmacologic intervention.

CpG DNA

Bacterial DNA has a higher content of the CpG dinucleotide than does vertebrate DNA, and, in contrast to vertebrate DNA, the CpG is not preferentially methylated. The unmethylated CpG DNA sequences provides a strong stimulus for the immune system. CpG DNA stimulates the secretion of IL-12 by macrophages and dendritic cells and thus provides a potent stimulus for type 1 immune responses. It also directly stimulates B cells to proliferate and differentiate into immunoglobulin secreting cells. A cellular receptor for CpG DNA has not been identified. The DNA appears to enter the cell via endocytosis, and some of the DNA escapes the endosomes into the cytoplasm of the cell where it activates various signaling pathways.

Applications for oligonucleotides containing unmethylated CpG sequences (CpG–ODN) are being explored in various areas of immunotherapy. Administration of CpG–ODN to mice protected against subsequent challenge with the intracellular bacteria *Listeria monocytogenes* and the intracellular protozoa *Leishmania major*. In addition, the CpG–ODN cured established *L. major* infections. The strong type 1 immunostimulatory property of CpG–ODN makes this compound a good candidate for vaccine adjuvants. Indeed, coadministration of CpG–ODN with antigen markedly boosts the humoral and cell-mediated immune responses. Allergic diseases such as asthma and atopic dermatitis are caused by type 2 immune responses directed against otherwise innocuous antigens. Treatment with CpG–ODN cleared established disease in a mouse model of airway hyper-reactivity, suggesting a CpG-induced reversal to type 1 immune responses. CpG DNA may also have a place in immunotherapy of cancer because of its ability to activate NK cells through the induction of IL-12. Administration of CpG–ODN in combination with monoclonal antibodies directed against tumor antigens greatly enhanced the survival of mice that had been inoculated with tumor cells.

Cytokines

Cytokines play a critical role in the regulation of the immune and inflammatory response, and they are potential targets for therapy. Important limitations, however, are the pleiotropy and redundancy in the cytokine system and the short half-life and short action range of most cytokines. In spite of these limitations, considerable effort is spent on developing reagents that either block or enhance the activity of a specific cytokine. Two remarkable successes of cytokine therapy are the treatment of multiple sclerosis with interferon-β and the treatment of rheumatoid arthritis and inflammatory bowel disease with tumor necrosis factor-α inhibitors.

Interferon-β

Clinical trials have demonstrated that subcutaneous injections of recombinant or natural interferon-β reduces the rate of exacerbation of relapsing-remitting multiple sclerosis. The mode of action of interferon-β has not been determined. Interferon-β reduces the production of tumor necrosis factor-α and increases the secretion of IL-10 in vitro. TNF-α is a proinflammatory cytokine that may contribute to demyelination in multiple sclerosis. IL-10 suppresses macrophage function and the production of TNF-α. In addition, interferon-β may reduce the entry of leukocytes into the central nervous system, a critical component in the inflammation that causes the lesions in multiple sclerosis.

Tumor necrosis factor-α inhibitors

Tumor necrosis factor-α (TNF-α) is a cytokine with multiple biological effects. It is produced as a transmembrane precursor molecule by various cells in the body. It is cleaved by the TNF-α-converting enzyme and forms trimeric aggregates that bind to either the TNF-receptor (TNFR) I or the TNFR II that are expressed on many different types of cells. The extracellular domains of the TNFR can be cleaved by enzymes and can inhibit TNF-α activity by preventing binding of TNF-α to cell-bound receptors. Recent studies have demonstrated that inhibition of TNF-α activity resulted in significant improvement of the clinical condition of many patients with rheumatoid arthritis and inflammatory bowel disease. These studies clearly demonstrate an important role of TNF-α in rheumatoid arthritis and inflammatory bowel disease, although the precise mechanisms remain to be determined. The inhibition of TNF-α activity is achieved by treatment with anti-TNF-α monoclonal antibodies or with soluble TNFR-fusion protein. To reduce the induction of antibodies against the mouse monoclonal antibodies, the monoclonal antibodies are chimeric (i.e., the constant portion is derived from human immunoglobulins and the TNF-α-specific variable portion is derived from mice) or humanized (all of the immunoglobulin is human except for the complementarity determining regions that fold into the TNF-α-binding region). The TNFR-fusion protein is constructed from the extracellular domain of TNFRII and the Fc portion of human immunoglobulins. This construct has a much longer half-life than does the naturally occurring soluble TNFR.

Challenges in Future Vaccine Formulations

Recent advancements in microbial pathogenesis, immunology, genetic engineering, plant genetics, and expression vector technology have formed the foundation for a new generation of vaccines and other pharmaceutical products. New developments in the delivery system have provided us with novel ways to enhance the immunogenicity of subunit antigens or nucleic acids by their controlled release and reduced degradation.

For more convenient and more effective immunization, current vaccine-delivery technologies need to be improved. Currently, vaccination of many inactivated or subunit antigens requires booster doses because of the lack of inherent immunogenicity found in the natural organism. Thus, reducing the number of doses is one of the primary goals in vaccination. Theoretically, various controlled-release technologies can be used to release antigens over time in a sustained or pulsatile manner and to direct antigens to specific antigen-presenting cells for increased vaccine efficacy. In addition to controlled-release technology, the single-shot vaccination requires development of better adjuvants. The mechanism of action of such adjuvants should be known so that reproducible results can be obtained in a mass vaccination program. The requirements and problems of immunizing immunocompromised, immature, older, or pregnant hosts need to be addressed effectively. Further improvement in our understanding of how to modulate Th1 and Th2 responses effectively would certainly help us design better vaccines. Another means of improvement is to combine a number of vaccines into multivalent vaccines. This will improve the immunization compliance in people living in developed or developing countries. Because the majority of pathogens enter their hosts via mucosal routes, the new-generation vaccines should have the advantage of providing effective protection at the mucosal sites. An ideal vaccine would be one that provides life-long protection with a single inoculation. The new-generation vaccine formulations should also have high stability, thus avoiding the problems commonly observed during storage.

8

THERAPEUTIC PROTEINS

Since the introduction of recombinant DNA techniques, it is possible to produce proteins on a large scale. These include proteins that are identical or nearly identical to endogenous human proteins, but also foreign proteins like streptokinase and asparaginase. Not only foreign proteins, but also recombinant human protein therapeutics are potentially immunogenic, and indeed most of these products induce antibodies in some patients after a certain period of treatment. Patients will first develop binding antibodies (BAbs), and this can be followed by the formation of neutralizing antibodies (NAbs). BAbs usually do not cause major complications, but NAbs bind to the active site of the protein and may interfere with the therapeutic effect. NAbs sometimes also cross-react with the endogenous protein, which can lead to serious complications.

Table 8.1. Examples of recombinant therapeutic proteins with reported immunogenicity

Type of Protein	*Protein*
Hormones	Insulin
	Growth hormone
Cytokines	Interferon alpha
	Interferon beta
	Interleukin 2, 3 and 12
Enzymes	Factor VIII
	DNase
	Tissue plasminogen activator
Antibodies	Anti-CD3 (murine antibody)
	Anti-Her2 (humanized antibody)
	Anti-IgE (humanized antibody)
	Anti-respiratory syncytial virus (humanized antibody)
	Anti-IL-2 receptor (humanized antibody)
Growth factors	G-CSF
	GM-CSF
	Erythropoietin
	Thrombopoietin

This chapter gives an overview of the current knowledge about the immunogenicity of therapeutic proteins. First the mechanisms by which antibodies are formed will be discussed, followed by the factors that can influence the immune response. An assay strategy for the detection of antibodies in human sera is discussed. The biological and clinical consequences are summarized, and the U.S. Food and Drug Administration (FDA) procedure to handle immunogenicity concerns of novel products is explained. Next, we give some examples of therapeutic proteins with immunogenicity problems, followed by the final conclusions.

Immune Mechanisms

Depending on the type of therapeutic protein, antibodies can be formed via two pathways: a classic immune response to foreign proteins and breaking of immune tolerance to self-proteins.

Classic Immune Response

A classic immune response occurs after administration of foreign proteins. Antigen-presenting cells (APCs) will take up the protein, digest it, and present peptides on major histocompatibility complex (MHC)-molecules on their surface. T cells will recognize these peptides in combination with the MHC-molecules and will activate B cells to produce antibodies against the foreign protein. This type of reaction is observed when proteins of animal, microbial, or plant origin are administered to patients. The antibody formation is usually fast, within days to weeks, and often occurs after a single injection. The antibodies are mostly NAbs and persist for a long time. A classic immune response can also occur on administration of recombinant human proteins to patients with an innate deficiency, e.g., children lacking growth hormone. These children lack the immune tolerance that normally exists for self-proteins.

Breaking of Immune Tolerance

Most recombinant human proteins are homologous to their endogenous counterparts. The immune system of the patients will therefore recognize the protein as a self-protein, for which the patient is tolerant. Antibody formation against self-proteins can occur through breaking of this immune tolerance. The antibody formation via this process is slow and often becomes apparent only after months of chronic administration of the protein to the patient. Usually the antibodies disappear when treatment is stopped. The exact mechanism of breaking of immune tolerance is not known. Multimeric antigen presentation with a narrow (~5–10 nm) spacing, however, is known to break immune tolerance, possibly by cross-linking of B-cell receptors. The only natural proteins showing this closely spaced multimeric antigen presentation are microbial antigens, and apparently during evolution, there was a strong selective pressure to react vigorously to this type of antigen presentation.

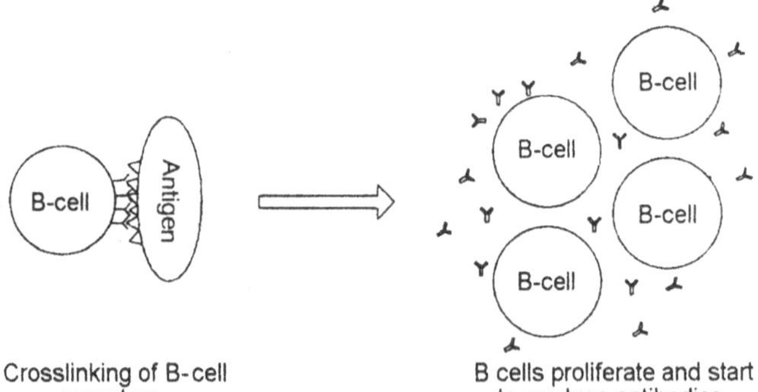

Fig. 8.1. Schematic representation of a possible mechanism of breaking B-cell tolerance.

Factors Influencing Immunogenicity

Many factors influence the immune response induced by therapeutic proteins. These can be divided into product, patient, and treatment characteristics, and several factors are still unknown.

Product Characteristics

Proteins are complex structures consisting of primary, secondary, tertiary, and sometimes quaternary structures. Changes in one of these structural levels might influence the immune response. How a protein is formulated influences the chemical and physical stability of the protein. Therefore the formulation can also influence the immunogenicity. Moreover, contaminants and impurities play an important role.

Primary sequence

Based on amino acid sequence, no definite predictions about the immunogenicity of a product can be made. A single amino acid change in insulin was enough to elicit a strong immune response. Consensus interferon alpha (co-IFNα), on the other hand, has several amino acid changes as compared with the naturally occurring human IFNαs (10–23 amino acid differences and on average 89% homology with naturally occurring IFNαs), but it has no increased immunogenicity. Foreign proteins, such as streptokinase, staphylokinase, bovine adenosine deaminase, and salmon calcitonin will elicit a classic immune response in patients.

Chemical changes of the primary structure, such as oxidation or deamidation of amino acids, can lead to novel epitopes, which can induce a classic immune response. Moreover, the chemical change can induce aggregation leading to multimeric antigen presentation and, thus, breaking of immune tolerance.

Glycosylation

Glycosylation is a common posttranslational modification and is cell and species specific. The glycans can differ in chain length, sequence, and linkage position to the peptide backbone. Endogenous proteins often consist of several glycosylated isoforms. The carbohydrates can play a role in molecular stability, *in vivo* activity, serum half-life, and immunogenicity. Carbohydrates can decrease the immunogenicity of therapeutic proteins, by shielding immunogenic epitopes or by increasing the solubility of the protein and thereby preventing aggregation.

Production of therapeutic proteins in plants is being developed, but concerns are raised about the immunogenicity of plant glycans. Glycosylation of proteins in plants and humans differ in fine detail. Especially the plant-specific α(1,3)-fucose and β(1,2)-xylose groups are considered immunogenic in humans. Metabolic engineering of the plant N-glycan biosynthesis pathway is being pursued to prevent the insertion of these sugars in the glycan chains.

PEGylation

The most successful approach to increase the mean plasma half-life of proteins is by chemically coupling poly(ethylene glycol) (PEG) moieties to the protein. The attachment of PEG (PEGylation) decreases the overall rate of clearance of the protein, shields the protein from proteolytic enzymes, and masks immunogenic sites. The PEG molecules can differ in conjugation type, molecular weight, and conformation (i.e., linear, branched, or multiple-branched). PEGylation can decrease the immunogenicity of a therapeutic protein by blocking antibody binding sites, promoting solubility, and permitting less frequent dosing. Branched PEG is more effective than linear PEG in improving the immunological properties of the protein. Although in most cases PEGylation decreases the immunogenicity of a therapeutic protein, two examples of therapeutic proteins are known in which the PEGylated protein was more immunogenic than the non-PEGylated variant: PEGylated recombinant human megakaryocyte growth and development factor (PEG-rhMGDF) and recombinant methionyl human tumor necrosis factor binding protein PEGylated dimer. The reason for this increased immunogenicity is not known, but it might be related to the increased plasma half-lives, which leads to prolonged exposure to the immune system.

Impurities and contaminants

Recombinant proteins can be produced in different expression systems, each having advantages and disadvantages. Impurities from the expression systems can be of influence on the immunogenicity of the final product. They can act as adjuvants or be immunogenic themselves. Patients receiving *Escherichia coli*-derived granulocyte-macrophage colony-stimulating factor (GM-CSF) were shown to develop antibodies to GM-CSF as well as *E. coli* proteins.

Secondary structure

Many studies have shown the importance of aggregation in inducing and/or increasing an immune response. Aggregation usually occurs after partial unfolding of the protein due to, e.g., shear/shaking or high temperature. Aggregation may expose new epitopes on the surface of the protein for which the immune system is not tolerant. This will lead to a classic immune response. Aggregation can also lead to multimeric antigen presentation, which is known to break B-cell tolerance. Therefore, assessing the presence of aggregates in protein formulations is considered to be very important, although not all aggregates will induce an immune response as was shown in our laboratory.

Patient Characteristics

Patient characteristics, such as genetic background and the disease status, are known to influence rate and type of immune reactions. Hemophilia patients with severe genetic defects are more prone to antibody formation than patients with minor genetic defects. Eprex associated pure red cell aplasia (PRCA) was only observed in patients with renal failure and not in cancer patients.

Treatment Characteristics

Also the treatment characteristics can have an influence on the immuno genicity of therapeutic proteins. Usually antibodies are only induced after prolonged treatment of the protein. The intramuscular (i.m.) route of administration is less immunogenic than subcutaneous (s.c.) administration. Intravenous (i.v.) administration usually is the least immunogenic route of administration.

Other Factors

When evaluating the immunogenicity of therapeutic proteins, one also has to consider the immunomodulatory effects of the protein. For instance, IFNα may increase the antibody production because of its innate immunomodulatory effects. The timing of blood sampling may influence the amount of antibody present in the sera. If a blood sample is taken too early after the administration of the protein, antibodies can still be complexed to the antigen and the sample may prove to be false-negative. If the sample is taken too long after the last injection, antibodies may already have disappeared.

Detection

Detection of antibodies can be done by several methods. As there are no standardized assays for antibodies to most products and laboratories mostly use their own in-house methods, comparison of results from different studies is in principle impossible. Ideally, a combination of standardized assays should be performed to ensure that all possible types (low affinity and high affinity, classes and isotypes, binding and neutralizing) of antibodies are detected.

Assays

Antibody assays can be divided into two main categories: binding assays and bioassays. The binding assays detect in principle any antibodies with sufficient affinity for the therapeutic protein. A bioassay tests whether the antibodies detected by the binding assay can neutralize the biological effects of the therapeutic protein. In most cases, BAbs have no clinical effect, but the binding assay is used as a screening tool to identify samples with possible neutralizing activity.

Binding assays

Several binding assays are available that can detect antibodies against therapeutic proteins, with solid phase binding assays being the most commonly used for antibody detection. The advantage of surface plasmon resonance over the other methods is the possibility to measure the binding of the antibodies in real time, which gives information about the affinity of the antibodies. A Western blot gives information about the specificity of the antibodies in the serum and may show antibodies to impurities as was shown in patients receiving GM-CSF.

Neutralizing assays

The detection of neutralizing antibodies is performed in assays that can show inhibition of the biological activity of the therapeutic protein. In general this will be a bioassay. The therapeutic protein is incubated with the serum to be tested, and the mixture is tested in the bioassay. If the antibodies in the serum have neutralizing capacities, the biological activity of the mixture is reduced, as compared with the pure therapeutic protein.

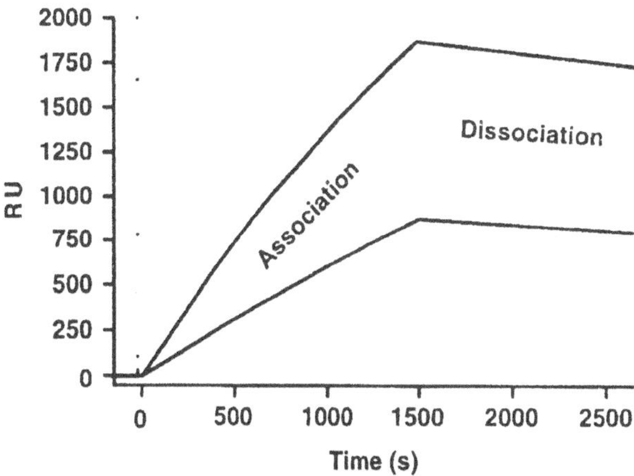

Fig. 8.2. Sensorgram obtained with BIAcore 3000 using anti-rhIFNα2b sera with different association and dissociation profiles.

Design of an Assay Strategy

Long-term studies are needed to fully assess the immunogenicity of a product. Also, the timing of sampling is important. A pretreatment blood sample should be taken, and several time points should be considered because antibodies may be induced only after prolonged treatment. If a sample is taken too early after administration of the therapeutic protein, the circulating protein may interfere with the antibody assay. Conversely, if the sampling is too long after the last administration of the protein, antibody levels might already have dropped below the detection limit of the assays. Both situations will lead to an underestimation of the incidence of antibody positive patients.

To fully assess the immunogenicity of a therapeutic protein, a combination of assays is necessary. In general, sera are screened first by an enzyme-linked immunosorbent assay (ELISA) or radioimmunoassay (RIA) type of binding assay, which have a high through-put and are easy to perform. A screening assay is optimized for sensitivity and therefore suffers from a relative high number of false-positive results. So, all initial positive sera should be confirmed, e.g., by showing a reduced binding after adding the product to the serum. The confirmed positive sera are then tested for neutralizing activity. Further characterization of the antibody response may follow to determine isotype, affinity, and so on. Whatever approach is used, it is important to validate the assays to show reproducibility, precision, robustness, and so on. International reference preparations are only available for a limited number of assays, but they are crucial for making comparison between different laboratories possible.

Predictive Models

Most of the data about immunogenicity of therapeutic proteins come from clinical trials or postmarketing surveillance. It would of course be better if the immunogenicity of a product could be predicted before the clinical phase of development.

Conventional animals

Conventional animal models may be useful to predict the immunogenicity of microbial products as staphylokinase and streptokinase, which are foreign proteins for humans as well as animals. Conventional animals can also be used if the therapeutic protein shows a high degree of intraspecies sequence homology. An example is human thrombopoietin, which induced neutralizing antibodies in animal models as well as in patients. However, most recombinant human therapeutic proteins are foreign proteins for animals that will elicit an immune response in all cases. So their predictive value for the immunogenicity of human proteins in humans is low. Nonhuman primates that share a higher level of sequence homology with humans have been shown to be excellent models for some products such as human growth hormone and lys-pro insulin, but for other proteins, their predictive value has shown to be limited.

Immune tolerant animals

In most cases, the induction of antibodies to human therapeutic proteins in patients is based on breaking B-cell tolerance. This process makes animals tolerant for the protein the best model for predicting immunogenicity in humans. Mice are the species of choice to induce tolerance, which can be achieved by chronic administration of the protein in large quantities or by making the animals transgenic for the gene expressing the protein. Obvious drawbacks of the first method are the large quantities of protein required and the need for testing the tolerance of each animal. Mouse lines expressing the transgene only need to be evaluated for immune tolerance once and only need testing by polymerase chain reaction (PCR) to identify transgene positivity after breeding. Transgenic animals, immune tolerant for insulin, tissue plasminogen activator (tPA), IFNα2, and IFNβ are available. The insulin and tPA models were used to evaluate whether amino acid substitutions in the protein introduced new epitopes. The interferon models were used to study the effect of aggregates and other degradation products on immunogenicity.

Some therapeutic proteins might have immune modulatory effects that influence the induction of antibodies. If the human protein lacks this effect in mice, their predictive value may suffer. This deficiency can be prevented by challenging both the human as well as the murine homologue. Braun et al. showed that mixtures of murine and human IFNα2a caused an increase in immune response in wild-type mice to the human protein. Another point of consideration when using transgenic mice as predictors for immunogenicity is the difference between mouse and human MHC and their presentation of T-cell epitopes. Also, important individual patient characteristics, such as disease burden and concomitant therapy influencing the antibody response, are difficult to reproduce in the transgenic immune-tolerant animal model. Although these models will never become predictors of the individual patient's antibody response, they will be very useful in the development phase of a new protein therapy or after a formulation or production change. The transgenic immune-tolerant mice can also be used to study the mechanism of antibody induction, because they share tolerance for the protein with patients.

Prediction on Basis of Structure and Sequence

Other strategies, based on structural analysis, have been described to predict the immunogenicity of therapeutic proteins. Immunogenic epitopes can be predicted based on amino acid sequence analysis and MHC-binding. Modifications in an immunodominant T-cell epitope by a single amino acid was reported to reduce the immunogenicity of rhIFNβ-1b in BALB/cByJ mice. Analysis of B-cell epitopes is more difficult, but it is also ongoing. These types of analyses may help to reduce the immunogenicity, in case the product is a foreign protein inducing a classic immune response. As discussed, in most of cases, the induction of antibodies in patients is based on breaking B-cell tolerance. Although the exact mechanism is still unknown, we know that the product quality, independent of the amino acid sequence, plays an important role.

Biological and Clinical Consequences

The clinical effects of antibody formation vary from no effect to severe life-threatening situations. Binding antibodies can alter the pharmacokinetic properties of the therapeutic protein. Neutralizing antibodies cannot only affect the pharmacokinetics but also block the pharmacological effect of the therapeutic protein. Severe side effects occur if NAbs cross-react with an endogenous protein, as was observed for PEG–rhMGDF and recombinant human erythropoietin (epoetin). Patients receiving PEG–rhMGDF developed NAbs cross-reacting with endogenous thrombopoietin, which resulted in a severe thrombocytopenia. Patients receiving Eprex (an epoetin formulation marketed in Europe, Canada, and Australia) developed NAbs that cross-reacted with endogenous erythropoietin, resulting in PRCA. The number of patients with antibody-mediated PRCA rapidly increased after a formulation change of Eprex, as will be discussed below. Besides the formation of antibodies, allergic reactions can occur.

Risk-based Approach of Imunogenicity

The FDA evaluates immunogenicity concerns of novel products in development and for major changes in manufacturing or clinical uses via a risk-based approach. Three elements are considered important for the risk assessment strategy: the severity of consequences of the immune response to a therapeutic protein, host-specific factors that impact the immunogenicity positively or negatively, and product-specific factors that impact the immunogenicity positively or negatively. Based on their expertise and literature data from marketed products, the FDA decides whether immunogenicity testing should be performed before or during clinical trials.

Epoetin: How a Formulation Change Increased the Immunogenicity

Erythropoietin is a protein produced by the kidneys that stimulates the production of erythrocytes. Epoetin is mainly used in patients suffering from anemia associated with chronic renal failure or cancer. Three forms of epoetin are commercially available, epoetin alfa, epoetin beta, and darbepoetin alfa, which is a hyperglycosylated analog. In 1997 the first patient with antibody-mediated PRCA was reported. Antibody-mediated PRCA is caused by antibodies induced by exogenous epoetin that cross-react with endogenous erythropoietin. In 2002, 13 patients were reported that had developed antibody-mediated PRCA, after administration of Eprex. These cases occurred after 1998. Since then, more patients with antibody-mediated PRCA were identified. In 1998 the formulation of Eprex was changed: Human serum albumin (HSA) was replaced by glycine and polysorbate 80. Several hypotheses have been postulated to explain the increase in PRCA cases.

Hermeling et al. hypothesized that some epoetin molecules were solubilized in micelles, which might have led to multimeric antigen presentation. Others claim that the polysorbate 80 extracted leachates out of the uncoated rubber stoppers, which had an adjuvant effect, leading to an increase in antibodies. An adjuvant, however, can only increase an existing immune response and cannot break B-cell tolerance by itself. It will be very diffcult to pinpoint the exact cause of the increased number of PRCA cases. In 2002, actions were taken to decrease the number of PRCA cases: emphasizing strict adherence to storage and handling conditions, the introduction of a contraindication for s.c. administration of Eprex in chronic renal failure in many countries and the introduction of coated rubber stoppers. These actions decreased the number of patients with antibody-mediated PRCA, but the question remains of what exactly caused the increased immunogenicity.

RhIFNβ: Immunogenicity of Glycosylated and Nonglycosylated Variants

Interferon beta is a cytokine with anti-inflammatory, antitumor, antiviral, and cell-growth-regulatory effects. It is mainly produced by macrophages and epithelial and fibroblast cells. Administration of rhIFNβ has been established as a treatment for relapsing-remitting multiple sclerosis. Natural hIFNβ is glycosylated, contains 166 amino acids, and has a molecular weight of approximately 25 kDa. Three forms of rhIFNβ are available on the market. RhIFNβ-1a (Rebif and Avonex) has an amino acid sequence similar to that of endogenous hIFNβ, is produced in Chinese hamster cells, and is glycosylated. RhIFNβ-1b (Betaseron) is produced in *E. coli* and thus not glycosylated. Moreover, Cys-17 has been mutated to Ser-17 and the N-terminal methionine is lacking.

All three formulations induce neutralizing antibodies of the IgG-type, reducing the efficacy of the therapy. The antibodies are usually detectable after the first 6 to 12 months of the treatment, but the clinical effects do not appear until after 18–24 months after the start of the treatment. RhIFNβ-1b induces antibodies in more patients than does rhIFNβ-1a. This increased incidence of immunogenicity of rhIFNβ-1b as compared with rhIFNβ-1a is probably due to the lack of glycosylation, which makes the protein more prone to aggregation. Size-exclusion chromatography showed that 60% of rhIFNβ-1b in Betaseron is heavily aggregated. It was shown that Betaseron can break the tolerance of transgenic immune tolerant mice, which suggests that these animals may be predictive for the immunogenicity observed in patients.

RhIFNα2: Reduction of the Immunogenicity by Optimizing Production and Formulation

RhIFNα2 is used for the treatment of a variety of malignancies and viral diseases. It inhibits viral replication, increases class I MHC expression, stimulates Th1 cells, and inhibits proliferation of many cell types. Two regular and two PEGylated forms of rhIFNα2 are on the market. The PEGylated forms are less immunogenic than the non-PEGylated forms. RhIFNα2a and rhIFNα2b only differ in 1 amino acid. RhIFNα2b is produced in *E. coli* cells, which implies that the protein is nonglycosylated. Natural hIFNα2 is O-glycosylated. Patients receiving rhIFNα2a initially produced higher levels of antibodies and at higher incidences than rhIFNα2b. This difference was shown not to be related to the difference in amino acid sequence. The antibodies induced by rhIFNα2a fully cross-react with rhIFNα2b and vice versa. Co-IFNα is a non-naturally occurring synthetic recombinant type I interferon. Its amino acid sequence (166 amino acids) is created by taking for each position the amino acid most commonly observed in 13 IFNα subtypes. Despite the nonsimilarity of co-IFNα with human IFNα species (10–23 amino acid differences and on average 89% homology with naturally occurring IFNαs), the number of patients producing antibodies against co-IFNα is similar to the number of patients producing antibodies after rhIFNα2b treatment.

Storing the formulation at room temperature leads to oxidation and increases the immunogenicity of a rhIFNα2a formulation. Better purification methods further reduce the immunogenicity. Recently it has been shown that not all aggregates, but only aggregates of rhIFNα2b with a native-like structure, can elicit an immune response in transgenic mice immune tolerant for hIFNα2. It was also shown that not the oxidation, but the aggregation, accompanying the oxidation was the reason for the immunogenicity.

Many factors influence the immune response against therapeutic proteins. Unfortunately, it is still impossible to fully predict the immunogenicity of a therapeutic protein before going into clinical trials. The presence of (native-like) aggregates in a formulation is one main factor known to increase the immune response. Formulation changes might have an effect on the immunogenicity as was observed for epoetin and rhIFNα2a. The effect of a for mulation change is also difficult to predict, but it can be evaluated in immune-tolerant transgenic mice. Although these tests will not fully predict the immunogenicity of a product, it can give information about the immunogenicity of a new formulation/product as compared with previous formulations/products. As most therapeutic proteins only induce antibodies in a small number of patients, postmarketing surveillance is important. Also basic studies to link physical–chemical properties with immunogenicity are important, and these studies may avoid animal testing in the future.

9

FLAVORS AND FLAVOR MODIFIERS

The use of flavors and flavor modifiers to improve the taste and aroma of foods and pharmaceuticals is an art that dates back several centuries. In large measure, the practice is still the same today and, except for the advent of new semisynthetic flavoring agents with improved stability, the field has remained relatively unchanged. In the analytical arena, the story is different. Sophisticated instrumentation methods have been developed to characterize, purify, and manufacture flavoring agents that are similar, in many respects, to those occurring in nature. The technology continues to evolve at an accelerated pace, resulting in several stable, potent, and unique flavors, which are now available to target both foods and pharmaceuticals. This article discusses flavors and flavoring agents typically used in industry and highlights formulation variables that could affect the performance of flavors in finished products. Where necessary, pertinent literature for further reading is cited.

DEFINITION OF FLAVOR

Flavor is the complex effect of three components: taste, odor, and feeling factors. It is usually associated with the pleasure of savoring food or beverages and has, subsequently, suffered from considerable imprecision in definition. Flavor is a sensation with multidimensional components involving subjective and objective perceptions. The sensory perceptions are both qualitative as well as quantitative and, therefore, can be measured. Webster's New Collegiate Dictionary defines flavor as the"... quality of something that affects the sense of taste, ... the blend of taste and smell sensations evoked by a substance in the mouth." This definition is correct, but incomplete, and should be redefined to include feeling factors.

Taste

Taste consists of four primary sensations: sweet, sour, bitter, and salty. Correspondingly, there are four different kinds of taste buds. These sensations are elicited by the tongue and interpreted by the brain. Certain areas of the tongue respond more readily to specific tastes than others. Sweet sensations are most easily detected at the tip of the tongue, whereas bitter ones are most readily detected at the back of the tongue. Sour sensations occur at the sides of the tongue, but salty sensations are usually detected at both the tip and at the sides of the tongue. During ingestion, taste buds react to soluble substances. The resulting sensations are transmitted to the brain by the ninth cranial (glossopharyngeal) nerve. The tenth and twelfth cranial nerves participate in this sensory reaction, but their role is limited.

Odor

The odor component of flavor is due to conscious or subconscious reactions to volatile substances, without which most foods would be lacking in taste appeal. By closing the nostrils while eating a mouthful of some flavored substance and immediately following this with another mouthful with the nostrils open, it may be shown that food could be rendered tasteless, as is often experienced by people suffering from the effects of a head cold.

There are many varieties of odorants, but a universally accepted structure–activity relationship of these has not been established. Yet, there is evidence that odor may involve specific receptor interactions, suggesting that structural properties of odorants may be important in eliciting specific odor sensations.

Feeling Factors

"Mouth feel" factors are critical in flavor perception. Examples include astringency, pepper bite, menthol cooling, and texture (e.g., softness or hardness as in candy). Sensations, such as crunch after biting into a crisp stick of celery or an apple, contribute to the overall flavor of foods. These mouth feel factors are also important in improving the organoleptic qualities of pharmaceuticals.

Flavoring Agents

Flavoring agents may be classified as natural, artificial, or natural and artificial (N&A) by combining the all- natural and synthetic flavors. Pharmaceutical flavors are available as liquids (e.g., essential oils, fluid extracts, tinctures, and distillates), solids (e.g., spray- dried, crystalline vanillin, freeze-dried cinnamon powders, and dried lemon fluid extract), and pastes (e.g., soft extracts, resins, and so-called concretes, which are brittle on the outside and soft on the inside). Liquid flavors are by far the most widely used because they diffuse readily into the substrate. They are available both as oily (e.g., essential oils) or non-oily liquids. Their texture is generally dependent on the solvent within which they are prepared. Fluid extracts may contain a single ingredient or a variety of compounded ingredients. Tinctures are obtained by maceration or percolation of specific herbs and spices in alcohol.

Essential oils boil at elevated temperatures, but many cannot be directly distilled without decomposition. Vacuum, steam, and fractional or molecular distillation are often used for their manufacture. Fractional distillation removes traces of water, resinous materials, colors, terpenes, and sesquiterpenes from the distillate. This process improves solubility and enhances flavor intensity. Sesquiterpeneless oils are more soluble than terpeneless oils because of the removal of head and tail fractions (e.g., waxy residues). Most common sesquiterpeneless oils used in the pharmaceutical industry include oil of orange and oil of lemon. Oils and juices are obtained from plant sources by expression. Citrus essential oils are almost exclusively obtained by this method. Thoroughly washed unripe citrus fruits are cold pressed manually, or mechanically, to rupture oil cells in the rind. The oil is collected by draining and centrifuging. Manual operation is labor intensive and has been replaced by machines.

Natural Flavoring Agents

Natural ingredients have been used since antiquity to flavor foods and to make early "*medicines*" palatable. Honey was and remains a sweetener and flavoring agent. Wine was used as a crude infusorial in medicinal herbs. Modern use of natural flavors in pharmaceuticals is limited, because they are often unstable and their quality is unpredictable from season to season. The most commonly used natural flavors are terpeneless citrus oils, which are stable if well protected from light and air. A variety of other natural flavors are used in the food and pharmaceutical industries.

Anise (*Pimpinella anisum*, Umbelliferae)

Anise is a herbaceous annual cultivated extensively in Europe. The essential oil is obtained by steam distillation of dried fruits (seeds). The distillate is a clear-to-pale yellowish oil. It solidifies at low temperatures and has a characteristic sweet licorice-like odor and flavor. Its main constituents include anethol (approximately 90%), methylchavicol, *p*-methoxyphenylacetone, and acetic aldehyde. Anise oil is used frequently at concentrations of up to approximately 3000 ppm in liquid preparations.

Cardamon (*Elettaria cardamomum*, Zingiberaceae)

Cardamon is cultivated in India and Sri Lanka. The essential oil is obtained by steam distillation of comminuted seeds to yield a greenish-yellow liquid with a warm, spicy, aromatic odor and flavor. The main constituents of the oil are limonene, cineol, D-α-terpineol, and terpinyl acetate. Cardamon is generally used at concentrations of approximately 5–50 ppm.

Wild Cherry (*Prunus serotina*, Rosaceae)

Wild cherry is a large tree, native to southern Canada. It is widespread in the United States and Europe. The bark, small branches, and twigs are used to prepare the fluid extract and tincture. The main constituent of wild cherry extract is the glucoside prunasin, which on enzymatic hydrolysis yields prussic acid, glucose, and benzaldehyde. Also present are coumarin, phytosterols, benzoic acid, and fatty acids (e.g., oleic, linoleic, and palmitic acids). It has a characteristic sweet, tart, cherry-like flavor. Wild cherry bark extract is commonly used at concentrations of approximately 50–800 ppm in foods and pharmaceuticals.

Lemon (*Citrus limonum*, Rutaceae)

Lemon is an evergreen shrub or tree native to the Far East; it was introduced to the Mediterranean regions at the time of the Crusades. The leaves, fruits, and rind are used either whole or pressed in foods and in liquid or solid pharmaceutical products. The essential oil of lemon is obtained by cold expression. Approximately 40 constituents have been identified, with 90% being limonene. Fluid extracts and tinctures are obtained from the dried peel. Lemon petitgrain is obtained by steam distillation of the leaves. For flavoring, it must be terpeneless. The main constituents are D-α-pinene, camphene, D-limonene, dipentene, L-linalol, nerol, and citral. Lemon petitgrain oil is used in a wide variety of applications. Typical concentrations range from 1 to 35 ppm. The essential oil and extract of lemon are generally used at higher concentrations that may range up to 1000 and 10,000 ppm, respectively. All lemon oil derivatives have the characteristic lemon odor and a slightly bitter flavor.

Orange, Bitter (*Citrus aurantium*, Rutaceae)

Bitter orange is a tall tropical tree that can grow up to approximately 10 m (33 ft.) high. The tree is native to the Far East and is cultivated extensively throughout the Mediterranean, Guinea, the West Indies, West Africa, and Brazil. The leaves and twigs produce essential petitgrain oil following steam distillation. *Neroli bigarade* essential oil is produced from the blossoms by steam distillation. The peel is expressed and steam distilled to produce essential oil of orange. The main constituent of orange oil is D-limonene, with various acids, aldehydes, and diesters. Essential oil of orange is widely used in foods and pharmaceuticals at concentrations of up to 500 ppm.

Orange, Sweet (*Citrus sinensis*, var. *aurantium dulcis*, Rutaceae)

Sweet orange is an evergreen tree that grows to approximately 6 m (20 ft.) high. It is generally of oriental origin and is cultivated extensively in the Mediterranean, Florida, and California. A petitgrain oil is obtained from the leaves and twigs, but its production is low because of limited use, primarily in the perfumery industry. Essential oil of sweet orange is obtained by expression. Its physical-chemical properties (e.g., specific gravity, optical rotation, and refractive index) vary according to origin. The oil contains more than 90% limonene, in addition to relatively high quantities of decylic, octylic, nonylic, and dodecylic aldehydes, and citral esters. It has a characteristic odor and a mildly bitter, astringent flavor; it is generally used at concentrations of up to 500 ppm.

Peppermint (*Mentha piperita*, Labiatae)

Peppermint is a herbaceous plant that grows to approximately 81 cm (32 in.) high. The essential oil is obtained by steam distillation of the flowering plant tops. It is cultivated in Europe, North and

South America, and Japan. The main constituents of the essential oil are α- and β-pinene, limonene, cineol, ethyl amylcarbinol, menthone, menthol, isomenthol, menthyl acetate, and piperitone. It has a strong mint odor with a sweet balsam taste masked by a strong cooling effect. It is widely used in foods, as well as in liquid pharmaceuticals, to 8000 ppm.

Artificial Flavoring Agents

Unlike natural flavoring agents, synthetic flavors are usually stable. The development of synthetic flavors paralleled the development of instrumental analysis, in which active ingredients in natural flavors are identified and reconstructed synthetically with reasonable accuracy. Exact duplication of a natural flavor is, however, difficult because often minor components are the most important contributors to the overall flavor profile. These minor components are not easily identified. For example, the major components of vanilla are vanillin and ethyl vanillin. However, the flavor nuances of the vanilla bean have never been successfully matched in artificial (synthetic) vanilla.

Natural and Artificial (N&A) Agents

In N&A flavor systems, natural flavors are combined with synthetic ingredients to enhance flavor balance and fullness. These flavors are generally classified according to type and taste sensation. Table 1 contains a list of N&A flavor components that elicit various sensory properties, all of which are commonly used in food and drug compounding. It is not an exhaustive list because manufacturers regard their flavor formularies as proprietary. Many N&A flavors may be chemically and structurally similar, but vary significantly in taste and aroma. Similar flavors from various vendors might vary significantly in composition. Of interest is the fact that a relatively small change in chain length can have a profound impact on flavor type. Minor changes, such as the conversion of allyl benzoate to cyclohexyl esters (e.g., a caproate or valerate), transform a basic cherry flavor to peach or pineapple.

In situ conversion of essential N&A flavor components from one molecular form to another, as a result of ion pairing, is common in food and drug products. Therefore, the inadvertent conversion of flavors between types during drug formulation studies (e.g., effect of pH, salts, and temperature) can present a serious challenge in flavor-quality assessment.

The fact that one and the same N&A flavor component can deliver several flavor and odor impressions implies that a blend of several flavor compounds would be preferable. Such blends show improved stability. In addition, flavor impressions from N&A flavor blends are usually not dominated by a single component. For these reasons, single natural and artificial flavor ingredients are seldom, if ever, used alone in a finished product. There has been a steady rise in the use of N&A flavors, in addition to their superior performance, when compared to natural flavors. Also, the quality and uniformity of the N&A flavor is greater than that of natural flavors, and lower concentrations of N&A flavors are often used to achieve the same effect as obtained with natural flavors. Table 4 shows a typical formulation of a commercial N&A strawberry flavor. It contains a small proportion of natural flavors; the bulk of the ingredients are synthetic.

Another advantage of N&A flavors is the broad spectrum of flavoring agents from which the formulator can develop an entirely new flavor system that is unique, not available naturally. A flavor extensively used in foods and pharmaceutical products is tuttifrutti—bubble gum.

In summary, there are a variety of flavor types: natural, synthetic, and semisynthetic. Appropriate use concentrations depend on many factors, including product characteristics, such as composition, physical state, shelf life, pH, processing temperature, storage conditions, and reactivity of components. Flavor concentrations also depend on the market sector for which the product is targeted. The age of the user and the mode of use are two examples of user-dependent variables that have significant bearing on the type, concentration, and nature of the flavor selected for product development.

FLAVOR SELECTION IN PHARMACEUTICAL PREPARATIONS

A number of criteria are used to select flavors during formulation. Different flavor concentrations produce highly subjective sensations. Specific requirements for balance and fullness are dependent, in part, on the drug substance and the physical form of the product. For this reason, when selecting a flavor system, the compounding pharmacist must take into account several variables upon which a desired response would depend. Some of these are product texture (e.g., viscosity of formulation, solid or liquid), water content, base vehicle or substrate, and taste of the subject drug. Notable specific examples to consider are:

1. Immediate flavor identity from the formulation as it is ingested.
2. Compatible mouth feel factors and rapid development of a fully blended flavor in the mouth during ingestion of the product.
3. Absence of "off" notes in the mouth and a mild transient aftertaste during ingestion of the product.

The selection of a flavor system, thus, requires an extensive evaluation of a number of organoleptic qualities. Vehicle components within which the drug is presented have a significant bearing on the performance of the flavor system. Of these, the sweetener is perhaps the most relevant.

Sweeteners

The most commonly used sweeteners are sucrose, glucose, fructose, sorbitol, and glycerin. Sweetness intensity changes with concentration. It has been estimated that the sweetness of glucose relative to cane sugar is 53 at a concentration of 8% but increases to 88 at a concentration of 35%. Sweetener intensity increases with concentration but reaches a maximum where feeling factors become more prominent. Sugar (sucrose), at a concentration of 30%, is intensely sweet. Yet, its sweet intensity at concentrations 50% or higher is not perceptibly different, although distinct mouthfeel characteristics (e.g., syrupy, salivation) become pronounced. This is due to osmotic effects on mucous membranes within the oral cavity.

Glycerin, glucose, sorbitol, and sucrose have limited use in solid dosage forms (e.g., tablets) because the materials are hygroscopic. Mannitol is used more often in tablet manufacture. Besides being less hygroscopic, it has a negative heat of solution. For this reason, chewable tablets containing mannitol have a pleasant cooling sweet taste, which complements flavor quality. The artificial sweetener saccharin is widely used in foods and pharmaceuticals. It is approximately 350 × as sweet as sugar. It is sweet at very low concentrations (equivalent to about 5–10% sugar) but bitter at higher concentrations. Approximately 20% of the population are "*saccharin sensitive*;" that is, they perceive saccharin to be bitter even at low concentrations.

Upon repeated tasting, saccharin becomes less sweet and increasingly bitter. By the third or fourth tasting, solutions of relatively low concentrations are often no longer sweet to the saccharin-sensitive person. The artificial sweeteners, cyclamate and aspartame, are about 30 × as sweet as sugar, but like saccharin, their sweet–bitter profiles are concentration dependent. Aspartame does not have a significant bitter aftertaste when compared to saccharin and has gained in popularity. Cyclamates were banned in the 1970s because of carcinogenic concerns, which have, subsequently, been shown to be overstated.

Monoammonium glycyrrhizinate has a lingering sweet aftertaste, which can be exploited for taste-masking products with a mildly bitter aftertaste. It is also effective in enhancing chocolate flavor. Glycerin is commonly used for its solvent effect on many compounds, as well as its humectant effect. Sugar syrups promote significant "*cap-locking*"—the crystallization of the sugar on the cap and bottle thread, but the addition of glycerin (10–20%) minimizes this effect. Glycerin is seldom used as a single sweetener in pharmaceuticals because it has a characteristic mouth-warming and burning effect.

Flavor Enhancers and Potentiators

Flavor enhancers are used universally in the food and pharmaceutical industries. Sugar, carboxylic acids (e.g., citric, malic, and tartaric), common salt (NaCl), amino acids, some amino acid derivatives (e.g., mono-sodium glutamate—MSG), and spices (e.g., peppers) are most often employed. Although extremely effective with proteins and vegetables, MSG has limited use in pharmaceuticals because it is not a sweetener. Citric acid is most frequently used to enhance taste performance of both liquid and solid pharmaceutical products, as well as a variety of foods. Other acidic agents, such as malic and tartaric acids, are also used for flavor enhancement. In oral liquids, these acids contribute unique and complex organoleptic effects, increasing overall flavor quality. Common salt provides similar effects at its taste threshold level in liquid pharmaceuticals. Vanilla, for example, has a delicate bland flavor, which is effectively enhanced by salt.

Taste-Masking Agents

The flavoring industry has many proprietary products purported to have excellent taste-masking properties, which have been used with some success. Yet, there are a number of natural and artificial flavors that can be generally described to possess similar taste-masking effects.

Of the many tastes that must be masked in pharmaceuticals, bitterness is most often encountered; to mask it completely is difficult. A tropical fruit has been used for centuries in central Africa to mask the bitter taste of native beers. This so-called "*miracle berry*" contains a glycoprotein that transiently and selectively binds to bitter taste buds. Due to stability challenges, attempts to isolate the compound for commercial exploitation have been unsuccessful. Yet, many fruit syrups are relatively stable in pharmaceuticals if formulated with antimicrobial preservative agents. Syrups of cinnamon, orange, citric acid, cherry, cocoa, wild cherry, raspberry, or glycyrrhiza elixir can be used to effectively mask salty and bitter tastes in a number of drug products. The extent to which taste-masking may be achieved is not usually predictable due to complex interactions of other flavor elements in these products. The degree to which bitterness may be masked by these agents ranks in a descending order: cocoa syrup is most effective, followed by raspberry syrup, cherry, cinnamon, compound sarsaparilla, citric acid, licorice, aromatic elixir, orange, and wild cherry.

Sour and metallic tastes in pharmaceuticals also can be reasonably masked. Sour substances containing hydrochloric acid are most effectively neutralized with raspberry and other fruit syrups. Metallic tastes in oral liquid products (e.g., iron) are usually masked by extracts of gurana, a tropical fruit. Gurana flavor is used at concentrations ranging from 0.001 to about 0.5% and may be useful in solid products as well (e.g., chewable tablets and granules).

Flavor Modification Technologies

Solubility-Limiting Methods

Many drugs are reasonably soluble in water and ionize extensively at physiologic pH. Drugs with an offensive taste usually demonstrate negative organoleptic properties after dissolving in saliva during ingestion. Chemical modification, such as derivatization or lipophilic counterion selection, where possible, may be an effective method for reducing aqueous solubility and taste. This is exemplified by erythromycin, a partially soluble, bitter-tasting macrolide anti-infective. The solubility of erythromycin monohydrate is approximately 2 mg/mL in water at a pH of approximately 7. When converted to erythromycin ethylsuccinate, the aqueous solubility of the drug is less than 50 μg/mL. This form is practically tasteless as a ready-made liquid or a chewable tablet. The rate of dissolution in body fluids (e.g., saliva) may be further reduced by controlling formulation pH, solids content, and temperature. This technique can be applied to a number of drugs whose taste profiles are dependent on aqueous solubility.

Vesicles and Liposomes

Host–guest systems (e.g., phospholipids and certain surfactants) form spherical or ellipsoidal, closed, bilayer structures called vesicles. These structures often comprise several compartments within which a drug could be trapped, either as a solution or a dispersion. Under various conditions, these vesicles form closed systems, which are ideal vehicles for taste masking or for modulated release of drug in vivo. It is a challenge to formulate drugs with these flavor-masking methods without altering the regulatory status of the product (e.g., chemical designation of the active substance, in vitro dissolution kinetics, physical or chemical stability, and bioavailability). Various manufacturers offer a complete line of phospholipids (purified and solubilized in various carrier systems) for use in the food and pharmaceutical industries.

Microencapsulation and Coated Systems

Recently, a great deal of attention has been focused on the usefulness of coated fine particles in achieving pharmaceutical objectives. By coating drug particles with an appropriate polymer system, desirable properties can be imparted to the dosage form, eliminating undesirable properties, such as taste. Coating drug particles significantly modulates drug release while improving taste, stability, and other handling characteristics (e.g., flow and compression). Commercial particle coaters make it possible to coat fine drug particles, achieving slow release and taste masking in oral formulations. Examples for which particle coating has been used to introduce unique line extensions to the marketplace include Theo-Dur and Depakote Sprinkle. In the case of Theo-Dur, theophylline is sprayed onto sugar beads followed by a polymer to control drug release. By encapsulating a drug substance, this process prevents interaction of the drug with taste receptors, thus eliminating bitterness. Other frequently used microencapsulation methods include spray drying, spray congealing, coacervation and phase separation, interfacial polymerization, and extrusion.

Complexation and Chemical Modification

The use of ion exchange resins to form drug adsorbates for sustained release was closely associated with Strasenburgh Laboratories, an affiliate of Pennwalt Corporation, which was granted several patents in this area. Their first significant application involved amphetamine adsorbed onto a sulfonic acid cation exchange resin (Biphetamine) for use in appetite suppression. Over the years, several products have been introduced commercially since the initial work with amphetamine; examples include Ionamin (phentermine), Tussionex (hydrocodone polistirex and chlorpheniramine polistirex), and a variety of cough-cold products, including phenylpropanolamine, chlorpheniramine, and dextromethorphan. This technology is applicable to taste masking as well.

The mechanism of drug release from the sustained-release complex (e.g., an ion exchange resinate consisting of a drug with a bitter taste) is ideal for liquids, when formulated either as granules for reconstitution or ready-made suspensions. By retaining a low counter- ion concentration in the product, almost all of the drug may be retained in the matrix, so that upon ingestion, ions of the body trigger the release mechanism through a dynamic equilibration process. Slow equilibrating complexes that provide low diffusivity of drug to the taste buds (e.g., low aqueous solubility of the drug) can eliminate bitterness and other offensive organoleptic drug properties. Other complexation phenomena employed in formulation work for flavor enhancement are: inclusion complexes (e.g., cyclodextrins and their derivatives), matrices, and physical complexes with waxy substances (e.g., polyethylene glycols).

More recently, pharmaceutical manufacturers have introduced various technologies for coating drug particles with semipermeable polymeric membranes designed to provide controlled release in vivo. Coatings of neat drugs and their adsorbates combined controlled-release characteristics with the benefit of taste masking, caused by the effective reduction of dissolved drug concentrations in the mouth.

Taste evaluation of a variety of these preparations showed a significant reduction in bitterness, suggesting that coatings and adsorbates have potential in the flavor enhancement of drugs with offensive tastes.

The use of flavors and flavor modifiers in pharmaceutical formulations is of considerable importance in promoting drug products. Flavors are also key factors in promoting patient compliance, because products with offensive taste are likely to be objectionable. Taste sensations are, however, wholly subjective, and of the many objective methods thus far used, none can adequately and completely characterize taste and aroma sensations without some bias. It is also certain that a fair proportion of the population is indifferent to taste and lacks the acuity necessary for distinguishing small differences in taste and aroma between samples. Furthermore, clear flavor performance differences can be obtained during pharmaceutical product development, by techniques designed to promote taste acceptance. The use of flavors, flavor modifiers, and other methods for flavor enhancement, such as physical and chemical manipulations of drugs, may be potential methods for the development of products with superior market preference characteristics.

10

Metabolism in Humans

The superfamily of cytochrome P450 (CYP) enzymes provides one of the most sophisticated catalysts of drug metabolism. These enzymes catalyze a wide variety of oxidative and reductive reactions and has activity towards chemically diverse substrates. Since only a small subset of the CYP enzymes is responsible for the majority of drug-metabolizing events, it is unavoidable that different drugs will compete for the active site of a given CYP. Several aspects of these enzymes, such as the rate and position of their metabolic attack, their inhibition and induction, and the specificity of the various isoforms, must be taken into account in the lead optimization process during the development of new therapeutic agents.

To this end, the pharmaceutical industry needs computational predictive methods to identify the major CYP enzymes responsible for the metabolism of a given drug, and to be able to avoid potential drug-drug interactions. Despite the large amount of information available on the functional role of these enzymes, the knowledge of their three-dimensional structure is still incomplete. At the time of writing, the only X-ray structure publicly available is that of human 2C9.

Although several papers report the development of computational models to predict cytochrome P450 inhibition, rate and position of metabolism, and selective interactions, this remains a major challenge due to the many different isoforms that can be involved in the metabolism of a single compound, the number of possible positions of metabolism for each isoform, and, as stated above, the lack of structural information about most human CYPs.

While in vitro screens for inhibition and metabolic stability can provide some of the above information, the experimental elucidation of the position (i.e., site) of metabolism is usually a high resource-demanding task which requires several experimental techniques and consumes large amounts of the compounds so investigated. Nevertheless, a recognition of the site(s) of metabolism could be of great help in designing new compounds with better pharmacokinetic profile and in avoiding the presence of toxic metabolites by chemically protecting the metabolic labile moieties. Another interest in predicting site(s) of metabolism is in prodrug design, where the compound needs to be metabolized to become active.

The aim of the present chapter is to describe a recent, fast, easy, and computationally inexpensive method to predict CYP2C9, 2D6, and 3A4 regioselective metabolism using ad hoc developed 3D homology enzyme models and the 3D structure of their potential substrates. The method requires only the 3D structure of the potential substrates and automatically determines the interaction of the virtual compounds with the enzymes using GRID flexible molecular interaction fields, providing the site(s) of metabolism in graphical output.

The computational procedure is fully automated and fast. The method thus appears as a valuable new tool in virtual screening and in early ADME/Toxicity evaluation, where potential drug–drug interactions and metabolic stability must be evaluated to facilitate drug design.

Description of the Method

The proposed methodology involves the calculation of different sets of descriptors, one for the CYP enzymes and one for the potential substrates. The set of descriptors used to characterize CYP enzymes is based on the GRID flexible molecular interaction field (MIF). The 3D structure of the CYP enzymes is required to derive the GRID-MIF interaction.

Structure of CYPs

The structure of a rabbit CYP2C5 was used as a template in homology modeling of the CYP2C9 enzyme. In fact, this enzyme shows a high degree of similarity (>82%) and identity (>77%) with the human CYP2C family. More recently, the crystal structure of human CYP2C9 was resolved and deposited in the Protein Data Bank. However, this structure appears biased by the cocrystallized substrate. The above-mentioned 3D structure from homology model was therefore used in our work.

The initial 3D structures of CYP2D6 and 3A4 were kindly provided by DeRienzo et al. The 3D models were built by restraint-based comparative modeling using the X-ray crystallographic structure of bacterial cytochromes P450 BM3, CAM, TERP, and ERYF as templates (PDB entries 2bmh, 3cpp, 1cpt, and 1oxa, resp.). Secondary structure predictions were obtained by the method of Rost and Sunders. The heme molecule, with its Fe-atom in the ferric (Fe^{III}) oxidation state, was extracted from the structure of P450-BM3 and fitted into the active site of each of the three cytochromes. The starting structures were submitted to dynamic runs, without any ligand, to select an average bioconformation for all the isoenzymes.

3D Structure of Substrates

The majority of CYP substrates contain flexible moieties. Since the conformation of the substrates had a sensible impact on the outcome of the method, two different protocols were used and tested to build their 3D structure. In the first method, a conformational search followed by energy minimization was performed for each substrate using the CONFORT program. The runs were constrained to obtain a population of diverse low-energy minimum conformations.

In the second method, which was implemented only later, each substrate was submitted to a conformational search followed by energy minimization by means of an in-house software. The runs were constrained to obtain a population of conformers with a 3D structure induced by the shape and the *interaction fields* of the CYP active site.

CYP Active Site Requirements

It is known that CYP2C9 binds compounds with large dipoles or negative charges. Thus, oxygen-rich compounds such as carboxylic acids, sulfonamides, and alcohols are substrates for CYP2C9. Site-directed mutagenesis experiments have demonstrated that lipophilic interactions are extremely important for binding in the enzyme cavity. The GRID force field applied to CYP2C9 shows that its side chains have a great flexibility and that the binding site can accomodate a variety of substrates. Side-chain flexibility, in turn, modifies the physicochemical enviroment of the cavity. H_2O Molecules were introduced or removed according to the relative position of side chains. GRID shows that the CYP2C9 cavity is ca. 600 $Å^3$ wide, with hydrophobic interactions filling 20–40% of the cavity volume depending on the 3D rearrangment of the side chains induced by ligand binding.

CYP2D6 binds compounds with a basic N-atom and/or a positive charge. Thus, nitrogen-rich compounds such as arylalkylamines are potential substrates for CYP2D6. It is known that the 3D pharmacophore of CYP2D6 substrates needs one site of oxidation and at least one basic N-atom at 5–7 Å from the oxidation site. However, several substrates do exist which show a greater distance between the oxidation site and the basic N-atom, e.g., tamoxifen (>10 Å). This example demonstrates the important role played by CYP flexibility in substrate recognition.

CYP3A4 tends to exhibit a broad substrate specificity. It binds low-molecular- and high-molecular-weight compounds and shows no pharmacophoric preferences or special structural constraints for its substrates, due to its large cavity. Since its substrates probably adopt more than one orientation in the active site, CYP3A4 attacks ligand positions mainly in function of their chemical reactivity.

In the resting state, the central Fe-atom of CYPs is hexacoordinated with a serine OH group. Furthermore, the exclusion of H_2O molecules from a functional water channel is essential for effective enzymatic function. Upon substrate binding, H_2O must be displaced from the active site to prevent electron uncoupling. It has been postulated that the water channel is located in the proximity of the thiolate side of the heme. Methods able to predict H_2O movement due to side-chain flexibility or substrate binding are essential for a correct prediction of CYP–substrate interactions.

CYP–Substrate Interactions

The molecular interaction fields (MIFs) in the binding site of CYP2C9, 2D6, and 3A4 are calculated by the GRID force field. Five MIFs are generated in this analysis: the DRY molecular interaction field simulating hydrophobic interactions, the N1-amide nitrogen probe simulating H-bond donor interactions, the O-carbonyl oxygen probe simulating H-bond acceptor interactions, and two charged probes (one positive, the other negative) simulating charge–charge electrostatic interactions. All MIFs are obtained using a 0.5 A grid and a self-accommodating dielectrical constant. The grid box size for the three isoforms is carefully placed around the active-site cavities. The active-site cavities range from ca. 600 $Å^3$ for 2C9 to 1100 $Å^3$ for 3A4. The MIFs are generated using the flexible mode in GRID (directive MOVE =1). With this option, some of the residue side chains can automatically move reflecting attractive or repulsive interactions with the probe. The side-chain flexibility in GRID can mimic this movement to accommodate different substrates depending on size, shape, and interaction pattern.

When a ligand approaches the side chains of residues, their movements are always influenced by neighbors and by the ligand. For example, the CH_2 groups in the side chain of lysine will tend to move toward the hydrophobic moiety of an interacting ligand. However, if the ligand contains a positively charged group, the charged N-atom of lysine will tend to move away from it. What actually happens depends on the overall balance between attractive and repulsive effects, and GRID is calibrated to simulate these movements. However, we point out that the flexible GRID map cannot take the large movements of the protein backbone into account.

Transformation of the Molecular Interaction Fields

In a first step, the regions close to the binding site but not accessible to the substrates are removed from the analysis. Then, the selected interaction points are used to calculate a new set of descriptors using the GRIND technology. For each CYP-probe interaction, this approach transforms the interaction energies at a certain spatial position (MIF descriptors) into a number of histograms that capture the 3D pharmacophoric interactions of the flexible protein (correlograms).

Substrate Treatment

The descriptors developed to characterize the substrate chemotypes are obtained from a combination of molecular orbitals calculations and GRID probe–pharmacophore recognition. Molecular orbital calculations are first performed to compute the substrate's electron-density distribution. All atom charges are determined using the AM1 Hamiltonian. The computed charges are used to derive a 3D pharmacophore based on the molecular electrostatic potential (MEP) around the substrate. Moreover, all atoms in the substrate are classified into GRID probe categories depending on their hydrophobic and H-bond donor and acceptor capabilities. Their intramolecular distances are then binned and transformed into clustered distances. One set of descriptors is computed for each atom-type category: hydrophobic. H-bond acceptor, and H-bond donor, yielding a fingerprint for each atom in the molecule. The distances between the different atomic positions classified using the previous criteria are then transformed into binned distances. In this case, the distances between the different atoms are calculated and a value of one or zero is assigned to each bin distance indicating the presence or the absence of such distance in the substrate.

Ligand–CYP Protein Comparison: The Recognition Component

Once the protein interaction pattern is translated from Cartesian coordinates to distances in the receptor and the structure of the ligand is described with similar fingerprints, both sets of descriptors can be compared. The complementarity of hydropobicities, charges, and H-bonds between the protein and the substrate are then computed using Carbo similarity indices. Finally, the different atoms in the substrate are ranked according to the computed total similarity index.

Reactivity Component

Cytochromes P450 catalyze oxidative and reductive reactions. Oxidative biotransformations are more frequent and include aromatic and side-chain hydroxylation, deamination, N-, O-, S-dealkylation, N-oxidation, sulfoxidation, dehalogenation, and desulfuration. The majority of these reactions can be rationalized considering a FeO^{3+} intermediate and a one-electron abstraction-rebound mechanism. This high-valent complex (FeO^{3+}, sometime written as $Fe^{IV}= O$) is electron-poor and abstracts either a H-atom or an electron from the substrate, generating an intermediate species. A subsequent collapse of the intermediate generates the product. Although many different reactions are possible, we have addressed only the most-common metabolic reactions. Less-frequent or exotic reactions will be probably addressed later. The major P450 reaction groups considered are carbon hydroxylation, homolytic heteroatom oxygenation, heteroatom release (dealkylation), heteroatom oxygenation (N-oxydation and S-oxydation).

Carbon hydroxylation is probably the most-common reaction. The mechanism requires the formation of a radical species. This basic metabolism can be extended to the oxidation of alcohols to carbonyl compounds and of hydrated aldehydes to carboxylic acids. In any case, for all the above reactions, the site of metabolism can be described by a probability function P_{SM} which is correlated to, and can be considered as, the free energy of the overall process:

$$P_{SM_i} = E_i \cdot R_i$$

where P is the probability of an atom i to be the site of metabolism, E is the accessibility of atom ito the heme, R is the reactivity of atom i in the actual mechanism of reaction. E_i is, thus, the recognition score between the CYP protein and the ligand when the latter is positioned in the CYP protein and exposes its atom i towards the heme. E_i depends on the 3D structure of the ligand, on its conformation

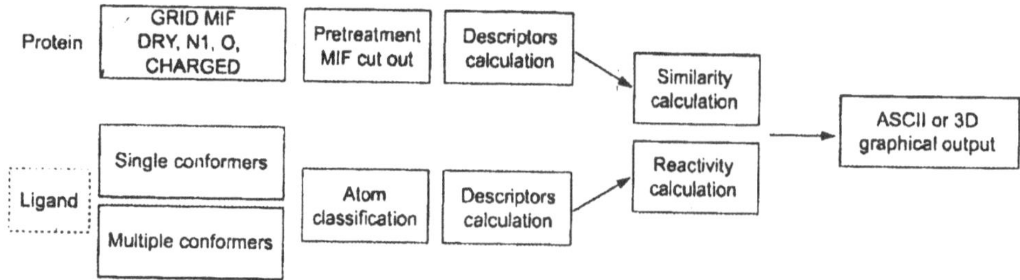

Fig. 10.1. The MetaSite computation flowchart.

and chirality, and on the 3D structure of the enzyme. The Ei score is proportional to the exposure of the atom ito the heme group.

Similarly, R_i is the reactivity of atom i in the appropriate reaction mechanism, and represents the activation energy needed to produce the reactive intermediate. It depends on the ligand 3D structure and on the reaction mechanism. For the same ligand, the P_{SM} function assumes different values for different atoms according to the E_i and R_i components.

Software Package

The procedure is called MetaSite (site-of-metabolism prediction). The MetaSite procedure is fully automated and does not require any user assistance. All the work can be handled and submitted in batch queue. The molecular interaction field for CYPs obtained from the GRID package are precomputed and stored inside the software. The semiempirical calculations, pharmacophoric recognition, descriptor handling, similarity computation and reactivity computation, are made automatically once the 3D structure of the compounds is provided. The complete calculation is performed in a few seconds in IRIX SGI machines and is even faster in the Linux or Windows environment. For example, processing a database of 100 compounds, starting from 3D molecular structures, takes ca. 3 min at full resolution with a R1 4000 Silicon Graphics 500 MHz CPU, less than 1 min in a Windows Pentium machine and ca. 30s in a Linux Pentium machine.

An Overview of Major Results

To validate the methodology in the three human enzymes, 120 metabolic reactions catalyzed by CYP2C9, 130 metabolic reactions catalyzed by CYP2D6, and 230 metabolic reactions catalyzed by CYP3A4, together with information concerning their sites of oxidation, were used.

The compounds show different metabolic pathways. Some are metabolized only at a single site, others present two sites of metabolism, and very seldom three. Moreover, substrates show a large structural diversity including rigid compounds (e.g. ,steroids) and very flexible ones with more than ten rotatable bonds, and a wide range of molecular weight and lipophilicity.

In more than 68% of CYP2C9 reactions, the first option selected by the methodology matches the experimental one. Moreover, in more than 13% and 5% of cases, the second and third atoms, respectively, are the ones that fit the experimental one. Therefore, in considering the overall ranking list for the multiple sites of metabolism, in ca. 86% of the reactions, the methodology predicts the site of metabolism for CYP2C9 within the first three atoms selected, independently of the conformer used.

In more than 68% of CYP2D6 substrates, the first option suggested by the methodology was in agreement with the reported site of metabolism. When the first three options suggested by the method were considered as the potential site of metabolism, 85% of the substrates were well predicted. In more than 50% of CYP3A4 substrates, the first option suggested by the methodology was in agreement with the reported site of metabolism. When the first three options suggested by the method were considered as the potential site of metabolism, 80% of the substrates were well predicted. A methodology has been developed to predict the site of metabolism for substrates of CYP2C9, 2D6, and 3A4. On average, for ca. 84% of cases, the method predicted the correct site of metabolism within the first three atoms in the ranking list.

The method is based on flexible molecular interaction fields generated by the GRID force field on CYP homology modeling structures that were treated and filtered to extract the most-relevant information. The methodology is very fast. To predict a site of metabolism for drug-like substrates, the method requires a few seconds per molecule. It is important to note that the method does not use any training set or statistical model or supervised technique, and it has proven to be predictive for extensively diverse validation sets examined in different pharmaceutical companies.

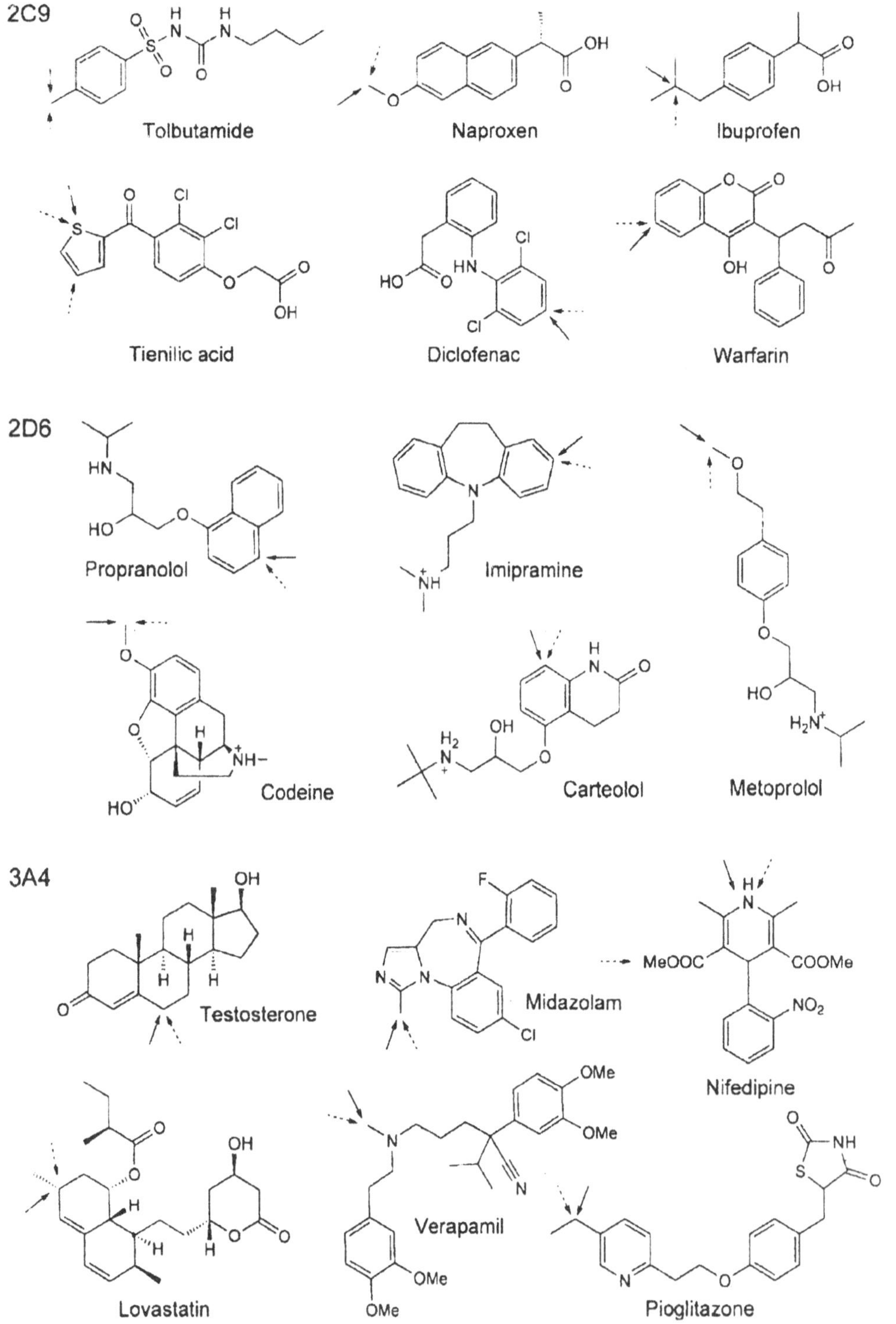

2C9

Tolbutamide

Naproxen

Ibuprofen

Tienilic acid

Diclofenac

Warfarin

2D6

Propranolol

Imipramine

Codeine

Carteolol

Metoprolol

3A4

Testosterone

Midazolam

Nifedipine

Lovastatin

Verapamil

Pioglitazone

Fig. 10.2. Some of the metabolic reactions used to validate the site of metabolism for CYP2C9, 2D6, and 3A4 with the experimental site of metabolism and the predicted site(s) of metabolism (dashed arrows)

The 3D structure of the substrate to be analyzed (the starting conformation) has an impact on the outcome of the method. Satisfactory results were obtained using an in-house conformer generation which takes the MIFs and the flexible shape of the active site of the enzymes into account. The latter procedure is automatically performed when a molecule or a set of molecules are provided in 3D coordinates. The methodology can be used either to suggest new positions that should be protected to avoid metabolic attack, or to check the suitability of a prodrug. Moreover, this procedure can be used to determine potential interactions of virtual compounds for early toxicity filtering.

11

BIOTERRORISM

The very fundamental characteristics of bioterrorism are presented, alongside with the distinct multidisciplinary configuration of the term and phenomenon. Some unique attributes are outlined that make bioterrorism an entity nourished by different essentials and bearing various, in part far-reaching, implications. Infectious diseases—the most effective extraneous regulator controlling the size of many animal populations in nature—are largely restrained in relation to mankind, thanks to the advancement of preventive and therapeutic medicine. The balance thus created is at any rate fragile, especially as human population density is steadily increasing, overall, whereas pathogens persist in acquiring drug-resistance. Pharmaceutical biotechnology is one major contributing arena to medicine, in that context; bioterrorism constitutes a counter-arena that unfortunately may amplify or substitute for the natural control mechanisms signified for by infectious diseases. Paradoxically, yet, pharmaceutical biotechnology in itself represents a potential key resource for bioterrorism. This is the case because pharmaceutical biotechnology is becoming an unparalleled front area, bearing a melting pot of remarkably sophisticated and multidisciplinary know-how, substances, and appliances. Large portions of which are dual use and may readily be exploited decently or viciously.

This built-in, intriguing duality is an essential feature, in that bioterrorism may imbibe extra potency from the very capacity destined to prevent and cope with bioterrorism. Although a very old way of sabotage, bioterrorism is presently, or soon to be, immeasurably more powerful, potentially, than ever, due to marked breakthroughs achieved in biopharmacology and biomedicine. Scientifically, this evolving, dichotomic course is inevitable, albeit significantly augmenting bioterrorism resources. The comprehension and practice allowing for combating pathogens and toxins may serve then, as well, to upgrade bioterrorism. It is becoming but a matter of their degree of availability of those bioagents. The same principle applies for pathogens of farm animals and plants, which form an additional dimension of bioterrorism—agricultural bioterrorism (agroterrorism). Also, the increasing availability of recreational drugs—mostly a sort of phytotoxins, in their essence—propels another terrorism variant—narcoterrorism.

In a sense, then, bioterrorism may embody the golem that rose against its creator. It can trigger a confined outbreak, an extensive epidemic, or a colossal pandemic, intentionally engined by man himself. The perpetrators may not even figure the anticipated impact—medically, psychologically, and logistically—which may immensely exceed what they want to achieve. Inversely, the in-effect impact may be but marginal, much less than that quested for. This uncertainty stems from various unknowns still marking the behavioral profile of infectious diseases. The interface between pathogens and man retains its enigmatic identity, although largely deciphered. At any rate, as James Woolsey, former CIA director has put it: "Germ terrorism is the single most dangerous threat to our national security in the foreseeable future." The magnitude of bioterrorism, yet, extends far beyond the boundaries of the United States. Man only can eradicate, either locally or globally, long-lasting formidable pathogens—as was the case with smallpox—by means of extraneous, far-reaching intervention, namely vaccination; antibiotics are not less important for wiping out certain bacterial pathogens. Yet man is, at the same time, the prime messenger of their possible reemergence, particularly through bioterrorism. Conceivably, his intelligence and impulse both shape, thus, a delicate balance, one that might branch unthinkable ramifications. It is, then, his own and absolute responsibility to pursue a steady state that would eliminate or minimize the risk of epidemic self-destruction. In general, calculated self-destruction is unsupprisingly, antagonistic to the very nature of most species.

The menace of terrorism at large, in its broad sense, is an unparalleled phenomenon that may be considered, basically, to be a sort of a limited self-destruction mechanism for mankind. In a way, it is even worse then wars, because of its inherent unpredictability, irrationalism, and wide scope, as well as the built-in, unapparent, vitality, and durability marking it. When the dimension of biological warfare is added to this featuring, it turns out to pose uncontrollable potentiality. Addressing the complicated domain of bioterrorism has to necessarily be conducted through a multidisciplinary approach. Therefore, the following chapter covers varitype aspects altogether, namely, microbiological, epidemiological, medical, technological, demographical, political, and strategic; the integration of which is essential, so as to comprehend the substance, complexity, and implications of bioterrorism. The entire issue of bioterrorism may thus gain a typical multidimensional structure and meaning.

Definition and Essence of Bioterrorism

Integrating two spheres that are innately unconnected to each other—terrorism and pathogens—the entity of bioterrorism reflects a complex, although in a sense fairly old, phenomenon of mankind. Given this starting point, the definition and essence of bioterrorism, together with its meaningfulness, are complicated. At the same time, the protean nature of bioterrorism endows it with uncommon attractiveness and advantageousness that may meet various courses. The two elements comprising bioterrorism, namely terrorizing by means of biological agents, represent two distinct spheres, each bearing multiple contents. Those two spheres form, thereby, a singular, mighty conjunction between strategic studies and life sciences. Terrorism at large, can be variedly featured, according to the following parameters:

1. Conducted by a country, organization, group, or individual.
2. Against a country, organization, group, or individual.
3. By threatening and/or attacking.
4. Covertly or overtly.
5. Terror may be the goal or a by-product of an in-effect damage.
6. The direct impact may be the ultimate objective or propel the occurrence of the ultimate objective.
7. The impact is intended to form in the short, medium, or long run.
8. With or without taking responsibility by the perpetrator.

Biological agents include, basically, pathogens and toxins, which may be classified in the following ways:

1. Live—hence reproducing—agents (pathogens) or nonviable agents (toxins). Prions, as reproducing molecules, constitute a notable, exceptional intermediate.
2. Lethal or sublethal (not a clear-cut division).
3. Transmissible—hence epidemic—pathogens or nontransmissible pathogens.
4. Natural or modified/engineered pathogens and toxins.

5. Abruptly or gradually affecting the target.
6. Affecting humans, husbandry, crops, or materials.
7. The vehicle may be natural (infected arthropod, animal, or human being) or artificial (man-made disseminator, i.e., sprayers and envelopes).
8. The route of penetrating the body is the respiratory system, alimentary tract, or skin.

Remarkably, almost any combination of the various mentioned parameters featuring terrorism and biological agents is feasible. That is one main attribute underlying the attractiveness and potential might of bioterrorism. Another one is the outstanding ratio between the amount of biological agent to be used and the resulting impact, especially with reference being made to epidemic pathogens. At the extreme, which is certainly feasible, an individual saboteur can disperse a scarcely existent, unapparent amount of a fully epidemic, virulent pathogen, be it pestilence, smallpox, or influenza, and give rise to a transgressing, questionably controllable, lethal plague.

Biocrimes, biosabotage, and biowarfare are terms appreciably dovetailing with bioterrorism, in different manners. Although biological crimes accentuate the illegal dimension of bioterrorism, they pertain, as well, to a variety of acts, such as the very holding or transferring of a certain microorganism, which are in violation of national or international rules and conventions. Biological sabotage is the in-effect employment of biological agents for whatever operational sabotage purpose, whether or not terrorism-oriented, usually by means of guerilla warfare. Biological warfare basically reflects a military confrontation in which biological weaponry is used; yet broadly, it may be waged against civilian target populations, thus explicitly having the quality of bioterrorism.

Bioterrorism may be perceived, overall, as the calculated, deliberate use of pathogens or toxins (or threat of using them) against civilian populations or economic/logistical infrastructures, in order to attain goals that are political, social, religious, financial, ideological, or personal in nature; this is done through intimidation or coercion or instilling fear. It may still be subclassified, then, as follows:

1. The unlawful release of biological agents or toxins with the intent to intimidate or coerce a government or civilian population to further political or social objectives. Humans, farm animals, and cultivars are often targets.
2. Use of microorganisms or toxins to kill, sicken, or cause other malfunction in people, animals, plants, or useful materials.

In its broad scope, thus, bioterrorism includes, beyond its classic targeting against humans:

1. Agroterrorism, which may involve anti-plant pests, in addition to anti-plant and anti-animal pathogens.
2. Narcoterrorism, namely the constant on-purpose input of recreational drugs onto a target population.
3. Any other type of sabotage achievable by means of microbes, such as fuel-eating bacteria, asphalt eating-bacteria, and alike.

In a way, the core of bioterrorism, both objectively and subjectively, is horrifying, whereas the involved weapon in itself consists in, absurdly, some of the most powerful natural foes of humanity, and can in practice bring about a very significant direct impact, far beyond horror. Hence, it may regretfully be regarded, in a sense, as the potential promoter of various infectious diseases that are currently being suppressed, pharmacologically and medically, just waiting for their opportunity to come.

One chief character of bioterrorism is, nonetheless, the conceivably immeasurable disproportion between effort and outcome, particularly when the latter is at its maximum. It thus poses a strong temptation. Any other weapons, terror means— and apparently any other context—are not competent in sustaining such disproportion. Technically, then, this attribute mostly represents the essence of bioterrorism, such that nears a legendary identity. The distance from reality is at any rate secondary, especially as it can readily be bridged over, in affect, quite soon. In that concern, recent breakthroughs made in the field of genetic engineering amplify at the same time, paradoxically, both imagination and practicality.

All in all, within the sphere of terrorism at large, three distinctions typify the essence of bioterrorism:

1. The distinction between bioterrorism and conventional terrorism.
2. Between bioterrorism and other unconventional terrorism (chemical, radiological, nuclear).
3. Between bioterrorism and biological warfare.

The projection of those three distinctions altogether reflects the whole substance of bioterrorism, as aimed, among other things, to be shown in this chapter.

Concept and Incentives

Several common denominators are outlined, which mark both terrorism-oriented states and terror organizations, on their way to resorting to bioterrorism. Other elements of their concept and incentives regarding bioterrorism comparatively differ, naturally, owing to their dissimilar essences. Various motives and objectives may then underlie their encouraged attitude toward bioterrorism. The roots are at any rate historical, appreciably shaping during time. Intuitively, not having any concrete knowledge in terms of toxinology and bacteriology until the nineteenth century, man adopted poisonous and infective substances for attacking rivals. It was mainly practical common sense that guided him. Much later, paving its way toward scientific horizons, man gradually mastered the related technical fundamentals. The recognition of infective microorganisms and naturally produced toxic molecules accumulated and ripened. It reached the level of having the full capacity to operate them as warfare agents.

But, anthropologically, the concept underlying bioterrorism extends far beyond technical and operational features, whether state or non-state sponsored. The very notion of afflicting passive civilian populations with infectious diseases seems to be, objectively, profoundly evil, even if accompanied by different considerations and calculations. In its simplest form, then, bioterrorism reflects but an extreme way of malevolence. Variably, the dimensions of governance and insidiousness may certainly play a roll, in conjunction. *A priori*, the power to generate epidemics was possessed only by God and nature. Thus, biblically, God waged, initially, the epidemics included within the Ten Plagues of Egypt. Later on, comprehending the principal mechanism and impact of epidemics, man tried to emulate and immobilize that route against adversaries. As a matter of fact, it was around 1500 bc, when the Hittites sent plague victims into the lands of their enemies.

The fundamental incentive and concept of bioterrorism did not substantially change, up to these days. What did alter, obviously, are the know-how, the technical tools, and the strategic approach. Strategically, there are three basic alternatives shaping the concept of bioterrorism acts:

1. The perpetrator (either state or non-state sponsored) would seek to remain unidentified.
2. The perpetrator would be indifferent as to its identity.
3. The perpetrator would seek to be identified.

The first and third alternatives have each two variants, respectively:

1. Anonymity would rely on objective inability to epidemiologically determine whether the event was an act of bioterrorism.
2. Anonymity would rely on objective inability to trace the perpetrator by means of investigation or intelligence (even if epidemiologically affirmed to be an act of bioterrorism).
3. Identification would rely on direct announcement, either before or subsequent to the act of bioterrorism.
4. Identification would rely on investigative and intelligence findings—either evidential or, deliberately, merely circumstantial (hence less valid)—without taking responsibility.

Several technological, political, and psychological explanations underly the quest of terrorists and terrorism-oriented states to opt for acquiring weapons of mass destruction (WMD), particularly biological agents, among them are the cheap cost of such weapons and the sense of prestige and security they grant to the owner. Parallel to offensive considerations, the inverse dimension of deterring capacity also plays a roll. All in all, terrorists or terrorism-oriented states may choose bioterrorism among many options, both conventional and unconventional. Preference may be given to bioterrorism due to various reasons. In terms of a pragmatic, clinical feasibility study, bioterrorism is, at least potentially, the most efficient form of sabotage, particularly when conducted indistinguishably from a natural event. Moreover, it may have a fully strategic impact; hence, it is often reckoned to be the ultimate mode of terrorism. Notably, most biological agents are not contagious; yet they might generate extensive outbreaks, if not epidemics, due to their transmissibility in other ways.

A terrorist group or terrorism-oriented state, intending to employ biological agents, will likely be attracted to their mass killing potential. In addition, their delayed impact may also enable the saboteur to escape detection. Also, an attacker might reckon the resemblance between a natural and an unnatural epidemic to be close enough to divert suspicion, or at least make it extremely difficult to trace. That would make it difficult to retaliate with a massive punitive strike, the expectation of which ordinarily serves as deterrent to an unconventional assault. Thus, the subsequent intimidation and chaos resulting from the inherently unknowable may make biological agents the terrorist weapon of choice. On the whole, the related line of terms accentuating the significance and potential impact of bioterrorism at large include, then: high consequence terrorism; catastrophic terrorism; total terrorism; asymmetric terrorism; superterrorism; ultraterrorism, and so on. Beyond, terrorists and terrorism-oriented states are certain to decide for themselves whether the conduction of bioterrorism serves their cause. Moreover, it is believed that biological weapons are preferable for terrorist groups, and that the allure for terrorists of biological weapons is currently intensifying due to the increase in availability of biotechnologists and sophistication of manufacturing methods.

Overall, one fundamental motive of bioterrorism (within the context of WMD at large), then, is the will to generate what is currently called high consequence terrorism, total terrorism, or catastrophic terrorism. Under certain circumstances it may be regarded as pure asymmetric terrorism, the purpose of which is not to take lives or destroy property. It is rather the mechanism by which the attacker seeks to achieve weakening of the sense of cohesion that binds communities together, to reduce its social capital, and to sow distrust, fear, and insecurity. Within this narrow course, it is but a method of waging a sort of social and psychological warfare. The availability of pathogenic agents, alongside with technical feasibility and operational modality of bioterrorism at large, are basically rather in favor of the saboteur or terrorism-oriented state. Still, the bioterrorism events that already took place overall, seemingly exhibit but a portion of its potentiality, whereas the essence of the related threshold of proliferation is vague. Resultantly, built-in limita tions interfere with thoroughly comprehending and foreseeing the course of bioterrorism.

Bioterrorism-patterned Natural Epidemics

The apparent resemblance. between natural epidemics and induced ones mostly leads to recognizing the relevance of bioterrorism-patterned natural epidemics as prime demonstrative occurrences. Let alone, that various infectious diseases, chiefly viral, are emerging or reemerging in an unpredictable, often overwhelming, manner. It would therefore be advisable to diligently observe some prominent natural epidemics that took place during the recent decade. The most distinct bioterrorism-patterned natural epidemics are typically those concerned with water- and food-borne infectious gastroenteritis, stemming from the contamination of a current collective source. Such epidemics would include, principally, two phases:

1. The first wave of infections is generated directly by the consumption of the collective source.
2. An additional wave is brought about, dependent on the degree of ongoing communicability or contagiousness of the causative agent toward potential secondary victims that are prone to be exposed, irrespective of the initial collective source.

This type of epidemic locally occurs very often, worldwide, in the form of relatively restricted innocent outbreaks. They bear the potency to expand, however. And they are quite easy to be produced deliberately, in practice. But, at any rate, they represent the simplest bioterrorism-patterned natural epidemics. Bioterrorism-patterned natural epidemics might be by far more complex and hazardous, nonetheless. It so happened that the past 10 years were marked by some outstanding epidemic events perfectly illustrating the tremendous potentiality of biological agents at large, as well as the candidature of certain pathogens for acts of bioterrorism, in particular. Those events are presented here in detail, then, so as to demonstrate the general effectuality of various bioterrorism-patterned scenarios. They include six virus- and germ-propelled catastrophic epidemics.

Ebola Hemorrhagic Fever

The 14th of April, 1995, Zaire (now the Democratic Republic of Congo). A 36- year-old laboratory technician checked into the medical clinic in Kikwit, complaining of a severe headache, stomach pains, fever, dizziness, weakness, and exhaustion. Surgeons did an exploratory operation to try to find the cause of his illness. To their horror, they found his entire gastrointestinal tract was necrotic and putrefying. He bled uncontrollably and within hours was dead. By the next day, the five medical workers who cared for him, including an Italian nun who assisted in the operation began to show similar symptoms, including high fevers, fatigue, bloody diarrhea, rashes, red and itchy eyes, vomiting, and bleeding from every body orifice. Less than 48 hours later, they, too, were dead, and the disease turned to form a deadly, uncontrollable epidemic.

As panicked residents fled into the bush, government officials responded to calls for help by closing off all travel, including humanitarian aid into or out of Kikwit, about 400 km from Kinshasa, the national capital. Fearful neighboring villages felled trees across the roads to seal off the pestilent city. No one dared enter houses where dead corpses rotted in the intense tropical heat. Boats plying the adjacent Kwilu River refused to stop to take on or discharge passengers or cargo. Food and clean water became scarce. Hos-pitals could hardly function as medications and medical personnel became scarce. Deadly tropical fevers are an unfortunate fact of life in Central Africa but rarely are they this contagious or lethal. The plague that afflicted Kikwit was Ebola hemorrhagic fever, a viral disease for which there is no known treatment. Within a few weeks, about 400 people in Kikwit had contracted the virus and 350 were dead. Where a 10% mortality rate is considered high for most infectious diseases, Ebola kills up to 90% of its victims, usually within only a few days after exposure. Still, contagiousness seems to be low.

The Kikwit Ebola outbreak was neither the first nor the last appearance of this dread disease. The first recognized Ebola epidemic occurred in 1976 in Yambuku, Zaire (near the Ebola River, after which the virus was named), where at least 280 people died. Three years later, 22 patients died in Sudan from a slightly different and less virulent form of Ebola. In 1996, about 100 people were killed by Ebola in two separate episodes in Gabon, and in 1999, an outbreak in the gold mining town of Durba in the Democratic Republic of Congo killed at least 63 people.

Ebola is one of two members of a family of RNA viruses called the Filoviridae (the other one being Marburg fever). No host or vector is known for Ebola, but it has been observed that monkeys and other primates can contract related diseases. Why viruses remain peacefully in their hosts for many years without causing much more trouble than a common cold, but then erupt sporadically and unpredictably into terrible human epidemics, is a new and growing question in environmental health and risk assessment. Although certainly a formidable pathogen, this virus exhibits changing rates of virulence (which is at times extremely high, more than any other pathogen), communicability, and, hence, epidimicity, the latter being rather restrained, in effect (400 infected and diseased people, out of 600,000 residents in Kikwit). Therefore, a shift in the transmissibility level of Ebola virus may be crucial and is immensely feared.

AIDS

AIDS, or acquired immunodeficiency syndrome, is a fatal disease caused by a rapidly mutating retrovirus that attacks the immune system and leaves the victim vulnerable to infections, malignancies, and neurological disorders. It was first recognized as a disease in 1981. The virus was isolated for the first time not long ago, in 1983. It is steadily spreading. During 2004, as a representation, around five million adults and children became infected with HIV (human immunodeficiency virus), the virus that causes AIDS. By the end of the year, an estimated 39.4 million people worldwide were living with HIV/AIDS. The year also saw more than three million deaths from AIDS, despite the availability of HIV antiretroviral therapy, which reduced the number of deaths in high-income countries. African and South-American tropical regions are heavily afflicted in particular for long periods of time.

But in certain regions the disease has risen remarkably swiftly during recent years. One of those arenas is Leningrad, were a notably exponential AIDS epidemic started in 1997. Beginning in that year and proceeding up to 2001, all patients in the Narcology Hospital of Leningrad Regional Center of Addictions (LRCA), were tested for HIV antibody. These clinical records (i.e., serostatus, gender, age, and addiction) and data from the HIV/AIDS Center in the Leningrad Region were reviewed. It has thus been shown that HIV prevalence at the LRCA increased from 0% to 12.7% overall, 33.4% among drug-dependent patients, and 1.2% among alcohol-dependent patients. During the same 5-year period (1997–2001), 2826 persons were registered at the HIV/AIDS Center: 6, 6, 51, 780, and 1983 persons in 1997, 1998, 1999, 2000, and 2001, respectively.

So, HIV infection is exploding in the Leningrad Region, currently in injection drug users, but potentially more broadly. The known high-per-capita alcohol intake in Russia heightens concern regarding the sexual transmission of HIV. Overall, the number of HIV-infected people in the Leningrad Region has risen to 2929 by the beginning of 2001, which is 2.3 times more than in 2000. Young people aged from 14 to 30, mostly drug addicts, account for 85% of the overall number of HIV-infected people. The number of teenagers sick with AIDS has risen by 2.5 times since last year. Particular concern was caused by a 10-fold increase in the number of AIDS victims among pregnant women. A total of 350 births given by HIV-infected mothers has been registered in the past year, and in 10 cases, parents gave up their babies. However, the AIDS pandemic, in its broad essence, is actually a global long-term eroding factor toward mankind at large. Caused by a type of attritional bioterrorism agent, analogicolly, its ultimate real impact is expected sometime in the future, unforeseeably. For now, and in relation to the magnitude of humanity, it is just crawling, slowly yet steadily. It may be regarded as an inherent, low-rate—although undefeatable, for the time being—cryptic, ostensibly overt pandemic, accumulating its critical mass.

SARS

The SARS (sever acute respiratory syndrome) virus emerged—and possibly rather formed, somehow, little earlier, in reality—on the 16 of November 2002. In Foshan, southern China, on the Pearl River Delta, the first case of SARS involved a man, a "*super-infector*" who subsequently infected four others.

It soon exploded. By November 31, 2002, a deadly outbreak of SARS carried on in China and has killed at least 34 people in the south and three in Beijing. Hundreds have been infected. Clearly an infectious disease, the illness was named and registered only clinically, owing to the unidentified nature of its casual agent. It was certainly recognized to be a virulent virus, at any rate. At that stage, the new virus seemed to be fairly confined. But during December, the disease "hitch-hiked" 200 km to Heyuan city, the provincial capital of Guangzhou. Virus spread to five hospital workers. Panic ensued in Heyuan, and the local authorities tried to calm the people with news that there was not epidemic. Within days, the alarm subsided. Somewhere during this time, provincial party leaders curbed the media from publishing details of the disease, hindering further efforts to contain the virus. By the end of December 2002, Guangdong had reported at least 300 cases.

Although showing to be a new virus, a comprehensive genomic analysis has established that the relationship between SARS Coronavirus and group 2 CoVs is monophyletic. Apparently, then, the SARS virus evolved as a strange zoonotic offshoot of group 2 CoVs, bearing greatly enhanced infectivity toward man. Actually, SARS is the first major novel infectious disease to hit the international community in the twenty-first century. It originated in southern China in November 2002 and spread rapidly thereafter to 29 countries/regions on five continents. At the end of the epidemic, the global cumulative total was 8098 with 774 deaths. Seven Asian countries/regions were among the top 10 on the list. It has alarmed the world with its infectivity and significant morbidity and mortality, its lack of a rapid, reliable diagnostic test, and lack of effective specific treatment and vaccination. The adverse impact on travel and business around the world, particularly in Asia, has been enormous. The consequences of the SARS epidemic were remarkable. In Taiwan, as an example, the impact of the SARS epidemic on the utilization of medical services was studied. Using interrupted time-series analysis and National Health Insurance data between January 2000 and August 2003, this study assessed the impact of SARS epidemic on medical service utilization in Taiwan. At the peak of the SARS epidemic, significant reductions in ambulatory care (23.9%), inpatient care (35.2%), and dental care (16.7%) were observed. People's fears of SARS appear to have had a strong impact on access to care. Adverse health outcomes resulting from accessibility barriers posed by the fear of SARS are significant.

West-Nile Encephalitis

In late August of 1999, an unusual cluster of severe cases of encephalitis was noted in an area around Queens in New York City. An epidemiologic investigation by the New York City Department of Health identified eight such cases and revealed that all of the patients had been previously healthy, had resided within the same 16 square mile area, and had recently engaged in outdoor activities. All but one had developed severe acute flaccid paralysis in the setting of encephalitis. At that point, the ethological agent had not yet been deciphered, though it seemed to be a basic virulent virus.

Both before and during the human encephalitis investigation, an epizootic among birds associated with a high fatality rate had been noted in and around New York City. Pathologic assessment of the dead birds displayed involvement of multiple organs, including evidence of encephalitis; however, common avian pathogens were not detected. The diseased birds were initially felt to be unrelated to the human epidemic. But genomic analyses using polymerase chain reaction and genome sequencing with specimens from New York City birds, infected mosquitoes collected in Connecticut, and human brain tissue from a fatal case of encephalitis, as well as expanded serological testing of specimens from suspected human cases identified WNE virus, a mosquito-borne pathogen, as the etiologic agent of this outbreak—4 weeks after the outbreak in humans was first reported to New York City public health officials! By the end of the summer of 1999, 62 patients with serologic evidence of acute WNE virus infection, including 59 ·hospitalized patients, had been identified. Seven died. Similar to more recent outbreaks of the virus, the epidemic seemed to be associated with a high rate of CNS involvement and a preponderance of cases in patients older than 60 years.

The introduction of WNE virus in North America was followed by progressive spread throughout the United States. During the summer of 2000, 21 cases of human WNE virus illnes, were identified,

2 died occurred among 10 counties in northeastern states. The following year, 66 cases were detected among a much more widespread geographic area, involving 38 counties in 10 states. The spread of human cases seemed to follow avian deaths; thus, avian death surveillance and, to a lesser extent, mosquito pool surveillance became important parts of public health efforts to track the virus and predict potential human cases. In addition to avian and human illness, a substantial number of equine cases were documented throughout the United States, a pattern also being observed in other parts of the world. An eco-epidemiological critical mass has been neared in 2002. During the summer of 2002 the number of WNV cases in North America ascended, and was the largest outbreak of arboviral meningoencephalitis ever documented in the Western Hemisphere. The WNE virus expanded its geographic range from the Mississippi River area at the conclusion of the 2001 season to the Pacific Coast by the end of 2002. Virus activity considerably increased and then found expression in the following figures: 2002—1460 cases; 66 deaths; 2003—9862 cases; 264 deaths; 2004—2470 cases; 88 deaths.

Avian Influenza

During 1997, an epidemic in Hong Kong of avian influenza in chickens and ducks occurred and was—merely marginally, then—transmitted to humans. Fortunately, the virus did not move from person to person and seemingly died out after the reservoir of domestic birds was completely depleted by the killing of approximately 1.6 million chickens, ducks, and geese by Hong Kong authorities. A variant of the type A H5N1 flu virus has been identified to be the cause of that event. It was but an ostensible defeat of that epidemic H5N1 variant. In actuality it silently proliferated spatially, and then catastrophic outbreaks of influenza H5N1 took place among poultry in many countries in Asia during late 2003 and early 2004. At that time, more than 100 million birds in the affected countries either died from the disease or were killed to try to control the outbreak. (Thailand 36 million, Vietnam 36 million, Indonesia 15 million, China 5 million, Pakistan 4 million) (Cambodia, Laos South Korea, and Japan have been less affected, so far.) By March 2004, the outbreak was reported to be under control. Beginning in late June 2004, however, new deadly outbreaks of influenza H5N1 among poultry were reported by several countries in Asia (Cambodia, China, Indonesia, Malaysia [first-time reports], Thailand, and Vietnam). These outbreaks—since extended— have been ongoing, and in 2005 reached Europe. They reached Africa in 2006.

The H5N1 virus does not usually infect humans. In 1997, however, the first case of spread from a bird to a human being was observed during the outbreak of bird flu in poultry in Hong Kong. The virus caused severe respiratory illness in 18 people, 6 of whom died. Since that time, there have been other cases of H5N1 infection among humans. Most recently, human cases of H5N1 infection have occurred in Thailand, Vietnam, and Cambodia during large H5N1 outbreaks in poultry. The death rate for these reported cases has been about 50%. Most of these cases occurred from contact with infected poultry or contaminated surfaces. Remarkably, however, it is thought that a few cases of human-to-human spread of H5N1 have occurred.

So far, spread of H5N1 virus from person to person has been rare, and proliferation has not continued beyond one person. Yet, because all influenza viruses have the ability to change, there is a great concern that the H5N1 virus could one day be able to become contagious and spread easily from one person to another. Because these viruses do not commonly infect humans, there is little or no immune protection against them in the human population. If the H5N1 virus were able to infect people and spread easily from person to person, a new flu pandemic could probably begin. It is impossible to foresee when a pandemic might occur. However, experts from around the world are watching the H5N1 situation in Asia very closely and are preparing for the possibility that the virus may begin to spread more easily and widely from person to person. Still, the H5N1 strain is but one variant within an immeasurable natural gallery of avian flu viruses. A few of them have already infected man, whereas the majority are taking their time, for now. A highly communicable derivative of them or of the H5N1 type will most probably generate the next colossal pandemic.

Until now, the most demanding flu pandemic that has been documented was the "*Spanish Flu*" (also known as "*Swine Flu*"), which killed 40–90 million people during just two years (1918–1919). The virus was of the H1N1 subtype. Later on, in 1957 a new serotype, H2N2, emerged and generated another pandemic, substituting the H1N1 virus. The next pandemic was given rise to in 1968 by the serotype H3N2, which replaced the H2N2. In 1977, a mild H1N1 virus resurfaced, bringing about another pandemic, but it did not substituted the H3N2 virus, and they are both prevailing currently. As a matter of fact, all pandemic and any other influenza virus strains are derived from avian viral strains. Moreover, at least some of them are likely preserved in perennial lake ice, mostly in the Northern Hemisphere, and may reintroduce—sub sequent to ice thawing—genes or entire genomes onto the current genetic pool of that protean virus. In regard to the current H5N1 strain, which is considerably virulent but noncontagious, for now, it may attain transmissibility by even a minor genetic alteration, the full essence of which is not yet clear.

In case this virus would retain its ongoing high communicability and virulence toward farm birds (currently chickens and ducks mainly) concomitantly with such genetic alteration, then an unparalleled pathogen, both pandemic and epizootic, may rise. Theoretically, it could disease pigs and horses as well, as the influenza A virus is in general infective and at times virulent toward those domestic mammals. But apparently this cannot occur in actuality, because there is, in all likelihood, some inherent viral incompetence to have such amplified affinity toward more then one host simultaneously. The remarkable potentiality of influenza A virus to attack various farm animals signifies, at any rate, its distinct candidature in the context of agroterrorism. Yet even in terms of merely an anti-human bioterrorism weapon, this varitype virus has been reckoned to be an ultimate pathogen, in some respects even exceeding the formidability of the notorious smallpox virus.

Pandemic spread would presumably bring about 6 0–80 million deaths worldwide. According to US Homeland Security Council's estimates, 90 million people could be infected in the US alone in case a bird flu pandemic breaks out, of which 45 million will require medical care, 10 million will require hospital admission and 2 million people could die. A British government report warns that The health service will be plunged into chaos if Britain is struck by a bird flu pandemic. Faced with a possible 4.5 million victims, demand for hospital beds would outstrip supply and doctors might have to deny treatment to the sick and elderly to save younger, fitter patients.

Not casually, all of the above-detailed illustrative epidemics represent, basically, bioterrorism-patterned scenarios specifically propelled by viruses. Antibiotics, the main combat-tool against germs, are of no relevance against viruses. Antiviral drugs are very limited in their scope. Vaccines are efficient against most viruses, but they cannot cope with viruses that are currently dynamically altering. Antisera against viruses are of marginal pharmacological contribution, for now. Viruses pose, then, in a sense, the ultimate biological weapon, and can be used for bioterrorism purposes. Still, the cultivation and handling of viruses is complicated in comparison with bacteria, due to the necessity of host tissue, whereby viruses obligatorily propagate.

Cholera

But, beyond viruses, other classes of pathogens and toxins are not at all to be depreciated, certainly. The germ causing cholera—mostly a water-borne disease—is nowadays the most epidemic and demanding bacterial pathogen, with reference being made to acute illness (parallel to the inversely lingering course of illness of tuberculosis, another remarkably demanding bacterial disease). In contrast to viruses, the cardinal characteristic marking pathogenic bacteria is their interface with various antibiotics, which is a very tangled and dynamic one. Thus, during March and April 2002, a resurgence of the causative agent *Vibrio cholerae* O139 occurred in Dhaka and adjoining areas of Bangladesh with an estimated 30,000 cases of cholera. The reemerged O139 strains belong to a single ribotype corresponding to one of two ribotypes that caused the initial O139 outbreak in 1993. Unlike the strains of 1993, however, the recent strains are susceptible to trimethoprim, streptomycin, and sulphamethoxazole, but resistant to nalidixic acid. This alternating profile exemplifies a predominant intensifying property of various bacterial pathogens resisting antibacterial drugs in an unpredictable fashion.

In general, cholera is an acute intestinal infection caused by ingestion of contaminated water or food. It has a short incubation period, from less than 1 day to 5 days, and produces an enterotoxin that causes copious, painless, watery diarrhea that can quickly lead to severe dehydration and death if treatment is not promptly given. Vomiting also occurs in most patients. Man-made and natural disasters can intensify the risk of epidemics considerably, as can conditions in crowded refugee camps. Explosive outbreaks with high case-fatality rates are often the result. For example, in the aftermath of the Rwanda crisis in 1994, outbreaks of cholera caused at least 48,000 cases and 23,800 deaths within one month in the refugee camps in Goma, the Congo. Although rarely so deadly, cholera outbreaks continue to be a major public health concern, causing considerable socioeconomic disruption as well as loss of life. In 2001 alone, the WHO and its partners in the Global Outbreak Alert and Response Network participated in the verification of 41 cholera outbreaks in 28 countries.

Throughout history, populations all over the world have sporadically been affected by devastating outbreaks of cholera. Records from Hippocrates (460–377 bc) and Galen (129–216 ad) already described an illness that might well have been cholera, and numerous hints indicate that a cholera-like malady has also been known in the plains of the Ganges River since antiquity.

Modern knowledge about cholera, however, dates only from the beginning of the nineteenth century when researchers began to make progress toward a better understanding of the causes of the disease and its appropriate treatment. The first cholera pandemic, or global epidemic, started in 1817 from its endemic area in Southeast Asia and subsequently spread to other parts of the world. The first and subsequent pandemics inflicted a heavy toll, spreading all over the world before receding.

In 1961, the seventh cholera pandemic wave began in Indonesia and spread rapidly to other countries in Asia, Europe, Africa, and finally in 1991 to Latin America, which had been free of cholera for more than one century. The disease spread rapidly in Latin America, causing nearly 400,000 reported cases and over 4000 deaths in 16 countries of the Americas that year. In 1992, a new serogroup—a genetic derivative of the EI-Tor biotype—emerged in Bangladesh and caused an extensive epidemic. Designated *V. cholerae* 0139 Bengal, the new serogroup has now been detected in 11 countries and likewise warrants close surveillance. Although no evidence is available to gauge the significance of these developments, the possibility of a new pandemic cannot be excluded. EI-Tor, for example, was originally isolated as an avirulent strain in 1905 and subsequently acquired sufficient virulence to cause the current pandemic.

The economic and social impacts of cholera are immense. In addition to human suffering caused by cholera, cholera outbreaks generate panic, disrupt the social and economic structure, and can impede development in the affected communities. Unjustified panic-induced reactions by other countries include curtailing or restricting travel from countries where a cholera outbreak is occurring or imposing import restrictions on certain foods. For example, the cholera outbreak in Peru in 1991 cost the country US$ 770 million due to food trade embargos and adverse effects on tourism.

The germ *Vibrio cholerae* is indeed a current unrestrained foe. Prominently transmissible among humans, this pathogen may readily be used for bioterrorism purposes.

Significance of Bioterrorism-Patterned Natural Epidemics

The principles and practicality of differentiating between epidemics stemming from bioterrorism acts and natural epidemics are outlined, to the extent attainable. The comprehension of bioterrorism-patterned natural epidemics thus turns out to be essential, and the related factors are presented in details, so as to facilitate the analysis of abrupt outbreaks.

The occurrence of epidemics, or outbreaks, at large, is the outcome of three alternative courses:

1. A natural biological process or move, such as the emergence of a new pathogenic variant, the spread of an infected vector onto a new biotope, and so on.
2. An innocent, either passive or active, artificial intervention, such as the arrival of an infected person at an epidemiologically virgin area/place, with relation to the pathogen harbored by him.
3. An act of bioterrorism (or a military biological war fare operation).

The significance of bioterrorism-patterned natural epidemics appears to be contributive in two major senses. It helps to appraise the profile and impact of bioterrorism scenarios, and it may facilitate the differentiation of an epidemic (or an outbreak), being a natural or man-made—either intentional or unintentional— occurrence. Hence, the recognition of a bioterrorism act is thus facilitated as well. This paradigmatic axis is vital for the very basic classification and handling of any epidemic or outbreak of an infectious disease or poisoning. In certain cases of diseased individuals, it ought to be applied as well, so as to arrive at the respecting differentiation. Thereby, the field of forensic microbiology plays an important roll.

In practice, classification and handling of various occurrences and events of concern ought to rely on the following elements:

1. Biotlogical and chemical analysis of specific markers related to the pathogen/ toxin involved, so as to trace its provenance.
2. Epidemiological analysis through which gauging of the event being a natural, innocently man-made, or deliberately man-made one, is allowed for.
3. Information obtained or assessment made by intelligence sources regarding identified or possible perpetrators, if any.

One essential trait of bioterrorism, then, is the degree of resemblance of a natural event. The perpetrator might be trying to emulate a natural occurrence—so as to mask his act—or might be indifferent in that respect. Being an artificial intervention, bioterrorism can rarely or scarcely initiate an infectious course that would otherwise take place naturally in the same way of appearance. Yet this incriminating disadvantage would in most cases remain uncertain owing to ambiguity, let alone events of innocent human intervention. To minimize that gray area, the mechanisms underlying natural epidemiological phenomena ought to be meticulously and thoroughly recognized. In general, they are rather gradually evolving, mostly unapparent, although their outcome may be abrupt and drastic, eventually. Acts of bioterrorism, even if looking similar in their resultant impact, lack the preceding evolving links that mark the natural apparatus. Of paramount importance, then, is the formation of a formulated, multifactorial epidemiological profile with respect to every infectious disease or toxin of special concern. This is particularly important regarding the deciphering of unexplained biological invasions of new pathogens, toxins or infected vectors/carriers.

A proper case study is the totally unexpected appearance of West Nile encephalitis (WNE) in New York City, which reflected, actually, a much broader and fundamental phenomenon, namely the introduction of a pathogen prevailing for long in the Eastern Hemisphere onto the Western Hemisphere (or vice versa). In that case, inherent difficulty emerged in both identifying the etiological agent and deciphering, later on, its provenance. Although a well-known disease in the Eastern Hemisphere, it was impossible, subjectively, to clinically identify, or even suspect, WNE. This means, instantly, that the inventory of diseases being looked into ought to be, *a priori*, perfectly global, even in terms of initial symptomatology. The term "exotic" (disease or pathogen)—hence less likely, ostensibly—largely loses its essence, therefore. As the primary suspicion was that of an arthropod-borne virus (arbovirus) encephalitis, early testing was directed at common eastern North-American arboviruses. The synchronic mortality of collocated birds could have been instrumental for postulating that the concerned virus is basically an avian pathogen. Early serologic testing displayed IgM antibodies against the St. Louis encephalitis virus by enzyme-linked immunosorbent assay, a basically correct finding that later turned to be misleading, showing a built-in limitation in identifying a pathogen new to a given locality.

Misdiagnosis is at times worse than lack of diagnosis, particularly with respect to infectious diseases, let alone in the context of epidemiological tracing intended to gauge bioterrorism-patterned events. Deliberate introduction of an encephalitic virus has been considered, among other possibilities, and has emerged to be more specific when it became clear that the etiological agent is WNE virus. It was a conjunction of three elements that propelled such assessment:

1. Information indicating that Iraq cultivated WNE virus as a biological agents.
2. An Iraqi intention to strike the United States by whatever means.
3. Ostensible infeasibility of WNE virus natural transfer from the Western to the Eastern Hemisphere.

Sensibly, however, the possibility of bioterrorism was not regarded to be a prime one, in this case. The probability of a natural or accidental event still appeared to be higher. Although the mechanism of the introduction of the WNE virus into North America remains unknown, it seems clear that the source of the WNE virus strain detected in New York City originated in the Middle East. A similar avian epizootic among domestic geese in Israel during 1997 and 1998 had been attributed to WNE virus. Human cases of WNE virus occurred simultaneously in Israel and New York in August 1999, and when the genomic sequences of WNE virus isolates or infected human brain tissue from the New York City outbreak were compared with various non-U.S. strains, the greatest homology was found with a WNE virus strain isolated from a goose from the Israeli 1998 epizootic and subsequently with a strain detected in the brain tissue of an Israeli patient who died of WNE in 1999. In addition, both the pattern of high avian mortality previously not associated with WNE virus outbreaks as well as the severity of human CNS disease seen in New York City and Israel were similar during the 1999 outbreaks. In between 1998 and 1999, this specific strain of WNE virus could have probably been harbored by certain migrating avian host species (transfected by mosquitoes) along an axis extending from the Western Hemisphere, through Greenland, and, later, onto New York.

Deliberate introduction or release of infected birds or mosquitos compatible with the above-described natural apparatus could be equally feasible, conceivably; yet certainly extremely sophisticated, somewhat beyond the expected capacity of a terror organization or even a terrorism-sponsoring state. On the other hand, the employment of a current epidemic strain of cholera, for instance, through introducing it into food supplies or water systems, even if conducted far away from an ongoing epidemic, could generate a wide outbreak that by all means may seem natural, resembling an infected traveler that innocently took a transcontinental flight. The chain of transmission in such cases is much simpler; hence, they are liable to be followed, untraceably, in the form of an act of bioterrorism. Furthermore, concentrating on AIDS and Ebola, an elaborated analysis inquired into those aspects, and aroused certain viewpoints that illustrate the significance of bioterrorism-patterned natural epidemics.

Notably, a recent outbreak of mumps (June 2006, Kansas)—a viral, often epidemic disease—is expected to help health officials prepare for an act of bioterrorism or a flu pandemic. The Kansas Health and Environment Department had found 761 confirmed or suspected cases of mumps around the state. In dealing with the outbreak, the department for the first time used its incident command system to spread information to agencies around the state. The same system would be used in the event of a natural or intentional disease outbreak.

Once the bioterrorism-employed pathogen has been introduced into the targeted site, the subsequent epidemiological featuring of the resultant events may expectedly be entirely futile, in terms of pointing to an act of bioterrorism, because those events would be shaped by whatever environmental, medical, and demographic circumstances prevailing at any rate in the targeted site. In the absence of direct evidence witnessing an act of bioterrorism, the only potentially incriminating indications can stem from the very specificity of the pathogenic strain involved, the particular manner of introduction, and the existence or lack of collateral factors such as natural vectors, carriers, or reservoirs, including natural abiotic vehicles, like rivers, of the pathogen in concern. Currently, the only fully reliable way to establish specificity is sequence analysis of both genomic and extragenomic DNA/RNA. This would be a necessary, yet usually insufficient, precondition/ prerequisite for deciphering the provenance of a pathogen used in an act of bioterrorism.

Therefore, diligent modeling is vital. Evaluating surveillance systems for the early detection of bioterrorism is particularly challenging when systems are designed to detect events for which there are few or no historical examples. One approach to benchmarking outbreak detection performance is to create semisynthetic data-sets containing authentic baseline patient data (noise) and injected artificial patient clusters, as signal. This useful pattern has very recently been developed.

It has thereby been pointed out, indeed, that doctors in training had difficulties diagnosing diseases associated with bioterrorism. The study involved 631 doctors, mostly medical residents—doctors still in training—in 30 internal medicine residency programs in 16 states and Washington, D.C.; it was found that half of the doctors surveyed misdiagnosed botulism, 84% misdiagnosed plague, and chickenpox was misdiagnosed as smallpox 42% of the time.

Yet beyond the clinical domain, various, at times crucial, gaps still prevailing within our overall knowledge about the biology of pathogens may play a significantly negative roll in that they can possibly bring about false incrimination or, inversely, false discrimination, referring to bioterrorism-resembling events. That is but one reason, even if a major one, for deepening our research and understanding of the essence and pronunciations of the complex mechanisms underlying the emergence and prognosis of infectious diseases. Mankind, at large, would expectedly endeavor to be most familiar with its prime extraneous foes, especially as their might is currently and steadily increasing.

Spectrum of Applicable Pathogens and Toxins

A general featuring of the spectrum of pathogens and toxins applicable for bioterrorism is given. Basic distinctions among various bioterrorism warfare agents, together with the implications they bear, are thereby presented. Basically, then, any epidemic pathogen may be regarded, potentially, as a candidate for carrying out a bioterrorism act, the germ causing plague, for example. To those agents should at any rate be added many nonepidemic—namely, incommunicable—pathogens, such as anthrax, and a large variety of toxins. The spectrum thus formed is in a way misleading in its amplitude. In actuality, a much narrower range of pathogens and toxins that may be used, practically, as weapons is notable, although but a marginal fraction, quantitatively, of the entire class of bacteria, viruses, fungi, and other infectious agents plus numerous different toxins found in nature. This being the case, their characteristics should meet, one way or another, at least part of the following fundamental criteria:

1. Infective/toxic and virulent.
2. Procurable or reproducible.
3. Conveyable and stable.
4. Introducible into the targeted area and people.

Still, the spectrum of agents applicable for bioterrorism acts is broader than those applicable for armed conflicts, due to the greater vulnerability and wider variety of civilian infrastructures that may be targeted. Qualitatively, however, this specific offense-oriented range of pathogens and toxins is marked by very potent and aggressive biological agents, some of which are extremely contagious and medically untreatable. Preferring, mostly justifiably, a comprehensive approach, the United Kingdom recently increased the number of biological agents that must be secured to ensure they are not obtained and used for acts of terrorism. The government boosted, thus, the number of restricted agents listed in the 2001 Antiterrorism, Crime and Security Act from 47 to 103. The list of controlled bioagents includes 45 viruses, 21 bacteria, 2 fungi, 13 toxins and 18 animal pathogens.

It seems, then, as if the most significant distinctions can be made between epidemic and nonepidemic agents, on the one hand, and, independently, between treatable and untreatable agents, on the other hand. Although the former distinction relates equally to bacterial and viral pathogens, the latter reflects a fundamental difference between those two major classes. Regardless of antisera, antiviral preparations are of limited efficacy, although they are expectedly being upgraded. Connectedly, within the sphere of toxins, the related spectrum may basically be divided into specifically treatable—protein toxins, hence may be coped by antitoxins—and specifically untreatable ones, which are otherwise chemically structured, like alkaloids. Vaccines, as prophylactic measures, are in principle efficient against viruses, bacteria, and protein toxins. At the same time, it would be insensible to refer to those distinctions as absolute categorizations, because some pathogens represent intermediaries, to a certain degree. Other distinctions such as between lethal and sublethal pathogens are rather artificial, although of course not meaningless. Influenza, as one example, is generally regarded as an incapacitating disease, while potentially much more virulent, in reality. A genuine distinction, obviously, is the one categorizing self-reproducing agents—hence a multiplying mass of weapon—as against unviable agents, meaning toxins. The former, if effectively applied, constitute an infectious apparatus that intensify itself; the latter rather resemble, in that sense, chemical warfare agents, bearing their own immense capacity.

Bacterial Agents

Varitype pathogenic germs may be used for bioterrorism purposes through different modes, and they are here represented by four entities: plague, brucellosis, Legionnaires disease, and tuberculosis. Their heterogeneity with respect to source of infection, impact, as well as short-, medium-, and long-term endurance is thereby accentuated. Within the context of bioterrorism, bacterial pathogens are signified for, foremost, by the germs responsible for the diseases of plague, anthrax, and alimentary tract infections (the latter group already typified above in the form of cholera). Other bacterial pathogens, such as those causing tularemia, brucellosis, glanders, Legionnaires disease, Klebsiella-associated pneumonia, and Q-fever, are of secondary—certainly not negligible—importance. A third category of potential microbial agents may be added, in case the perpetrator chooses to employ a slow-acting, scarcely traceable type of germ. Those three categories are here visited, then, through four representatives, namely, the causative agents of plague, Legionnaires disease, brucellosis, and tuberculosis. Anthrax is separately covered.

Plague

The plague bacterium is an old, salient foe to mankind. Posing three significantly different forms of an aggressive disease—bubonic, pneumonic, and septicemic plague—this germ is chiefly marked by two hosts, prior to man infection, namely rat and flee; hence, it can in principal be employed as a bioterrorism agent through each of those three modes, namely, inhalable air-borne bacteria, infected rats, or infected flees. Naturally, the humane plague cycle is usually initiated by the bite of a rodent flea or occasionally by the human flea. The bubonic plague is the common form, so called because of the buboes or swellings, which are the obvious visible symptom, communicated by flea bites and attacking the human lymphatic system. Simple bubonic plague may kill within 5 days, if antibiotic is not applied. It is regarded as the "true" or classic form of the disease. Pneumonic plague occurs when a victim develops pneumonia as a consequence of first getting the bubonic plague. The pneumonic variant occurs when the bacilli colonize the alveoli and cause latent suppurative pneumonia. This results in hemorrhagic sputum that can spread the disease via aerosolized droplets. In that case, the infection is then communicated by exhalation and affects the bronchial system of the next host directly. The pneumonic variant kills within 1-3 days. The third variant, the septicemic plague, is extremely rare and occurs where the bloodstream is directly affected raising the concentration of bacilli in the bloodstream to a level at which it can be transmitted directly by the human flea without passing through the intermediary host of the rat. This plague variant can kill within hours and explains contemporary accounts of people who went to bed apparently well and when they awoke in the morning they were, like the biblical Assyrians (also victims of a god-sent plague), all dead men.

The bubonic form of the plague is the one most widely described by chroniclers and, contrary to popular belief, can be survived, especially if the buboes burst or are lanced, although this was not understood at the time. Both the pneumonic and the septicemic varieties were fulminant and 100% lethal. The pneumonic variety, however, could be transmitted only by close human contact, in the same way as influenza today, but it accounted for the high mortality among monks, priests, and others tending to the dying, putting their faces close to the patient. As those infected in this way were unlikely to get far in the period between infection and death, the pneumonic plague remained localized within families and communities, for example, monasteries where it could spread like wildfire. Henry of Knighton, a regular Canon in the Abbey at Leicester and opponent of the Franciscan Order, reported the death of the entire population of 150 Friars in a Franciscan monastery in Marseilles, adding as a malicious afterthought, a good thing too. The bubonic version also kills its hosts, but more slowly, especially in the case of the flea that can survive dormant for weeks, even months, in the goods of a traveling merchant. The causative agent, *Yersinia pestis*, will, however, die off when it has itself killed off all accessible and susceptible hosts, whether human, rat, or flea. To sustain itself the bacillus must find a host that is not affected by it or that reproduces faster than the bacillus can kill the host.

Legionnaires Disease (Legionellosis)

The particular significance of *Legionalla* sp. as a human pathogen was not recognized until 1976, when a mysterious epidemic of pneumonia struck members of the Pennsylvania American Legion. Indeed, the most common presentation of *Legionella pneumophila* is acute pneumonia (legionellosis); potentially any species (about 40, allover) of *Legionella* may cause the disease. Extrapulmonary disease (e.g., pericarditis and endocarditis) is rare. Less often, the disease presents as a nonpneumonic epidemic, influenza-like illness called Pontiac fever.

Remarkably, *Legionella* bacilli are primarily waterborne. They reside in surface and drinking water and are usually transmitted to humans in watery aerosols. The pathogenesis of *Legionella* infections begins with a supply of water containing virulent bacteria and with a means for dissemination to humans. Person-to-person transmission has never been observed, and *Legionella* is not a member of the bacterial flora of humans. Infection starts in the lower respiratory tract. Alveolar macrophages, which are the primary defense against bacterial infection of the lungs, engulf the bacteria; however, *Legionella* is, unlike most bacterial pathogens, a facultative intracellular parasite and multiplies freely in alveolar macrophages. Recruited neutrophils and monocytes, as well as bacterial enzymes, produce destructive alveolar inflammation. Direct inoculation of surgical wounds by contaminated tap water has been described.

In most cases, the initial infective link is an aerosol of water contaminated with the organisms. Evaporative condensers and cooling towers are proven sources of outdoor infection. Indoors, nebulizers, and humidifiers filled with contaminated drinking water have disseminated *Legionella* to susceptible patients. The automatic misting devices that keep supermarket produce fresh have even been fingered as culprits in outbreaks of pneumonia. Notably, aerosols are produced in numerous ways in our environment, from taking a shower to flushing the toilet. An epidemic of Pontiac fever caused by *Legionella anisa* was associated with an ornamental fountain in a public place. Clusters of *Legionella* pneumonia have occurred after exposure to whirlpool spas in hotels or cruise ships. In most cases, the source of the infection remains unknown. Direct infection of surgical wounds has been linked to washing of patients with tap water that harbored pathogenic *Legionella* organisms.

Legionella infections may be sporadic or epidemic, community acquired, or nosocomial. There is great geographic variation in the frequency of infection even within communities, presumably reflecting the presence of suitable aquatic environments and susceptible subjects. Both sporadic and epidemic cases are more common during summer than winter months, apparently because of increased use of air-cooling equipment that generates aerosols. As a bioterrorism agent, this prominent bacterium is prone to be applied, then, in both water sources and air circulating systems.

Brucellosis

Brucellosis represents a narrow, uniquely significant category of diseases combining proximate and lingering effects altogether. This clinical profile may meet, then, certain needs of both short- and long-term warfare. In the short run, it is featured by an acute phase. After a relatively long and variable incubation period (1–8 weeks), it most often manifests as an acute bacteremic disease, and it may be complicated by secondary hematogenous localization in almost every organ. Inversely, chronic brucellosis is defined as a disease evolving for more than a year, without evident secondary localization. During asymptomatic infection, the pathogen is sequestered in lymphoid tissues, bone, and liver. It would tend to persist for many years, at times in a steadily debilitating incurable state. Four bacterial species are responsible for human brucellosis: *Brucella suis* (from pigs; high pathogenicity), *Brucella melitensis* (from sheep; highest pathogenicity), *Brucella abortus* (from cattle; moderate pathogenicity), and *Brucella canis* (from dogs; moderate pathogenicity). Many animals are potential reservoirs for various *Brucella* species.

Epidemiologically, brucellosis is a zoonotic infection transmitted from animals to humans by ingestion of infected food products (milk and dairy products are the main sources for human contamination), direct contact with an infected animal, or inhalation of aerosols. This last mode of transmission is remarkably efficient given the relatively low concentration of organisms (as few as 10–100 bacteria) needed to establish infection in humans and has brought renewed attention to this old disease. Descriptions of the disease date back to the days of Hippocrates, although the organism was not isolated until 1887, when British Army physician David Bruce isolated the organism that bears his name from the spleens of five patients with fatal cases on Malta. The disease gets its additional names from both its course (undulant fever) and location (Malta fever, Crimean fever).

Given the ease of effectiveness of aerosol transmission of *Brucella* species, researchers attempted to develop it into a biological weapon beginning in 1942. In 1954, it became the first agent weaponized by the old U.S. offensive biological weapons program. Field testing on animals soon followed. By 1955, the United States was producing *B suis*-filled cluster bombs for the U.S. Air Force at the Pine Bluff Arsenal in Arkansas. Not much later, it was weaponized and standardizes by the USSR. The pathogen may meet both large-scale and guerilla warfare purposes.

Tuberculosis (TB)

Although AIDS represents an attritional viral disease, as described, tuberculosis is, in parallel, a bacterial disease of a long-lasting debilitating course, both individually and demographically. Migration of contagion within community and the course of the disease in itself are very clumsy, yet consistent, aided by fortified stability toward antibacterial drugs. A staggering 1.9 million around the globe die of tuberculosis each year—another 1.9 billion are infected with the causative agent, *Mycobacterium tuberculosis*, and are at risk for active disease. It's sobering to realize that this ancient scourge, which has been found in 2000-year-old mummies (but much earlier evolved), remains a severe global health threat despite modern medicine. In fact, TB is a leading infectious disease killer in the world, alongside AIDS and malaria.

Millions of people—fully one third of the world's population—are infected with TB. Five to 10% of those will develop the active disease, for reasons only partially understood. This is, certainly, a key trait. The bacteria can lie dormant for many years and become active when the host is weakened by factors such as stress, poor nutrition, diabetes, or HIV infection. Once active, TB destroys tissue in the lungs and becomes contagious. Because it is airborne, there is little that can be done to protect against infection.

Antibiotics and public health measures failed to wipe out TB, although until the mid-1980s its rates had been brought very low, even in the developed world. Then the TB bacteria acquired immunity to many drugs, spreading rapidly among homeless people, AIDS patients, and other vulnerable groups worldwide. Several drugs can cure TB, but only if they are taken for many months. With abbreviated treatment, bacteria that have evolved ways of evading the drugs can escape eradication and proliferate as a resistant strain. Then, even when treated with the strongest drugs for 2 years, the resistant TB is fatal about 60% of the time.

Russian prisons are a major source of multidrug-resistant TB. As tens of thousands of infected inmates reenter the civilian world every year, TB spreads when they cough and sneeze. Some experts fear that with the speed and frequency of modern travel, the resistant epidemic could spread to Europe and the United States. To counter the threat of a worldwide epidemic, the costly second-line drugs are supplied, and prison health workers are being helped to ensure that infected inmates take their entire course of drugs—even if it means the prisoners have to remain in confinement for up to 2 years past the start of treatment.

In 2005, in Japan, the Tuberculosis Prevention Law was set to be abolished so that bacteria that cause the disease can be included in counterterrorism regulations in an updated Infectious Disease. The Tuberculosis Prevention Law does not contain counterterrorism pro visions or regulations requiring the quick investigation of an epidemic. The change is aimed at restricting transfer of the disease (alongside with other ones), allowing inspections, and requiring registration of ownership of samples. The bacterium causing TB is regarded, in a sense, as an attritional bioterrorism agent.

Viral Agents

In addition to the viruses mentioned above, some other viral pathogens are noticeable, of which several are profiled herewith as varitype representatives: Rift Valley fever, yellow fever, Norwalk, and hepatitis A. The smallpox virus is presented later. Notably, the handling of viruses is much more complicated then that of bacteria; hence, it is less likely to be mastered by terrorist organizations, individuals, or perpetrators, with reference being made to the viruses mentioned below as well as others.

Rift Valley Fever (RVF)

The RVF virus typically represents a zoonotic hemorrhagic pathogen equally potent against man as well as various mammalian farm animals (such as cattle, buffalo, sheep, goats, and camels). For viruses, this wide spectrum featuring is rare, making this pathogen a biological agent of appreciable uniqueness. This trait characteristically found expression in the late 1970s, in Egypt. After an initial epizootic of RVF in Egypt in 1971, the first recorded epidemic of RVF in Egypt, in 1977–1980, inflicted an estimated 200,000 human cases, with some 600 reported deaths, plus enormous losses of farm animals. An epidemic of the disease occurred again in Egypt in 1993. RVF virus is naturally a mosquito-borne pathogen, but it is adequately infective in the form of an air-borne aerosol, making it a biological agent applicable through those two modes. It is found in the Old World only, principally in Africa. In September 2000, an RVF outbreak was reported in Saudi Arabia and subsequently Yemen. These cases represent the first RVF cases identified outside Africa. Fortunately, it is not carried by migrating birds, as is the case with many other arboviruses (including the parallel mosquito-borne West Nile virus) and with influenza A virus. RVF virus, then, is basically a geographically slowly crawling virus of notable potentiality, particularly with respect to tropical and subtropical regions. It may be employed as a bioterrorism agent in the context of both antihuman bioterrorism as well as agroterrorism. Basically a mosquito-dependent tropical virus, it could doubtfully colonize temperate regions, however.

RVF is generally observed during years in which unusually heavy rainfall and localized flooding occur. The excessive rainfall allows mosquito eggs, usually of the genus *Aedes*, to hatch. The mosquito eggs are naturally infected with the RVF virus, and the resulting mosquitoes transfer the virus to the livestock on which they feed. Once the livestock is infected, other species of mosquitoes can become infected from the animals and can spread the disease among other hosts, including man.

Yellow Fever

The Yellow Fever virus is another mosquito-borne pathogen, in that case affecting both man and primates. In the past, it was mass-accumulated as a biological weapon, in the form of infected mosquitoes, by the U.S. Army. Although somewhat complex, this is an effective way of employing this virus as a weapon either through guerilla or apparent warfare. It so happened that this standardized weapon-form resembled and reestablished the first human virus ever isolated. It was in 1901 that the pathogen causing yellow fever was proved to be a filterable virus carried by mosquitoes.

Yellow fever is a viral hemorrhagic fever. There are three types of transmission cycle: sylvatic (or jungle), intermediate, and urban. All three cycles exist in Africa, but in South America, only sylvatic and urban yellow fever occur. Sylvatic yellow fever occurs in tropical rainforests where monkeys, infected by sylvatic mosquitoes, pass the virus onto other mosquitoes that feed on them; these mosquitoes, in turn, bite and infect humans entering the forest. This produces sporadic cases, the majority of which are often young men working in the forest, e.g., logging.

On occasion, the virus spreads beyond the affected individual. The intermediate cycle of yellow fever transmission occurs in humid or semi-humid savannahs of Africa and can produce small-scale epidemics in rural villages. Semi-domestic mosquitoes infect both monkey and human hosts and increased contact between man and infected mosquito leads to disease. This is the most common type of outbreak observed in recent decades in Africa. Urban yellow fever results in large explosive epidemics when travelers from rural areas introduce the virus into areas with high human population density. Domestic mosquitoes, most notably *Aedes aegypti*, carry the virus from person to person. These outbreaks tend to spread outward from one source to cover a wide area.

Norwalk

The Norwalk virus is an enterovirus with pronounced eco-epidemiological traits. It causes acute gastroenteritis with nausea, vomiting, fever, and myalgia that lasts 24–48 hours. The virus is transmitted through fecal-oral contact. The Norwalk virus is well established as the chief cause of viral gastroenteritis epidemics. The disease occurs throughout the year without a seasonal predominance. Norwalk virus was first associated with gastroenteritis in 1972. For a long time, it was an unnoticed, although extremely important, pathogen. It was identified by electron microscopy of stool samples that had been saved from a 1968 gastroenteritis epidemic that occurred in Norwalk, Ohio. In a 2-day period, acute gastroenteritis developed in 50% of 232 students or teachers in an elementary school. The virus initially was labeled as a small, round, structured virus, and it was named after the city in which the outbreak occurred. The virus is transmitted through contaminated food, water, or infected contacts. After ingestion, the virus infects the mucosa of the proximal small intestine, damages microvilli, and causes mal absorption. Although no histopathological lesions can be found in the stomach mucosa, the virus causes abnormal gastric motility and delayed gastric emptying.

In the United States, the Norwalk virus is estimated to cause approximately 40% of cases of nonbacterial gastroenteritis. The Norwalk virus is, then, the leading cause of viral gastroenteritis in the United States. January 1, 2002, to December 2, 2002: Norwalk virus was attributed to 9 of the 21 outbreaks of acute gastroenteritis on cruise ships reported to the U.S. Centers for Disease Control and Prevention's Vessel Sanitation Program in this time period. The Norwalk virus brings about approximately 23 million cases of acute gastroenteritis each year and is the major cause of outbreaks of gastroenteritis. An extensive outbreak has been recorded in Europe (Finland). As a bioterrorism weapon, this enterovirus is a typical incapacitating agent.

Hepatitis A

Inversely a water/food-borne virus of a relatively long incubation period (several weeks) and a causative agent of a lingering incapacitating infectious disease, hepatitis A virus (HAV), has been intended mainly for attrition warfare purposes and has apparently been employed by the Soviet army in Afghanistan, through contaminating water or food sources. Also, hepatitis A virus is reported to have been studied as a possible bioterrorism agent by South Africa.

Infectious hepatitis caused by HAV is common worldwide and is usually spread as a result of poor personal hygiene and can be a problem in day care centers, refugee camps, and among troops in the field. The virus is hardy and can withstand relatively harsh chemical treatments and can survive outside the body for days. It attacks humans only, invading the liver and generating, hence, a systemic debilitating illness.

The disease has an incubation period that is relatively long for a biological weapon at 3–4 weeks, but the onset of the disease is abrupt and victims become exhausted and develop jaundice as their livers lose function. Victims typically take about 10 weeks to recover. The disease is rarely fatal, and victims have lifelong immunity. Overall, hepatitis A virus may be regarded, then, as a representative of a class of water/food borne antihuman viruses, in that case, a pathogen of a rather attritional nature. Lasting for more than 3 months, the entire course of the virus since contracted by a victim produces a fairly chronic infection.

Toxins

Overall, about 400 toxins have been identified, which are certainly but a small proportion of what is actually found in nature. Out of this remarkable inventory, several are reckoned as typical bioterrorism agents. Presented here are few prominent toxins: two protein toxins (botulinum and SEB)—hence detectible and treatable by anti-toxins—and three non-protein toxins (T-2 toxin, aflatoxin and aconitine), hence hardly detectable or treatable by antidotes. Etiological diagnosis of toxins is often extremely complicated.

The realm of toxins is a very wide one. Those microbial, fungal, plant, and animal biomolecules exhibit an unthinkably diversified inventory of natural substances, all poisonous toward man, by definition. They are extremely variable chemically and physically. But dosage plays a cardinal role, both in terms of its great differential among toxins, as well as the delicate transition onto the tangential domain of toxin-based pharmacological applications. Moreover, most usable for man—as proteins, chiefly—in preparing toxoids and antisera, toxins are inwardly inert—sometimes rather immensely beneficial—within their own toxinogenic biosystem, or extremely poisonous, outwardly, as natural toxicants. Fundamentally, they constitute the pristine form of biochemical warfare in nature, much earlier to the emergence of mankind. Thus, for instance, Hydrogen cyanide, reckoned as a classical chemical warfare agent, is found in various toxic plants, thereby equipping them with a powerful poison.

Overall, about 400 toxins have been identified, which are certainly but a small proportion of what is actually found in nature. They include, however, bacterial toxins-49; plant-36; fungal-26; algal-22; (other) marine organism-111; snake-124; insect-22; amphibian-5; and in total-395. Out of this remarkable inventory, several are reckoned as typical bioterrorism warfare agents. Presented here are few prominent toxins: two protein toxins (botulinum and SEB)—hence detectible and treatable by antitoxins—and three nonprotein toxins (T-2 toxin, aflatoxin, and aconitine), which are hardly detectable and treatable by antidotes. Ricin, an outstanding bioterrorism toxin on its own, is covered separately. Other notable toxins, such as tetradotoxin, saxitoxin, mamba toxin, and many others are not discussed, although certainly potential candidates for bioterrorism tasks, particularly state-sponsored ones. Mamba toxin, as one example, has been developed as a weapon in South Africa. Also, various plant and fungal psychotoxins—part of which constitute important psychopharmacological agens—have in some countries been exploited experimentally, to the least, as a major means to attain compelled mind control over normal human beings—an act of governance regardable as bioterrorism.

Botulinum Toxin

Botulism toxin, a bacterial protein, is reputed as the most known toxic molecule. It is produced by *Clostridium botulinum*, a gram-positive spore-forming anaerobe germ that dwells in the soil. There are 7 different antigenic types of this toxin: A through G. Disease in humans is caused by types A, B, E, or F. Aerosol exposure studies in rhesus monkeys indicate that type F is the most toxic and that it is 60× more toxic than type B, the least toxic. Extrapolations from primate studies predict that the fatal dose of Botulinum toxin in humans is on the order of:

1. 70 μg by mouth
2. 0.7–0.9 μg via the respiratory route
3. 0.09 μg by intravenous or intramuscular routes

The toxin is a 150-kDa zinc-dependent metalloproteinase that cleaves proteins involved in the docking and fusion of synaptic vesicles to the membrane at the neuromuscular junction. The toxin consists of two chains: a heavy chain (100 kDa) and a light chain (50 kDa) linked by a disulfide bond. The crystal structure of the molecule has been solved to 3.3-A resolution. The protein structure revealed a 50-residue belt that partially obscures the active site access channel; the authors note that this unusual feature makes rational inhibitor design more difficult.

The deadly toxin irreversibly blocks acetylcholine release from peripheral nerves resulting in muscle paralysis. It has been developed as a biological weapon by many government research programs, including the United States, Russia, and Iraq. Currently, public health services classifies botulinum toxin as a Category A Bioterrorism Agent, indicating that it is a high-priority risk to public health. As a bioterrorism weapon, it is a potent substance that is easy to produce and transport. A large population of victims requiring intensive care could easily overwhelm health-care systems. It can be introduced into the food and water supply or be aerosolized. The toxin is unstable after a few days in surface water, and it cannot withstand chlorine treatment. Although it is more stable in packaged foods, it is inactivated by normal cooking practices (heat > 85°). Aerosolization is technically difficult but would bring about the poisoning of a large number of people. At the conclusion of the Gulf War, the Iraqis reported that they produced 19,000 L of pure botulinum toxin to a UN team. A total of 19,000 L of botulinum toxin is estimated, just arithmetically, to be sufficient to kill three times the current human population by inhalation. Overall, 10,000 L of the toxin had been loaded into weapons. They loaded botulinum toxin into thirteen 600-km missiles and one hundred 400-lb bombs. Some of the toxin has not been accounted for. The JAMA consensus statement points out that it is "note worthy that Iraq chose to weaponize more botulinum toxin than any other of its known *biological agents.*"

Incubation times vary according to the amount of toxin ingested and the toxin type. The range reported from natural infections is between 6 hours and 10 days. Symptoms most commonly present between 12 and 36 hours of eating contaminated food. Inhalational exposures are predicted to progress more rapidly. Regardless of the route of intoxication, the neurological symptoms are similar. Gastrointestinal cases may also display nausea and vomiting. Botulinum toxicity presents as a febrile, descending paralysis. In cases of severe exposure, it is possible that respiratory failure will occur suddenly. Without treatment, the cause of death is respiratory failure due to obstruction from the pharyngeal muscles and failure of the diaphragm to move adequate volumes of air.

The standardized antitoxin is equine in origin, and of high efficacy, provided that it is administrated quite early. When treatment is administered promptly, the risk of death is significantly decreased. In the past 50 years, the mortality has decreased from 50% to 8%. It is important to note that the antitoxin prevents worsening of the condition, but recovery may not occur until after several weeks to months of intensive care. Complications such as long-lasting weakness, aspiration pneumonia, and nervous system dysfunction may occur. This would at any rate make botulinum toxin a deadly and/or medium-term debilitating agent. The toxoid is highly efficient as prophylaxis.

Most experts predict that a terrorist attack with botulinum toxin would attempt to distribute the agent via aerosolization to intoxicate the largest number of people. The toxin does not survive long in the water supply. In fact, there are no reported cases of water-transmitted botulism. The food supply is at some risk, but the agent can be inactivated by food preparation. Weapons programs, such as the one in Iraq, have demonstrated that it is not difficult to produce and store large amounts of concentrated toxin.

Staphylococcal Enterotoxin B (SEB)

One of seven staphylococcal enterotoxins, this bacterial protein is the best studied potential bioterrorism weapon of a group of molecules described as superantigens; others include two streptococcal pyrogenic toxins, and the toxic shock syndrome toxin. Superantigens create stable bonds across class II molecules of major histocompatibility complex (MHC) and specific variable (Vβ) T-cell receptors on TH cells, causing a release of disease-producing cytokines. Naturally, SEB intoxication occurs due to consumption of contaminated foods or drinks. SEB may be aerosolized or used to sabotage food supplies. As a weapon it would induce substantial, prolonged morbidity (up to 2 weeks) with little mortality.

From 1 to 6 hours after aerosol exposure to SEB, a distinct syndrome of high fever, chills, myalgias, nonproductive cough, dyspnea, and severe substernal chest pain may appear. Headache is also common, and nausea, vomiting, and anorexia may occur. Illness usually lasts for a few days, but it is rarely fatal. Physical examination may be unremarkable or reveal inspiratory and/or expiratory rales. After SEB ingestion, symptoms are primarily vomiting and diarrhea; fever only occurs in about one quarter of ill persons and respiratory involvement is absent. Although symptoms may be quite severe and lead to dehydration or even shock, illness usually lasts less than 12 hours. Physical examination may be unremarkable or reveal inspiratory and/or expiratory rales. Were Toxic shock syndrome toxin-1 (TSST-1) or streptococcal pyrogenic exotins to be used, they would likely cause acute erythroderma followed by desquamation and multiorgan failure. Differential diagnosis is complicated by many other diseases. Yet although toxin is transient in serum, it accumulates in the urine and is detectable for several hours postexposure. Antibodies generally develop within 6 days of exposure. SEB, a very potent and enduring protein toxin, was included in the past U.S. BW program and standardized as a powerful biological warfare agent. Although reckoned to be an effectual incapacitating agent, it has not been connected, so far, with terror organizations.

T-2 Toxin

The Soviet military discovered—and later on materialiged—the potential use of the fungal trichothecene toxins—chiefly T-2 toxin—as aggressive bioterrorism agents shortly after World War II, when many Russian civilians ate bread baked from flour, naturally contaminated with extremely toxinogenic species of *Fusarium* mold. During this vast epidemic, numerous victims developed a protracted lethal illness characterized by initial symptoms of abdominal pain, diarrhea, vomiting, and exhaustion followed within days by fever, chills, muscular pain, and an imbalance of the red and white blood cells accompanied by pus-forming or other disease-causing organisms or their toxins in the blood or tissues. It was then named Alimentary Toxic Aleucia. The trichothecene mycotoxins are nonvolatile compounds produced by molds. They are very stable and resist heat- and ultraviolet light-induced inactivation. Only after heating at 500°F for 30 minutes will the toxins inactivate.

This discussion focuses on the hemorrhagic T-2 mycotoxin, a highly toxic agent that causes several illnesses in humans and animals, as described. From the 1970s and 1980s, trichothecene mycotoxins surfaced in the press as bioterrorism warfare agents in incidents labeled "*yellow rain*" attacks against civilians in Southeast Asia. Although such attacks have not been verified officially, it has been observed that trichothecene mycotoxins, T-2 in particular, have been produced in the USSR, weaponized, transferred to North Vietnam, and employed by North Vietnamese airplanes. The impact was vast and terrorizing, owing to many civilians that were vulnerably exposed, and then suffered a prolonged course of conspicuous pathological effects, with high mortality rate. Somehow, the evident employment of trichothecene mycotoxins in Southeast Asia, destined for bioterrorism—as well as live human field experimentation—purposes, turned into a saga involving alternative, natural explanations for the "*yellow rain*" phenomenon, which are certainly legitimate but do not refute the coexistence of the two—vicious and naive—occurrences.

Reportedly, the Egyptian Air Force employed trichothecene mycotoxins during the Yemen War (in the 1960s) against Yemenis civilians—the main impact being terrorizing. Later on, the Iraqi Air Force allegedly employed trichothecene mycotoxins against Iranian soldiers during the Iraq-Iran War in 1984. According to UNSCOM, the Iraqis researched trichothecene mycotoxins, including T-2; they probably weaponized the T-2 toxin.

Unlike most biotoxins and microorganisms that do not affect the skin, T-2 toxin is an aggresive dermal irritant and can severely harm an unprotected person's skin and eyes. The pain associated with the exposure occurs within seconds to minutes. Larger doses produce incapacitation and death within minutes to hours. A larger amount of T-2 toxin is required for a lethal dose than of the chemical warfare agents VX, soman, or sarin. Comparisons with blister agents such as sulfur mustard show the T-2 toxin is about 400 times more efficient in producing blisters: It takes approximately 50 ng of T-2 toxin to produce the same injury to the skin as 20 μg (20,000 ng) of mustard. The T-2 toxin has a diverse effect depending on the manner and amount of exposure with vomiting and diarrhea noted at exposure doses one fifth to one tenth the lethal dose.

Exposure causes skin pain, itching, redness, blisters, and sloughing (shedding) of dead skin. Effects on the airway include nose and throat pain, nasal discharge, itching and sneezing, cough, shortness of breath, wheezing, and chest pain; the victim spits blood as a result of pulmonary or bronchial hemorrhage. The T-2 toxin also produces effects after ingestion or eye contact. Severe poisoning results in prostration, weakness, jerky movement, collapse, shock, and death. The only protection against T-2 toxin effects is the individual protective mask and chemical protective overgarment. No chemotherapy, vaccine, or specific antidote is available. Altogether, the trichothecene mycotoxins are reckoned as primarily blister agents that, at lower exposure concentrations, would cause extreme skin and eye irritation, and at larger doses would produce considerable incapacitation and death within minutes to hours.

Aflatoxin

As a public health hazard, the major routes for aflatoxin exposure are inhalation, pulmonary mycotoxicosis, especially of grain dusts, and ingestion as a result of eating food made with contaminated grains. The aflatoxin problem was first recognized in 1960, when there was a severe outbreak of a disease referred to as "Turkey 'X' Disease" in the United Kingdom, in which over 100,000 turkey poults died. The cause of the disease was due to toxins in peanut meal infected with *Aspergillus flavus*, and the toxins were called aflatoxins. The potentialities of aflatoxins as toxic carcinogens, mutagens, teratogens, and immunosuppressive agents are well documented [58]. They are produced as secondary metabolites by the fungus *Aspergillus flavus* and *A. parasiticus* on a variety of food products. Chemically, aflatoxins normally refer to the group of difuranocoumarins.

Two forms of illness have been observed:

1. (Primary) Acute aflatoxicosis is produced when moderate-to-high levels of aflatoxins are consumed. Specific, acute episodes of disease may include hemorrhage, acute liver damage, edema, alteration in digestion, absorption and/or metabolism of nutrients, and possibly death.
2. (Primary) Chronic aflatoxicosis results from ingestion of low-to-moderate levels of aflatoxins. The effects are usually subclinical and difficult to recognize. Some common symptoms are impaired food conversion and slower rates of growth with or without the production of an overt aflatoxin syndrome. In the long term, exposure to aflatoxin is thought to explain the high rates of primary liver cancer in Africa and parts of Asia. Pooled data from Kenya, Mozambique, Swaziland, and Thailand show a positive correlation between daily dietary aflatoxin intake (in the range of 3.5- to 222.4-ng/kg body weight per day) and the crude incidence rate of primary liver cancer (ranging from 1.2 to 13.0 cases per 100,000 people per year).

Iraq developed and weaponized aflatoxins, chiefly as a bioterrorism agent. It has then been noted that "The discovery (by UNSCOM, during the 90s) that Iraq was researching aflatoxin, not a traditional BW candidate, was a cause for some surprise. It is a carcinogen, the effects of which manifest themselves only after many years, and several Western experts have rationalized this Iraqi program only in terms of genocidal goals. If aflatoxin were used against the Kurds, for instance, it would be impossible definitively to prove the use of BW once the symptoms emerged. Another possible explanation is its potential use as an immune suppressant, making victims more susceptible to other agents. However, the aflatoxin declaration may also hide other aspects of Iraq's BW program: according to Iraq's depositions, the production program never encountered any mishap (as other parts of the BW program had) and, to judge from the declared time-frame for the total amount produced, production could never have stopped, even for cleaning of the equipment. This raises the suspicion that Iraq declared an excessive amount of aflatoxin in order to disguise the fact that other, more destructive agents had been produced in greater quantities."

Iraq developed and produced aflatoxin as a long-term debilitating bioterrorism agent, intended to be used against the Kurds. There is documentary evidence and statements obtained by UNSCOM that Iraq was mixing aflatoxin with riot-control gas. Although seemingly peculiar, some rational can be figured out regarding this type of weaponization.

Aconitine

This relatively unnoticed plant toxin is an intensely poisonous alkaloid obtained from aconite root. It occurs in colorless crystals. Aconite tubers are most toxic wild plants distributed from Asia to western Europe. It achieved some notoriety in the nineteenth century as an agent for homicides and suicides. In modern times, aconite has been used as Chinese herbal medicine, which is freely purchased from herb shops and consumed as a doctation by a herbal practitioner for pain control in the Northern Hemisphere. In Japan, some cases of aconite poisoning appeared as a result of committing suicide or accidental ingestion, which were mistaken for edible grass. However, aconite alkaloids have the potential for serious and even fatal cardiotoxity, which management has continued to fail save patients with therapeutic resistant fatal arrhythmia.

Serious aconitine poisoning is characterized by hypotension, palpitations, shock, delay in myocardial conduction, and dysrhythmia beginning within 6 hours of ingestion. Respiration is progressively depressed by the effect of aconitine on the bulbar respiratory center. Tingling of the tongue, mouth, and skin, followed by numbness and anesthesia, are characteristic signs of aconitine poisoning. Excessive salivation is a characteristic sign of poisoning. The skin becomes cold, clammy, sweaty, and pale. Initial bradycardia is due to vagal stimulation. Soon after ingestion, aconite causes a tingling, burning sensation on the lips, tongue, mouth, and throat, which is followed by numbness and constriction of the throat. When applied to the skin, aconite causes a tingling sensation and then numbness. Blurring of vision occurs. Initial miosis is followed by mydriasis. There is a feeling of constriction in the throat.

According to some reports, Egyptian Armed Forces Commander-in-Chief Field Marshall Mohammed Abd el Hakim Amer, who headed the defeated Egyptian Army in the 1967 Six Days War, was later poisoned, institutionally, by this substance. Allegedly, he committed suicide by means of aconitine that had been introduced to him while arrested. An unidentified toxicant, possibly the same plant toxin, was used to replace the antidote with which Egyptian autoinjectors were filled, for personal assassinations.

Another trivial, yet peculiar episode, involved an English doctor who used aconitine to murder his crippled 18-year-old nephew for his inheritance. Percy Malcolm John was a resident at Blenheim School in Wimbledon and owned a small property that would go to his uncle on his death. Lamson visited the boy, bringing a cake and a capsule that he said was medicine. A few hours later he died in agony from aconitine poisoning. Reportedly, aconitine toxin has been adopted by some states for assassination purposes.

Availability of Infective Agents and Toxins

A broad spectrum of availability of pathogens and toxins is discussed, especially pertaining to potential resources worldwide. Still, the spectrum is much narrower regarding weaponized agents, making the course of the attacker complicated, unless "raw" infective agents or toxins are to be employed. Different episodes illustrating that variability are presented. The common nonstate-sponsored scenario of a just-graduated microbiologist cultivating a pathogenic germ in a rudimentary household laboratory, so as to produce it as a weapon for bioterrorism acts, is partially feasible. It is much less likely with regard to weaponizing or engineering bioterrorism agents. A significant advantage emerges concerning state-sponsored bioterrorism, because the relevant pathogens and toxins are appreciably more procurable, reproducible, and conveyable for a state, generally speaking. Therefore, the inventory of agents, their handling and the feasibility of conducting bioterrorism are scaled up when a state is involved, either intending to carry out an act of bioterrorism on its own or to assist a terror organization. Any step made by a country may basically be institutionalized, hence be more legitimate compared with an unaffiliated or noninstitutionalized body, element, or person.

Overall, the wide range of bioterrorism agents is reflected by considerably varying degrees of availability. Ricin toxin can readily be produced, roughly, by unqualified saboteurs. Conversely, an expedient way to meet the need for high-leveled know-how often faced by terror organizations would be in the form of "*scientific mercenaries.*" At large, varitype availability of pathogens and toxins is demonstrated though the following episodes.

In Japan, in 1965, outbreaks of typhoid and dysentery were intentionally induced by a local bacteriologist, with professional direct access to those germs. In 1972 two men affiliated with the U.S. group "Order of the Rising Sun," who eventually fled to Cuba, had conspired to contaminate the water supplies of some large U.S. Midwestern cities with stocks of typhoid fever germs cultivated by one of them. Up to 40 kg of bacteria cultures were found in a college laboratory.

In 1973, the American leftist terrorist group, the Weather Underground, reportedly attempted to blackmail a homosexual officer at USAMRIID into supplying organisms that would be used to contaminate municipal water supplies in the United States. The plot was discovered when the officer requested several items "unrelated to his work."

In 1975, the Symbionese Liberation Army was found in possession of technical manuals on how to produce bioterrorism weapons. Moving to Europe, in 1980, police raided a German Red Army Faction apartment in Paris and found a miniature laboratory containing a culture medium of the germ that produces botulinum toxin. Notes about bacteria-induced diseases were found in the apartment as well. Once again in Europe, several Muslim terrorists affiliated with the Algerian "Armed Muslim Group" were arrested in Belgium, holding a lot of information about biological (and chemical) weapons and about the World Cup football games.

Outstandingly, protesters claimed to have taken infected soil from the Scottish island of Gruinard and placed it at the Microbiological Defence Establishment at Porton Down, Britain. The island has been closed to the public since germ warfare experiments on sheep were conducted there in 1941. The anthrax spores used in the experiments can remain dangerous for decades.

The American Type Culture Collection (ATCC) has often been approached. Two Canadians attempted to procure botulinum and tetanus cultures from the ATCC. Reportedly the first phone order, of less deadly cultures, was fulfilled, and it was not until the second order that ATCC employees became sufficiently suspicious to notify authorities.

A member of the white supremacist Aryan Nation acquired freeze-dried bubonic plague bacteria from the ATCC. In May 1995, in the United States, Larry Wayne Harris was arrested for illegally obtaining the plague bacteria *Yersinia pestis*. Using his previous employer's certification, Harris obtained the samples through the mail from the ATCC. He was sentenced to 18 months probation and 200 hours of community service. Harris was again arrested in 1998 when he and another individual were found allegedly in possession of anthrax cultures, which were later determined to be anthrax vaccine. Due to the ease of obtaining dangerous pathogens, the CDC established rigorous guidelines for shipment of specific pathogens that may be used as bioterrorism agents.

Yet, as a matter of fact, a wide variety of pathogens and toxins serving the Iraqi BW program during the 198 0s has been freely procured from different Western and Eastern sources, mostly the ATCC. The Iraqi case study provides remarkable demonstration, indeed, of repeated procurements of highly dangerous pathogens and toxins that readily took place albeit an integral part of the past Iraqi BW program. And beyond, paradoxically, anti-bioterrorism programs worldwide bring about academic, commercial, and industrial institutionalization of numerous new pathogens-holdings labs which constitute potential resources for pathogens seekers. It so happened, that 245 facilities are now authorized to work with live anthrax in the US, and about 100 actually do so, compared to roughly 12 prior to the 2001 anthrax mailings.

Inadequately secured state-held stockpiles of BW constitute a potential resource. Reportedly, bin Laden's associates managed to receive anthrax and plague cultures or weaponized agents, from former

Soviet facilities in Kazakhstan, or elsewhere. This has not been evidenced, although attempts to obtain those and other germs have certainly been made by al-Qaeda, perhaps fruitlessly. Still, assuming that al-Qaeda is responsible (together with Iraq) for the Sept. 2001 anthrax letter attacks, its members were at least involved in the final step of the envelope posting, thus possessing, temporarily, this pathogen. Also, aerosol-released bioterrorism weapons were often in the possession of Spetsnaz operatives who were believed to be involved with terrorists, especially those associated with bin Laden. A typical example demonstrating an endeavor to exploit an institutionalized researcher as a 'scientific mercenary' was the case in which al-Qaeda had direct connections with a senior Pakistani microbiologist, Dr. Abdur Rauf, who attempted to support al-Qaeda's pursue of BW.

Adriana Stujit, an acknowledged Dutch journalist, contended that radical Muslims have gotten control over South Africa's biological weapons stockpiles. Quantities of anthrax, Ebola, Congo fever, and other agents are missing from South Africa, with the only explanation being theft. There has been no explanation or accurate documentation of the amounts, locations, and contents of the stockpiles. This is not at all surprising, considering the picture described below regarding South Africa.

Obtaining pathogens and toxins from their natural environment is another sensible, though skill-demanding mode. In 1993, the Japanese cult Aum Shinrikyo sent a group of 16 cult doctors and nurses to Zaire, on a supposed medical mission. The actual purpose of the trip to Central Africa was to learn as much as possible about and, ideally, to bring back samples of Ebola virus. In early 1994, cult doctors were quoted on Russian radio as discussing the possibility of using Ebola as a bioterrorism weapon. The attempt was fruitless. Also, they attempted to purchase a Q-fever culture from a Japanese academic researcher but were rebuffed. But they did obtain botulinum germs from earth in Japan, anthrax germs, and cholera germs. The anthrax strain was consistent with strain Sterne 34F2, which is used in Japan for animal prophylaxis against anthrax.

Domestic naive facilities may readily be contributive. In Israel, much concern was raised that regular microbiological laboratories—whether private or institutionalized, and particularly those located in the Palestinian-occupied territories—may be used as minifactories for producing biological agents in quantities sufficient for bioterrorism purposes. A broad spectrum of resources of pathogens and toxins is notable, then, especially pertaining to potential resources worldwide. Still, it is much narrower regarding weaponized agents, making the course of the attacker complicated, unless "raw" infective agents or toxins are to be employed in an act of bioterrorism. But, on the other hand, dozens of biotech firms now offer to synthesize complete genes from the chemical components of DNA, making it feasible, seemingly, that a bioterrorist, armed with only a fake e-mail address, could probably order such deadly biological components online and receive them by mail. He would doubtfully be able to transform, however, those components into a weapon, if not substantially assisted.

Technical Feasibility of Biosabotage Acts

Pragmatically, biosabotage acts are featured by high technical feasibility, making them attractive, in that sense. Various operational options allowing for such feasibility are presented and discussed. Still, an appreciable level of know-how is needed for all preparatory stages preceding the in-effect act of bioterrorism. The most plain, nearly self-evident; act of bioterrorism is demonstrated by one person emptying a tube into a water source so as to contaminate it with a water-borne pathogen. Against such an act stands mainly the level of water chlorination, which does not interfere, practically, with the distinct technical feasibility of this deed. It is, indeed, a simple thing to do.

But the technical feasibility of bioterrorism may extend much further. A fairly sophisticated practice involves the preparation and dispersing of a toxin or pathogen in an inhalable aerosol form, either dry or wet. Various advanced aerosol technology-based devices structured to dispersing inhalable aerosols of pharmacological quality are available and may likewise release a pathogen or toxin. Alternatively, dissemination may be achieved by infected insects. During an infamous biowarfare attack in 1941, the Japanese Military released an estimated 150-million plague-infected fleas from airplanes over villages in China and Manchuria, resulting in several plague outbreaks in those villages. The victims were, deliberately, merely civilians. The same principle may be applied for disseminating plague by the release of infected rats in an enemy's settlements. Another example, similarly complex, yet plainly feasible act of bioterrorism, rabid, pre-symptomatic dogs or other canines infiltrated covertly, steadily, and untraceably in the wild through borderlines, may then bring about the spread of rabies onto local dogs and farm animals plus humans, gradually elevating the overall level of rabies endemicity.

Currently, effective worldwide dissemination is achievable through postal systems. The following recent incident, although certainly a naïve one, illustrates the technical feasibility of biosabotage acts at large, as one, outstanding example: Thousands of scientists were scrambling at the urging of global health authorities to destroy vials of a pandemic flu strain sent to laboratories in 18 countries as part of routine testing. The rush, urged by the World Health Organization, was sparked by a slim, but real, risk that the samples could spark a global flu epidemic. The vials of virus sent by a U.S. company went to nearly 5000 laboratories, mostly in the United States.

Referring to the incident, WHO's influenza chief, Klaus Stohr contended that "The risk is relatively low that a lab worker will get sick, but a large number of labs got it and if someone does get infected, the risk of severe illness is high and this virus has shown to be fully transmissible. The risk is low but things can go wrong as long as these samples are out there and there are some still out there."

The 1957 pandemic strain, which killed between 1 million and 4 million people, was in the proficiency test kits routinely sent to laboratories. This strain has not been included in the flu vaccine since 1968, and anyone born after that date has no immunity to it.

Most samples were sent at the request of the College of American Pathologists, which helps laboratories do proficiency testing. A private company, Meridian Bioscience Inc. of Cincinnati, Ohio, is paid to prepare the samples. The firm was told to pick an influenza type A virus sample and chose from its stockpile the deadly 1957 H2N2 strain. The reason for choosing this past, mighty strain, and not a current strain, remains unclear. Still, some other test kit providers besides the college also used the 1957 pandemic strain in samples sent to laboratories in the United States.

The majority of the laboratories that got the test kits are in the United States. Fourteen were in Canada, and 61 samples went to laboratories in 16 other countries in Europe, Asia, the Middle East, and South America, according to the WHO. The test kits are used for internal quality control checks to demonstrate that a laboratory is able to correctly identify viruses or as a way for laboratories to get certified by the College of American Pathologists. The kits involve blind samples. The laboratory then has to correctly identify the pathogen in the vial in order to pass the test. Usually, the influenza virus included in these kits is one that is currently circulating, or at least one that has recently been in circulation. The WHO then notified the health authorities in all countries that received the kits and recommended that all samples be destroyed immediately. That same day, the College of American Pathologists faxed the laboratories asking them to immediately incinerate the samples and to confirm in writing that the operation had been completed.

Unintentionally, this demonstration of the technical feasibility of biosabotage operations marks both simultaneous, wide-range distributable shipment of a virulent—in that case, rather recoverably pandemic—pathogen in a stable infective form, as well as specifically, on-spot targeted sites intended to be attacked biologically. The two options are equally feasible. Actually, two events of unintentional postal distribution of smallpox—yet in that case generating epidemics in effect—happened to occur already in 1901. Smallpox had developed in a woman in Saginaw, Michigan, after she received a letter form her sweetheart, a soldier in Alaska.

He had written it while recovering from this disease. The infection subsequently spread to 33 other persons in Saginaw. Also in 1901, an outbreak of 5 cases of smallpox was recorded at the Mormon headquarters in Nottingham, England, apparently after receipt of "letters or other fomites" from Salt Lake City, Utah, where smallpox was widespread.

Heavily crowded facilities single out the technical feasibility of bioterrorism. Thus, the British army tested model bacilli spore powder released (1963) from a window of a tube train traveling in the London Underground. The trial concluded that the spores can be carried for several miles on the tube system, and locally can persist as an aerosol of high concentration for a considerable period. Also, widespread dispersal of bacteria was found in a May 1965 secret release of innocent bacilli at Washington's National Airport and its Greyhound bus terminal, according to declassified military reports. More than 130 passengers who had been exposed to the bacteria traveled to 39 cities in seven states in the two weeks following the mock attack. By 1966, in a similar trail in New-York Subway, bacilli powder-carrying light bulbs were dropped.

Water is an easy target, basically. The feasibility of water contamination has been pointed out to be concrete in Israel: Deliberate influx of sewage from Judea and Samaria hills onto the Israel Coast Plain was been observed during the 1990s, according to the Israel Minister for Environment Quality, causing the contamination of Israeli water systems. Objectively, this may become much more feasible as a result of the 2005 Israeli disengagement. It should be mentioned that, in the past, outbreaks of cholera occurred in Judea and Samaria as a result of sewage being routinely and innocently used for the irrigation of vegetables. Connectedly, the factual situation is that most streams found in Israel stem from the mountainous aquifers, which are mostly located in the Judean and Samarian Hills, parts of which are now outside of Israeli territorial control. The other Israeli water sources stem from the Golan Heights and Southern Lebanon.

Furthermore, rather unusual modes illustrating the technical feasibility of biosabotage acts have been noted in Israel: In the body of one person who survived suicide bomber sabotage, bone fragments were discovered that are believed to come from a suicide bomber. The bone fragments tested positive for hepatitis B. Medical experts believe "This is possibly the first report of human bone fragments acting as foreign bodies in a blast injury, and consequently all survivors of these attacks in Israel are now vaccinated for hepatitis B." The experts suggested that bone fragments embedded in attack victims should be routinely tested. Theoretically, bone fragments might also spread other diseases including HIV, dengue fever, syphilis, and Creutz-Jakob disease.

In August 2004, an Iranian-made unmanned drone launched from southern Lebanon by the Iranian-supported Shi'lte militia, the Hezbollah flew for about 15 minutes along Israel's northern Mediterranean coast until it reached the coastal resort of Nahariyah. "Iran has not only supplied Hezbollah with these UAVs but has also trained 30 of the group's members to operate them," an official (a senior commander in the Iranian Revolutionary Guards) told the London-based Arab daily *al-Sharq al-A wsat* 11 Nov 2004. The efficiency of UAVs as aerosol disseminators of biological agents is well known.

Drifted saboteurs may even be full residents of the country to be attacked. A terrorist state or organization might use such residents, particularly extremists, to carry out bioterrorism acts, thus considerably elevating the technical feasibility of those operations. The attacked might catch the extremists, but not understand they were minor figures, and present them instead as major figures. All in all, the practicability of bioterrorism is fairly plain, although a degree of professional knowledge is needed for planning and preparations.

It is also possible to disseminate infected insects or infected animals (like rats, for instance). Also, deliberate infection of contacts by an infected individual harboring a contagious disease (AIDS, for example—a plot already carried out not infrequently) is, in a sense, an act of bioterrorism. Water and ventilation systems may be targeted. During the First Gulf War, there were serious concerns in the United States, that the ventilation systems of buildings might be attacked by terrorists using BW agents.

According to Norqvist, terrorists might effectively and easily disseminate biological agents through water systems, resulting in a high number of casualties, the terrorism focusing either on large cities or military facilities. It has thereupon been pointed out that chlorination can be neutralized by using naturally chlorine-resistant microorganisms or constructing bacteria resistant to chlorine concentrations normally used in the municipal drinking water systems. Simple devices might be used to deliver biological agents into the ventilation systems of buildings. Open-air experiments carried out in the 1960s demonstrated that throwing a light bulb filled with biological agent before an incoming subway train during rush hour is sufficient to infect tens of thousands of people. Plausibly, state-supported terrorist groups would be the most likely of all terrorist groups to get a hold of biological weapons by the supporting government transferring entire systems from their national programs.

Operational Models

A wide variety of modes that may serve for operating bioterrorism is described. Essentially aimed at attaining advantage through asymmetric warfare, they may lead, at most, to an impact equaling catastrophic terrorism. They might be limited, inversely, to merely assassination. Hoax acts are visited as well. One-man operational mode can bring about any of the mentioned outcomes.

The operational modes marking bioterrorism are closely related to asymmetric and catastrophic warfare. Asymmetric warfare is a military term to describe warfare in which the two belligerents are mismatched in their total capabilities or accustomed methods of engagement such that the inferior side must press its special advantages or effectively exploit its enemy's particular weaknesses if they are to have any hope of *prevailing*. Thus, asymmetric warfare is a recipe for engaging an opponent who has superior military power at his disposal and where the main target is not the armed forces but the fabric of society itself. Catastrophic terrorism differs from the more traditional forms of terrorism because it has no closely defined political aim. It is based on the belief that the current world order is dominated by certain "*universal values*" that the terrorists despise and that this order must be destroyed.

Consequence management roles vary depending on whether the attack is a terrorist event or an act of war. Yet, the distinction between terrorist and military use of WMDs is increasingly problematic. State adversaries, perhaps acting through terrorist surrogates, may be inclined to use WMDs early, unconventionally, and if possible, anonymously. They may use WMDs against such military targets as ports, airfields, staging areas, and overseas bases to prepare the military battlefield by slowing logistics and power projection. Similarly, they may psychologically undermine public support or politically divide a coalition for an operation by attacking domestic or allied civilian targets. Eager to deter regional involvement while avoiding an overwhelming retaliatory response, perpetrators may try to obscure their identity. Under these circumstances, the line between terrorism and symmetric warfare may then vanish.

The stealthy qualities of BW further complicate the distinction between terrorism and war. An adversary with effective agent dissemination capabilities could employ BW as part of a covert attack nearly impossible to detect until casualties appear. Depending on the agent used, the attacked might not know whether an outbreak was natural, a terrorist attack, or the opening assault of a war. For all the legitimate concern about bioterrorism, systemized weapons are mostly still difficult to employ effectively without access to state-developed technology. Rogue states and well-financed terrorists with access to state-developed technology remain the most serious danger from the effective, large-scale use of biological agents through guerilla warfare.

The repertoire of bioterrorism modes is potentially an incredible one, extending from ricin-based assassination of one person to a worldwide smallpox pandemic, even if not aimed, a priori, to reach such magnitude. Those two edges may each take shape in actuality due to a seemingly slight act carried out by a single perpetrator. The former mode has practically been materialized through the murder of Markov, the Bulgarian journalist in London, whereas instead of ricin the lethal toxin used could variedly be of another type, as detailed above. The latter mode is a continuously floating menace, the possible realization of which is attentively being faced, in terms of both preventive measures and preparedness for handling such occurrence. The one-man mode was exemplified in 1998, when the British government issued a warning to all ports about an Iraqi attempt to bring large quantities of the deadly germs of anthrax into Britain (and other countries) inside cosmetics bottles, cigarette lighters, and perfume sprays, disguised as duty-free goods.

A bioterrrorism attack could consist, then, of nothing more than a person deliberately coughing on people and surfaces after being infected with a pathogen, as correctly pointed out in a study conducted by the Australian Strategic Policy Institute. This could happen by a terrorist knowingly infected and incubating an infection flying to Australia and then walking around a crowded shopping center for some hours, coughing near people and over surfaces. The study found that even without their knowledge, infected individuals could likewise be used as carriers for bioterrorism acts.

One major operational mode of massive bioterrorism may focus on endpoints of collective source reservoirs right before their physical division into much smaller to individually consumed portions. Such reservoirs may include blood, sera, or other preparations intended to be introduced into the body as well as foods, drinks, and water. Thus, certain collective infusion fluids may be contaminated before being packed: AIDS, hepatitis B, hepatitis C, arboviruses, and other blood-adapted pathogens.

Milk supplies, as another example, meet that very same biosabotage principle and have aroused much worry. About a third of an ounce of botulism toxin poured by bioterrorists into a milk truck en route from a dairy farm to a processing plant could cause hundreds of thousands of deaths and billions of dollars in economic losses, according to a scientific analysis.

The analysis considered what might happen if terrorists poured into a milk tanker truck a couple of gallons of concentrated sludge containing as much as 10 g of botulinum toxin. Because milk from many sources is combined in huge tanks holding hundreds of thousands of gallons, the toxin would get widely distributed in low, but potentially lethal, concentrations and within days be consumed by about 568,000 people, the report concludes. The researchers acknowledge that their numbers are very rough. But depending on how thoroughly the milk was pasteurized (which partially inactivates toxins) and how promptly the outbreak was detected and supplies recalled, about 400,000 people would be likely to fall ill, they conclude. Although only 6% of victims would generally be expected to die, the death rate could easily hit 60%, they conclude, because there would not be nearly enough mechanical ventilators or doses of antitoxin to treat so many victims.

A different mode of bioterrorism may aim to bring about the outward leakage of infectious microorganisms by physically damaging facilities containing them. A variety of installations may serve for such a mode, including P-3 and P-4 laboratories, vaccine factories, and institutionalized depositories. Such sabotage may questionably be regarded as bioterrorism, particularly if directed toward a facility engaged in biological warfare, even if but defensive. Yet the consequences and ultimate impact may be very severe. Hardly accusable may as well be bioterrorists choosing a mode of amplifying an ongoing outbreak or epidemic, especially if the very same causative pathogenic strain is concurrently employed by them for that purpose.

The various options of bioterrorism conducted as a sole operative mode or in conjunction with other sabotage acts add a further dimension. Bioterrorism acts may on the spot be accompanied by simultaneous conventional and/or unconventional—mostly chemical or radiological—sabotage. Such synchronism may form camouflage and be misleading, making the bioterrorism component scarcely thinkable or detectable. Spatial diversity may concomitantly increase the blurring effect. Combined employment of WMDs indeed drew the Pentagon's attention. The Pentagon has implemented, thus, a plan to expand its support of civilian authorities in the event of multiple domestic attacks involving chemical, biological, radiological, or nuclear weapons, The Virginia-based Joint Task Force-Civil Support was previously the Pentagon's only force dedicated to such a mission.

"We have identified capabilities within our force structure—beyond Joint Task Force-Civil Support—in order to ensure that we could respond not simply to a domestic attack involving a WMD, but to multiple attacks at diverse locations. several cities perhaps at once where terrorists might have employed weapons of mass destruction," Paul McHale, deputy assistant secretary of defense for homeland defense, said. "It is now the established policy of the Department of Defense that we will train and equip for the mission requirement of multiple WMD response," said McHale.

Two overt modes are notable:

1. Suicide by a person carrying a detectable contagion.
2. Bioterrorism combined with conventional terrorism, simultaneously serving for two advantages:
   (a) Temporary misleading (until infected cases present).
   (b) Increasing vulnerability to bioterrorism agents by conventional wounding.

Opposite in polarity to the extreme mode involving in-effect bioterrorism in conjunction with multi-WMDs, are bioterrorism hoaxes. Bioterrorism hoaxes—whether consisting of unviable or viable substances that are benign—constitute an increasing mode of bioterrorism. The anonymously angry of the world are creating serious trouble today with just a stamp, an envelope, and a household product. It takes only moments for someone to send a package containing a suspicious but ultimately harmless powder. Moreover, hoaxers often see the powder-filled letters as a way to send a message, without considering that they are committing a crime. The act, however, can force entire buildings to be locked down and tie up emergency personnel for hours. Each incident must be taken seriously in case the contents turn out to be anthrax rather than crushed aspirin.

It so happened that the uncertainty prevailing around a hoax caused Australian Prime Minister John Howard to say in the early hours of a crisis thereupon created due to an powder containing envelope received in the Indonesian Embassy (June 2005): "This is a very serious development for our country, and I can't overstate the sense of concern I feel that such a recklessly criminal act should have been committed." He added he believed the threat was meant as retaliation for the 20-year prison sentence Australian national Schapelle Corby received in Indonesia for smuggling drugs. Such acts could damage relations between the two nations and invite retaliations against Australians in Indonesia.

Actually, however, people were putting powder in the mail to scare others years before someone sent envelopes laced with anthrax that killed five American people in the fall of 2001. There were 22 incidents reported worldwide in 2000 involving faked biological agents, according to the Monterey Institute's Center for Nonproliferation Studies. The count jumped to about 730 in 2001, due largely to Clayton Lee Waagner's campaign against abortion providers.

Waagner was arrested late that year after sending roughly 550 powder-filled letters, and the number of bioterrorism hoaxes dropped to 70 in 2002. However, excluding his count, both 2001 and 2002 saw significant increases in such incidents from 2000, spurred by the anthrax mailings and the resulting media coverage, according to Sundara Vadlamudi, research associate for the center's WMD Terrorism Research Program.

Although certainly the most relentless, Waagner was not the first anti-abortion bioterrorism hoaxer or the last. More than 20 letters containing fake anthrax were mailed to abortion providers and abortion rights organizations in January 2002, several weeks after his arrest. Currently, however, the trend is increasing; notable receiving powder-filled envelopes since April 2005: the Israeli Embassy in Washington, D.C., the Danish embassies in Stockholm and Vienna, the New Mexico state capitol, a Slovenian government office, the office of Quebec Premier Jean Charest, a Vermont multimedia company, Israel Army Radio, the Bank of Israel, and NATD's Joint Warfare Center, Norway.

Spatially and Temporally Varying Impacts

The expected impact of bioterrorism acts, together with the featuring of their spatial and temporal variance, are configured. A typical multifactorial system is thus formed, the handling of which is remarkably complicated, demanding, and vital. It includes a far-reaching range of bioterrorism scenarios, some evident, some tentative, beginning with hoaxes scenarios, and ending in the form of a pandemic.

The impact of bioterrorism acts is appreciably varied, both spatially and temporally. Its variability is shaped by the following factors:

1. Initial area coverage (via air, water, food, or animal vectors/carriers)
2. Duration of pathogenetic course
3. Curability
4. Environmental stability of the pathogen/toxin
5. Contagiousness
6. Demographic conditions
7. Climatic conditions
8. Conduction and effectiveness of preventing measures (before and after the act of bioterrorism)

The multifactorial integral thus formed is complex. For automating the testing and validation of spatial and temporal cluster detection algorithms, and enabling the ready creation of datasets for benchmarking outbreak detection systems, a specific software tool has been developed. It allows for the creation of simulated clusters with controlled feature sets, varying the desired cluster radius, density, distance, relative location from a reference point, and temporal epidemiological growth pattern. This tool does not require the use of an external geographical information system program for cluster creation. Based on user-specified parameters describing the location, properties, and temporal pattern of simulated clusters, it creates clusters accurately and uniformly.

The impact is pronounced within several domains:

1. Personal illness that may lead to death
2. Paralyzed manpower
3. Logistical efforts needed to medically support and isolate the infected/sickened victims
4. Meticulous, extremely demanding managing of the apparently uninfected population
5. Demoralization that may ascend to total panic
6. Overall instability

The remarkable psychological responses subsequent to a bioterrorism attack were summarized as follows: horror, wrath, panic, paranoia, demoralization, magical thinking about germs and viruses, fear of invisible pathogenic agents, fright of contagion, anger at terrorists, government, or both, attribution of arousal symptoms to infection, scapegoating, social isolation, and loss of faith in social institutions. Panic is a power multiplier in itself. Some plead that the use of biological agents can cause severe panic and hysteria among the civic population. For example, during the Sept. 2001 anthrax letter attack, thousands of civilians came to hospitals, although only few of them were found to be suffering from exposure to the anthrax powder. When BW agents are used, there is a great fear that the number of civilians turning to get medical help will overload the health service systems and those who really need treatment will not be able to get it. This overload, besides keeping treatment from those who need it, will also cause mass hysteria. Mass hysteria is very significant. In case of contagious diseases, there is a grave concern that the mass hysteria and the urge to flee the scene will only cause the disease to spread. That is contrary to the proper way of fighting it, namely, closing and isolating the contaminated area.

A typically acute bioterrorism episode would be featured by a toxin or pathogen of a short incubation period, pronounced illness, recovery or death, absence of secondary epidemic waves, and the creation of long-lasting immunity of the surviving population, which would inhibit relapsing occurrences. Such a prototypic episode may at times not exceed a week, just as it had been designed by the perpetrator. But, contrastingly, attritional or demographically debilitating impact may result from a delayed, relapsing, or slowly progressing pathogenetic course that may prevail for many years in a given population.

Spatially, however, any combination with the above-mentioned temporal variations is possible, basically. This means that in a relatively confined area a several-weeks transient bioterrorism episode or a lingering impact stemming from a bioterrorism act lasting for years, may take place. Equally, a vast territory may be afflicted by a swiftly moving epidemic or, alternatively, by a clumsily evolving pathogen, in terms of epidemic rate and virulence, whether it is an incapacitating or deadly agent. The dynamics underlying this complex variability is foremost shaped by the nature of the toxin or pathogen employed in-effect, and the countermeasures to be specifically taken against it. Fundamentally, this fluctuating dynamics is well illustrated, both spatially and temporally, through the varitype bacteria, viruses, and toxins presented within the above corresponding sections. It prevails, thereby, for both the dimension of the individual victim as well as the demographic dimension at large.

On the other hand are the bioterrorism hoax incidents, of which the spatial and temporal impacts, though, are still significant. Even an absolutely empty post envelope bearing but one word, like "*biohazard*," would bring about those undesirable impacts. If not empty, it may contain but paper and/or innocent chemical, toxin, non-infective microorganism, infective yet attenuated microorganism, or pathogenic microorganism. In this order of possibilities, there is an ascending line of spatial and temporal impacts. (The envelope content may as well comprise insects, infected or naive.)

Three recent examples are herewith mentioned, then, resembling the spatial and temporal variance of impacts: After a harmless bacillus powder was found in an post envelope sent to the Indonesian Embassy in Australia, the Australian capital of Canberra sustained a barrage of bioterrorism hoax mailings beginning 1 June 2005 to its Parliament building, Prime Minister and Cabinet Department, and the embassies of Indonesia, the United States, United Kingdom, Japan, Italy, and South Korea. Emergency personnel in Canberra had to decontaminate 46 staffers at the Indonesian Embassy when it appeared some form of powered toxin had been sent to the building, according to Australian media reports. Tests later indicated the substance was not dangerous.

Some days later, continuation took place far away. On 10 June 2005, an employee in the collections department of Imperial Parking in Vancouver, British Columbia, opened an envelope containing a similarly suspicious white powder. Vancouver emergency services were quickly alerted. The affected section of the building was locked down—the air-conditioning system and elevators were shut off, and no one was allowed to enter or leave. Twenty-five workers were quarantined for several hours until tests determined the substance was not dangerous. Forty-eight emergency workers and 18 pieces of equipment were sent to the powder scare at the Imperial Parking office. Firefighters suited up in protective gear to retrieve a sample, whereas others managed the quarantine and organized decontamination for the hazardous materials workers. Emergency medical personnel examined firefighters before they entered the building and after they exited, and waited to see whether they would have to take anyone to the hospital. Police officers handled crowd control and traffic and provided an escort when the sample was taken for further testing at a laboratory. This occurred, unfortunately, while the city's emergency services were also handling a hotel fire, an injured person, and the nearby appearance of the Aga Khan, spiritual leader of Shia Imami Ismaili Muslims.

A third episode followed soon. An Israeli embassy employee in the United States checking mail at 5 p.m. 16 June 2005 opened one envelope that contained a small amount of a white powder. A section of the building was closed, and some employees remained inside until tests indicated at 11 p.m. that the substance was benign. The letter, which reportedly contained anti-Semitic language, was traced to a man jailed in North Carolina, according to the FBI. The logistical, mental (and medical) impacts would be much worse, certainly, both temporally and spatially, in case a mailed envelope contains a living pathogen, as was the 2001 anthrax letter attack.

History and Evolution

An old tool of mankind, the chronology of bioterrorism from 1500 BC to now is presented. It demonstrates the gradual, consistent transition from intuitive bioterrorism to knowledge-based bioterrorism. It shows, as well, the past, recent, and present trends of bioterrorism as an evolving course, the extrapolative featuring of which is troublesome. The evolutionary course of biological warfare at large is fascinatingly long. Almost as soon as humans figured out how to make arrows, they were dipping them in animal feces or sick persons so as to contaminate them. Practically, bioterrorism agents were the earliest weapons of mass destruction ever used by mankind. Long before having any idea regarding the in-effect nature of poisonous and infectious substances, man used toxins, feces, carcasses, and the like as effective weapons, in order to disease, kill, and terrorize opponents and enemies, thus following, from the very beginning, the three very basic fundamentals: incapacitating, killing, and intimidating. Rather a sort of intuitive bioterrorism, primarily.

Still, most of the ancient world liked to believe it fought with a code of honor. According to Adrienne Mayor, "Archers were disdained because they shot safely from afar: long range missiles implied unwillingness to face the enemy at close range. And long range missiles daubed with poisons seemed even more cowardly." Yet Odysseus, hardly a coward, returns home to kill his wife's suitors with poison arrows. The roots of repugnance toward contaminated weapons are deep. Such weapons were singled out for disdain more than 2000 years ago in Greek and Roman codes of conduct, as well as in Hindu writings. But the course of using pathogens and toxins for terrorism continued. The rulers of ancient India were no less conflicted than the Greeks about arrows "barbed, poisoned or blazing with flame." These instruments violated the "traditional Hindu laws of conduct for Brahmans and high castes, the Laws of Manu." But in the Arthashastra, the Brahman military strategist Kautilya advised his king to use whatever means necessary to attain his military goals, including poisons.

In the Near East, it was after the mythic Greek hero Hercules slew the multi-headed Hydra that he developed a technology at the heart of today's most pressing international issue. In her illuminating history of warfare, the acknowledged folklorist Adrienne Mayor argues, in a sense, that "by steeping his arrows in the monster's venom, Hercules created the first biological weapon."

Amazingly, then, the ancient world already made an important distinction between using disease weapons for purely defensive purposes as opposed to "first strikes." Although this constraint was rooted partially in ethics, Mayor contends it also reflected a shrewd understanding of epidemiology: "The principle of summoning plague for self-defense may be related to the reality that invaders are 'immunologically naïve' and therefore more vulnerable to epidemic diseases in foreign lands than the local population." Mayor is intrigued with the often fantastic devices the ancients used in war, but "Greek Fire" also excavates ancient attitudes toward biological arms and terrorism tools that are startlingly relevant today. Poisonous arrows were the Bronze Age's terror weapons. "Almost as soon as they were created," Mayor writes, "poison weapons set in motion a relentless train of tragedies for Hercules and the Greeks—not to mention the Greeks' enemies, the Trojans."

Similar, unrecorded biotterorism-like events followed, most probably. Yet, beyond Greek mythology, even earlier, the ancient world also contained examples of bioterrorism warfare against settled populations stretching back to 1500 BC, when the Hittites sent plague victims into the lands of their enemies. Later, it was in about 600 BC that Solon of Athens put hellebore roots in the drinking water of Kirrha to kill the inhabitants. At about the same time, the Assyrians used to poison enemy wells with a fungus that would make the enemy delusional. Around 500 BC, Socrates was poisoned by the juice of Conium, which was the state poison of the Athenians. Necrotizing germs were intuitively employed in 400 BC, whereas Scythian archers systematically used arrows dipped in blood and manure or decomposing bodies to prevent wounds from healing. There are accounts from 300 BC of parts of the dead bodies of humans or animals being used by the Romans to poison water supplies. There have also been instances of the dead bodies of those who died from plague being catapulted into besieged cities. Later on, by 200 BC, Carthaginians used Mandrake root left in wine to sedate the enemy. Furthermore, in 184 BC, Carthaginian leader Hannibal is credited with an interesting use of bioterrorism weapons. In anticipation of a naval battle with the Pergamenes at Eurymedon, he ordered his troops to fill clay pots with snakes. During the battle, Hannibal sent the pots crashing down on the deck on the Pergamene ship. The confused Pergamenes lost the battle, having to fight both Hannibal's forces and a ship full of snakes. The act brought about panic and injured enemy sailors. Pergamenes, a king in Asia Minor, remarked that "he did not think any general would want to obtain a victory by the use of means which might in turn be directed against himself." Honey bees are known to have been used as weapons since Roman times, as was then the case of Lucullus, who defeated Mithridates (74 BC) via bees.

As man expended onto the Far East and, later, the Americas, tropical plants became a common source for toxins. Thus, poisoned arrows are used widely throughout the jungles of Burma, Malaysia, and Assam. The principal sources of arrow poison are varieties of *Antiaris*, *Strychnos*, and *Strophanthus*. *Antiaris toxicaria*, for example, is a tree of the mulberry and breadfruit family, common in Java and the neighboring islands. The active agents in all of these are either contained within the milky sap or the juice of crushed seeds. This is smeared behind the arrow point on its own, or mixed with another plant latex. When introduced into the bloodstream, the active ingredient (either antiarin, strychnine, or strophanthin depending on the species) acts quickly, attacking the central nervous system causing paralysis, convulsions, and cardiac failure.

The story of the *Strychnos*-derived toxin Curare is remarkable, in that it perfectly embodies a complete bivalent evolutionary line, starting with a very old arrow-poison—still in its very same traditional use presently—and ending, for the time being, as an important muscle relaxant. Contemporarily, curare is usable for selected assassinations just like "modern" toxins. In the sixteenth century, a group of Spanish explorers traveled the Amazon River. During the voyage, one explorer was hit in the hand by an arrow and died soon after. The culprit was curare, used widely as an arrow poison by many Amazon Indian groups (as it is still used by a few today). The complex processes used to make curare were a guarded secret. Often 30 or more ingredients could be found in one recipe. Indigenous Amazonians often mixed plants of different genera to concoct their potent toxins; their skill and knowledge in safely preparing these poisons is a testimony to their incredible ingenuity. Amazonian curares are divided into two groups based on the container the plant is stored in: pots or tubes. Pot curare in the East Amazon is predominately from the species *Strychnos guianensis*. Tube curare in the West Amazon is from *Chrondrodendron tomentosum*. (The curare in modern medicine is made from the latter species, therefore, its name: tubocurarine.)

For many centuries, the exact content of curare remained a mystery to Western observers; not until 1800 did Alexander Von Humboldt witness and document the preparation of curare by the Indians from the Orinco River. In 1814, an explorer named Charles Waterton injected a donkey with curare. Within 10 minutes, the donkey appeared dead. Waterton cut a small hole in her throat and inserted a pair of bellows, and then pumped to inflate the lungs. The donkey held her head up and looked around. Waterton continued artificial respiration for 2 hours until the effects of curare had worn off. Curare was found to block the transmission of nerve impulses to muscle, including the diaphragm muscle, which controls breathing. Back to Europe, the Middle Ages, the use of infectious diseases to break sieges of castles and fortified towns is widespread. The most common method is to use catapults to hurl dead human or animal bodies over walls to spread disease. This same method is used to poison water sources. Plagued rats and infected flies were employed as well for introducing and disseminating the contagion. This was the case in 1155, when Barbarossa uses dead bodies to spread pathogens among the enemy during the battle of Tortona. About 200 years later, in 1340 attackers hurled dead horses and other animals by catapult at the castle of Thun L'Eveque in Hainault, in what is now northern France. The defenders reported that "the stink and the air were so abominable... they could not long endure" and negotiated a truce.

In 1346, Tartar forces led by Khan Janibeg attacked the city of Kaffa (now Feodossia, Ukraine), catapulting the plague-infected bodies of their own men over the city's walls, and forcing the defending Genoese to abandon it when plague spread. Connectedly, ships carrying plague infected refugees (and possibly rats) sailed to Constantinople, Genoa, Venice, and other Mediterranean ports and are thought to have contributed to the second plague pandemic. (The first plague pandemic in 541 ad spread from Egypt to other parts of the world and killed 50–60% of the world population). It was perhaps the trigger of a subsequent outbreak of Bubonic plague that swept medieval Europe, causing 25 million deaths. Using dead bodies and excrement as weapons continued in Europe during the Black Plague of the fourteenth and fifteenth centuries. Even as late as 1710, Russian troops fighting Sweden resorted to catapulting plagued bodies over the city walls of Reval.

During that era, three peculiar events took place, as well: In 1422, at Karlstein in Bohemia, attacking forces launched the decaying cadavers of men killed in battle over the castle walls. They also stockpiled animal manure in the hope of spreading illness. Yet the defense held fast, and the siege was abandoned after 5 months. In 1495, the Spanish tried wine infected with leprosy patients' blood against the French near Naples, and, in 1650, Polish artillery General put saliva from rabid dogs into hollow spheres for firing against his enemies.

In between, a sort of bioterrorism came to the New World in the fifteenth century, aimed to defeat the Indians. Spanish conquistador Pizarro gave clothing contaminated with the smallpox virus to natives in South America. During the French and Indian War (1754–1767) Sir Jeffrey Amherst, commander of British forces in North America, suggested the deliberate use of smallpox to "reduce" Native American tribes hostile to the British. An outbreak of smallpox at Fort Pitt results in the opportunity to execute Amherst's plan. On June 24, 1763, Captain Ecuyer, Amherst's subordinate, gives blankets and a handkerchief from the smallpox hospital to the Native Americans and records in his journal, "I hope it will have the desired effect." This was followed by an epidemic of smallpox among Native American tribes in the Ohio River valley, which may also have been spread by contact with settlers. Transmission of smallpox by fomites (on blankets) is inefficient compared with respiratory droplet transmission.

Still, although the ancient world's arsenal of primitive bioterrorism weapons was trivial compared with the horrors of the modern world, those weapons raised the same terrifying moral and political dilemmas then as now. Thus, the absence of brought out events whereby BW were employed throughout the nineteenth century was possibly the latency preceding proliferation. Let alone that the nineteenth century marked the first isolation of germs in science.

During the twentieth century, then, an ascending course took place. In modern times, BW was used first for sabotage by Germany during WWI. German forces reportedly spread glanders and anthrax to debilitate enemy cavalries.

In 1918, the Japanese formed a biological weapons section in the Japanese Army (Unit 731). Later on, in 1931, Japan expanded its territory into Manchuria and made available "an endless supply of human experiment materials" (prisoners of war, mostly civilians) for Unit 731. Biological weapons experiments in Harbin, Manchuria, continued until 1945. A post-World War II autopsy investigation of 1000 victims revealed that most were exposed to aerosolized anthrax. It is estimated that up to 3000 more prisoners and Chinese nationals may have died in this facility. During an infamous bio warfare attack in 1941, the Japanese Military released an estimated 150-million plague-infected fleas from airplanes over villages in China and Manchuria, resulting in several plague outbreaks in those villages. Overall, the Japanese Imperial Army experimented with and operated about 16 biological agents as tools of warfare and terrorism between 1932 and 1945. This took place in numerous locations in Asia, and it has been estimated that a total of 10,000 Chinese prisoners, U.S. prisoners of war, and British detainees were killed by some of the most gruesome human experimentation in history. The Japanese used BW agents such as anthrax, plague, tularemia, and smallpox.

During World War II, another effort, taken by Britain, was the production of over 5 million anthrax infected cattle cakes, which would have been dropped over Germany in an attempt to decrease meat stocks by some 30%. Events overtook plans to put these into operation.

Ken Alibek, formerly a chief scientist of the Soviet offensive biological warfare program, has alleged that the Soviets employed the germs causing tularemia during World War II. In his book *Biohazard*, he states that there is evidence tularemia was used by the Soviet troops to help stop the German panzer troops in the Battle of Stalingrad. The resulting tularemia outbreak may have halted the Nazi advance, but the Soviet troops also developed the disease because of what Alibek suspects was a sudden change in wind direction. Over 100,000 cases of tularemia were reported in the Soviet Union in 1942, a 10-fold increase in incidence experienced in 1941 and 1943. Seventy percent of the cases were the respiratory form of the disease, which is the form that would have been expected from a BW rather than a natural outbreak of the disease. Nonetheless, this episode may constitute a good example of biological warfare, rather than bioterrorism.

Avner Cohen, an expert on unconventional weapons proliferation, has catalogued reported uses of bioterrorism weapons by Jewish forces during the 1948 War of Independence in Palestine. Connectedly, the Israeli historian Uri Milstein alleged that "in many conquered Arab villages, the water supply was poisoned to prevent the inhabitants from coming back." Milstein states that one of the largest of such covert operations caused the typhoid outbreak in Acre in May 1948. Within that context, the Palestinian Arab Higher Committee reported in July 1948 that there was some evidence that Jewish forces were responsible for a cholera outbreak in Egypt in November 1947 and in Syrian villages near the Palestinian-Syrian border in February 1948. Fur thermore, in May 1948, the Egyptian ministry of defense stated that four "Zionists" had been captured while trying to contaminate artesian wells in Gaza with "a liquid which was discovered to contain germs of dys-entery and typhoid."

A pause took place for almost two decades (apart from minor or marginal incidents), but since 1965, the trend significantly changed. Multiple bioterrorism occurrences have been observed, as follows.

1965—In Japan, outbreaks of typhoid and dysentery were deliberately induced by a local bacteriologist.

1970—In Canada, several students became badly ill after eating food deliberately contaminated with the eggs of parasitic ringworm. During the 1970s, the Soviets used mycotoxins in Laos and Cambodia and hepatitis A virus in Afganistan.

1972—Two men affiliated with the U.S. group "Order of the Rising Sun," who eventually fled to Cuba, had conspired to contaminate the water supplies of some large Midwestern cities with stocks of typhoid fever germs cultivated by one of them. Up to 40 kg of bacteria cultures were found in a college laboratory.

1975—The Symbionese Liberation Army was found in possession of technical manuals on how to produce bioweapons.

1980—Assassination of CIA agent Boris Korczak in McLean, Virginia, Tyson's Corner, using a ricin weapon, possibly in umbrella configuration.

Police raided a German Red Army Faction apartment in Paris and found a miniature laboratory containing a culture medium of the germ that produces botulinum toxin. Notes about bacteria-induced diseases were found in the apartment as well.

Protesters claimed to have taken infected soil from the Hebridean island of Gruinard and placed it at the chemical defense establishment at Porton Down. The island has been closed to the public since germ warfare experiments on sheep were conducted there in 1941. The anthrax spores used in the experiments can remain dangerous for decades.

1983—The FBI obtained one ounce of ricin in a 35-mm film canister from an individual in Springfield, Massachusetts, who had manufactured it himself. This is believed to be one of several confiscations of ricin .

Some 750 people were sickened due to typhoid fever, consequent to bacterial contamination of restaurant salad bars in Oregon, conducted by a local cult attempting to affect the outcome of a local election.

1984—Australian authorities received an anonymous threat warning that foot- and-mouth disease virus would be released among livestock if reforms in Queensland Prison were not implemented.

A Cuban expert defected and testified that one third of the United States could have been contaminated if a stockpile of toxins held by Cuba were to be "strategically placed in the Mississippi River".

Two Canadians attempt to procure tetanus and botulism cultures from ATCC. Reportedly the first phone order, of less deadly cultures, was fulfilled, and it was not until the second order that ATCC employees become sufficiently suspicious to notify authorities.

1990-1995—Japanese cult Aum Shinriky attempted at least three times to disperse aerosolized botulinum toxin and anthrax in downtown Tokyo and at U.S. military installations in Japan. All attempts failed.

1990—In Scotland, a limited outbreak of giardiasis occurred as result of deliberate water contamination.

1991—During the Gulf War, there were serious concerns in the United States, that the ventilation systems of buildings might be attacked by terrorists using BW agents.

1993—An Arkansas man with survivalist group connections attempted to smuggle 130 g of ricin from Alaska into Canada to use as a weapon.

1994—An Iraqi scientist specializing in genetic engineering and implanted in New York by Saddam Hussein's regime intended to conduct an act of bioterrorism, due to having access to various local laboratories.

1995—Two members of the Minnesota Patriots Council were convicted of conspiracy to assassinate a deputy U.S. Marshal and International Revenue Service agents by ricin.

A member of the white supremacist Aryan Nation acquired freeze-dried bubonic plague bacteria from the ATCC.

1996—In Texas. 12 laboratory workers at a medical center became ill as a result of eating muffins and doughnuts intentionally contaminated by dysentery germs type 2.

1998—An Iraqi terrorist network was maintained in the United States, intending to conduct acts of bioterrorism and reportedly furnished with BW agents by Iraqi women that smuggle agents filled vials into the United States within their bodies.

The British government has issued a warning to all ports about an Iraqi attempt to bring large quantities of the deadly germs of anthrax into Britain (and other countries) inside cosmetics bottles, cigarette lighters, and perfume sprays, disguised as duty-free goods.

Several Muslim terrorists affiliated with the Algerian "Armed Muslim Group" were arrested in Belgium, holding a lot of information about biological and chemical weapons and about the World Cup football games.

1999—A group of medical workers, mostly Bulgarian, employed in the Benghazi children's hospital, Libya, were detained, subsequent to an explosive AIDS epidemic that apparently started in 1998 in that hospital, and involved, thereupon, hundreds of children. By the year 2000, the medics were charged with deliberately infecting 393 Libyan children in their care with HIV, by injecting them with infected products. The HIV type was the same in each case—a rare and previously unrecorded strain that originated in West Africa when two existing viruses combined. Ananalysis conducted by European experts suggested that the outbreak has the hallmarks of accidental cross-contamination, where poor hygiene and ineffective sterilization procedures allowed contaminated blood to be spread between patients from a single infected child. Highly involved in the affair, the charged medics were then sentenced to death, however. Libyan leader Muammar Gadhafisaid he believes the medics are guilty.

2001—The anthrax letters were sent in the USA, containing highly sophisticated militory-grade spore powder.

2003—Former Texas Tech professor Thomas Butler said that 30 vials of plague bacteria were missing from the university. In fact, he stole, smuggled, and illicitly transported the bacteria to Tanzania.

Further episodes have been discussed above. All in all, the various above-described episodes are at any rate but a small segment of the entire picture. By 1998, Carus undertook a comprehensive inventory and assessment of bioterrorism (together with biocrimes) in the twentieth century. He has documented 222 cases, categorizing the cases and number of reported cases:

1. Confirmed use of bioterrorism agents—24
2. Probable or possible use—28
3. Threatened use (probable or confirmed possession)—11
4. Threatened use (no confirmed possession)—121
5. Confirmed possession (no known attempts or threats to use)—5
6. Probable or possible possession—6
7. Possible interest in acquisition (no known possession)—13
8. False cases and hoaxes—14

Surprisingly, there have been only 222 bioterrorism-related incidents in a 100-year period and in only 24 cases have there been confirmed attacks—an average of 1 every 4 years worldwide. Most were abortive. Fourteen of the 24 confirmed cases of bioterrorism or biocrimes are food or agriculture-related; of these cases, 11 involved food poisoning and only 3 targeted commercial animals or plants.

Of the 222 documented incidents, only 6 appear to be clearly linked to attacks on commercial plants and animals.

Significantly, yet, the survey made by Carus points at 144 incidents that occurred in the 1990s, meaning nearly two thirds of the total. This may reflect better incident tracking and record keeping in recent years, or it may indicate a dramatic increase in the propensity of terrorists or criminals to employ bioterrorism agents. Available evidence supports the latter premise. For example, FBI statistics indicate that U.S. incidents involving weapons of mass destruction using chemical, biological, radiological, or nuclear materials have soared from 37 in 1996 to over 200 in 1999, with three fourths of the cases involving bioterrorism agents—usually the threatened release of anthrax. Notably, the vast majority of incidents have been directed against individuals or small groups, not mass populations. On the whole, if any sort of extrapolation can be made, then the next decade is supposed to be a disturbing one, at the least.

State-sponsored Bioterrorism

State-sponsored bioterrorism may be carried out by saboteurs either affiliated with the concerned state or acting on their own but institutionally assisted by some country specifically aware of the ultimate outcome. Biosabotage programs and projects, in part realized, have been identified mainly in Germany, Japan, USSR, the United States, South Africa, and Iraq. They are here presented in detail, illustrating the conceptual and practical paradigm of state-sponsored bioterrorism.

States running a methodical biological weapons program would usually adopt a collateral subsystem dealing with bioterrorism means and operations. But the opposite equation remains open, in that the absence of a methodical program may not at all impair an effectual framework in charge of developing, manufacturing, and deploying of terrorism-oriented biological agents. The perpetrators tasked for carrying out the biosabotage acts may equally be affiliated with the involved state, or with another state, be it a friendly or a hostile state, including the target country itself. State-sponsored bioterrorism may as well be directed against domestic opponents and carried out internally. Another variance lies between bioterrorism initiated by a state and such that is initiated by a terror organization (or a second state) but is crucially and knowingly assisted by the concerned state. All those modes may be categorized as state-sponsored bioterrorism and are looked into through the following case studies.

Germany

From 1915 to 1918, Germany waged an ambitious campaign of covert biosabotage on animals being shipped from neutral countries to the Allies. The program used the germs causing glanders and anthrax, and employed secret agents to administer the bacterial cultures to animals penned for shipment. The cultures were sometimes injected using needles dipped into the cultures, sometimes poured onto feed, or (later in the war) contained in capillary tubes embedded in lumps of sugar that were fed to the animals. Horses and mules were the main targets, but in some cases sheep and cattle appear to have been targeted as well. The programs were initiated nearly simultaneously in Romania and the United States. The Romanian campaign was administered by Major Nodolny of the German General Staff, through his Military Attaché in Bucharest. The agents disseminating the cultures were Bulgarian, run by the Bulgarian embassy. Cultures were shipped from Berlin. The program lasted until the August 1916 Romanian declaration of war against Austro-Hungary and the expulsion of German diplomats.

The campaign in the United States was operated by a U.S.-born, German-raised, physician, Anton Dilger. Dr. Dilger brought seed cultures with him to the United States in 1915 and set up a culture facility in the suburban Washington, D.C. home that he rented. He supplied cultures to the German merchant-ship captain Hinsch, stranded in the United States by the British naval blockade, who ran the agents, largely stevedores. Dr. Dilger returned to Germany in early 1916, and the campaign came to a halt a few months later. Similar campaigns were conducted concomitantly in Argentina, Mesopotamia, and Norway. During WWII, the only known conduction of biosabotage by Germany was the contamination of a large reservoir in Bohemia with sewage, in 1945. Throughout that war, however, the Nazis routinely used non-German-captured civilians for induced infection experimentations.

Japan

Civilians were the main object of mass terror attacks launched by the Japanese bacteriological Unit 731 on multiple Chinese targets during the 1930s and 1940s, various bombs and other disseminating devices being thereupon applied. Furthermore, if terrorism at large is a term of relevance with respect to enemy civilian prisoners, then the vast biological experimentations conducted by Unit 731 on thousands of arrested civilian Chinese during the 1930s and 1940s are certainly a sort of an extremely brutal bioterrorism. First-hand accounts testify the Japanese infected civilians through the distribution of contaminated foodstuffs, such as dumplings and vegetables. There are also reports of contaminated water supplies. Such estimates report over 580,000 victims, largely due to plague, anthrax, tularemia, smallpox, and cholera outbreaks. Plague was often induced through infected flees, as well. In addition, repeated seasonal outbreaks after the conclusion of the war brought the death toll to much higher. On one occasion at least (1939), the Japanese military contaminated Soviet water sources with typhoid bacteria at the former Mongolian border.

United States

Declassified documents reveal the past existence of at least two bioterrorism operations worked out, if not conducted, by the CIA against Cuba: Operation FULL-UP, the objective of which was to destroy confidence in fuel supplied by the Soviet Bloc by indicating it is contaminated. The operation was to be accomplished by introducing a known biological agent into jet fuel storage facilities. This agent flourishes in jet fuel and grows until it consumes all the space inside the tank.

Operation MONGOOSE: A document entitled "Project Cuba", dated 18 January 1962, sets forth the aims and the 32 original tasks of what sub sequently became known as "Operation MONGOOSE." For task 21, it states that, on 15 February 1962, the CIA would submit a plan to disrupt the harvest of food crops in Cuba. The following two sections of the declassified text of this document, which might be expected to clarify the method to be used in pursuit of this objective, appear to be censored: Clearly their content was so repugnant that even the officials responsible for declassifying the document saw fit to keep that part of it secret. However, in materials provided to the U.S. Senate Select Committee on Intelligence Activities by the CIA during the mid-1970s, the CIA acknowledged that it had developed methods and systems for carrying out a covert attack against crops and causing severe crop loss. The CIA denied that it had ever employed such systems.

The United States has repeatedly been accused by Cuba of biosabotage acts that allegedly occurred. Reportedly, in 1977, a U.S. intelligence source admitted that the United States used the swine-fever virus as biological warfare against Cuba. The agent told U.S. media he was ordered to transport the virus from a U.S. Army Base and CIA training center in the Panama Canal Zone to a group of right-wing Cuban exiles who in turn delivered it to operatives inside Cuba in March 1971. This may seemingly be connected to the outbreak of swine-fever virus in Cuba on 6 May, 1971—its first appearance in the Western Hemisphere. The highly contagious virus is lethal to pigs. Six weeks into the epidemic, the Cubans were forced to slaughter a half-million pigs to stem the spread of the epidemic. Also, the *New York Times* reported in 1983 how the head of a Miami-based anti-Cuban terrorist group admitted in a U.S. court that he had taken germs to Cuba in 1980.

Furthermore, Project MKNAOMI is notable as well. In the 1970s, the CIA publicly revealed that a U.S. Army team called the Special Operations Division (SOD) at Fort Detrick, Maryland, developed biological and chemical weapons for the CIA under a Top Secret project that would last almost 20 years. This project, MKNAOMI, was practically unknown at the CIA due to the extreme sensitivity of its mission. Few written records were kept. CIA personnel working at Fort Detrick used the cover of Special Support Staff of the Department of Defense. Indeed, on 23 October 1962, the U.S. Patent Office granted patent 3,060,165 to four persons "as represented by the Secretary of the Army." The patent was first filed 3 July 1952, Serial Number 297,142 for the use of ricin as a biological weapon. The strikingly honest descriptive language used to apply for this U.S. patent, in 1952, is very revealing: "Ricin is a protoplasmic poison prepared from castor beans after the extraction of castor oil therefrom. It is most effective as a poison when injected intravenously or inhaled. A very fine particle size was necessary so that the product might be used as a toxic weapon." Also, in the early 50s the SOD conducted—as revealed in a document partially declassified by the FBI—a biosabotage experiment, using the Pentagon building as a model target, so as to prove that all persons present therein would be unknowingly exposed within a relatively short period of time. Additional model targets where selected to simulate biosabotage operations, for example the Washington's National Airport and the New-York Subway during the 60s. The CIA and possibly other elements within the U.S. intelligence community apparently persisted in holding bioterrorism agents after the United States destroyed its biological weapons arsenal. Besides, an increasing debate has aroused as to the shear innocence of the US outstandingly growing research of virulent pathogens, referring to the fragile borderline separating between defensive- and offensive-oriented implications. However, the very same debate may equally pertain, in principle, to other states.

South Africa

Rather unexpectedly, an extremely meticulous biosabotage program has been uncovered in South Africa. Apparently, it constitutes an outstanding case of a state-sponsored bioterrorism paradigm that has been fairly brought out in details. The most characteristic feature of the South African biological (and chemical) terrorism program was undoubtedly the development, testing, and utilization of a wide array of hard-to-trace agents to assassinate "enemies of the state." As insider testimony and the notorious "sales list" of 1989 indicate, several of the highly poisonous substances produced at both Delta G and Roodeplaat Research Laboratories were actually deployed by clandestine units ADF and SAP "*death squads*," above all the Security Branch's C1 section (later renamed C10), housed at the Vlakplaas base, in covert assassination operations.

There is no doubt whatsoever that high-ranking officers within the SADF and SAP and other "*securocrats*" within the government were generally aware of these activities, many of which they in fact authorized. Some civilian Afrikaner paramilitary groups, whose pro-apartheid members remain violently opposed to black majority rule, have even publicly threatened to attack their enemies with biological and chemical agents.

In the mid-1980s, a higher level and more formalized assassination program formed when the Teen-Rewolusionêre Inligting Taakspan was created. Then, on the verbal instructions of a senior cardiologist, Colonel Dr. Wouter Basson—head of Project Coast: Apartheid's Chemical and Biological Warfare Program—a host of freeze-dried pathogens and highly toxic substances that had been produced either at Delta G or RRL—was secretly transferred and thereafter stored in a refrigerator inside a fireproof and bombproof walk-in safe in his own office to military and police personnel through various channels. The deadly agents were passed on, either to the aforementioned persons in innocuous public places like restaurants or to Basson himself in the latter's office at South African Medical Services (SAMS) headquarters in Centurion. The specific recipients of these lethal substances and contaminated items were operatives of the "*death squads*," officers who either deployed some of them personally or later distributed them to the so-called "hit team" members; an ex-psychologist who in 1988 assumed control over Systems Research and Development; a bioengineering company set up in part to manufacture special "applicators," i.e., arcane assassination devices such as rings, screwdrivers, walking sticks, and umbrellas that had been transformed into weapons by means of the addition of poison compartments and injectors or firing mechanisms for poisoned pellets; and Basson himself. Furthermore, holes were drilled in cans of Game orange soda, into which some substance was injected, and then closed by means of soldering so that they were no longer visible.

The actual substances included the viruses of Ebola, Congo, and Marburg; lethal toxins such as mamba toxin, botulinum, and ricin; bacterial agents such as plague, anthrax, brucellosis, salmonellosis, and bottles of cholera bacteria; and a wide variety of foodstuffs, beverages, household items, and cigarettes that had been contaminated with these biological agents. There can be little doubt that several of these materials, items, or devices were subsequently often used to murder or sicken opponents of the apartheid regime. If one excludes the hundreds of drugged and secretly disposed guerrilla opponents, the total number of victims appears to have been in the dozens.

International ties formed as well within that dark context. Dr. Wouter Basson, or other Coast personnel, may have transferred dangerous biological warfare materials and know-how to elements of a loose international network of right-wing extremists. Fears have been expressed that Basson and other Coast scientists were associated with an even broader international right-wing network, purportedly known as Die Organisasie, among whose members are said to be expatriate Rhodesians and South Africans who emigrated to other countries both during the apartheid era and as the apartheid system was collapsing. Basson also had strong bonds with Arabic elements, particularly Iraqi and Libyan.

Connectedly, according to a pair of Federal Bureau of Investigation (FBI) informants, in the mid-1980s, the American doctor Larry Ford transferred a suitcase full of dangerous "kaffir-killing" pathogens to Surgeon-General Knobel at the Los Angeles residence of the South African trade attaché, Gideon Bouwer. It has also emerged that at Knobel's request Ford lectured Coast scientists about the contamination of household items with biological agents. The whole apparatus was dismantled during the 1990s. Still, such a complex state-sponsored bioterrorism program, operating both inside South Africa and beyond, all over, has not elsewhere been uncovered publicly, yet certainly not an isolated one, worldwide; the Soviet, and later Russian parallel system did not—and apparently does not—lag far behind.

USSR and Russia

Two bioterrorism affairs, one momentary—the planned assassination of an opponent by ricin toxin in London—and the other one lasting for years—the relapsing employment of fungal toxins against civilians in South East Asia—were sponsored, in effect, by USSR, whereas Bulgaria and North Vietnam were involved as partners, respectively. Not singular (referring to the Soviet apparatus at large), those two affairs attracted much attention. Although the latter has been surreptitiously—yet massively—conducted by the Soviet MOD, the former was a fine product of the KGB.

Various modes of biosabotage have been specifically encountered with regard to the USSR and Russia, in the book titled *Biological Espionage*, written by former KGB officer Alexander Kouzminov who worked for the so-called "Department 12, Directorate S (the KGB Operational Technical Support Directorate)." This directorate oversees Moscow's "illegals" (i.e., Russian agents posing as Westerners, operating under deep cover). Department 12 (and Department 8) of the KGB were tasked with preparing "clandestine acts of biological sabotage against 'potential strike targets' on the enemy's territory." These potential targets include military research laboratories, combat units, weapon stockpiles, public drinking water, food stores, vaccine repositories, pharmaceutical plants, and the overall economy of the target country. These two departments would also assassinate, incapacitate, or kidnap foreign officials, political enemies, and "important persons" (where "important" is determined by the exigencies of war).

Department 12 was referred to in intelligence circles as the "Chamber" or "Kamera." KGB General Viktor Chebrikov, Andropov's closest subordinate in the KGB, was then the Director of this department. The "Chamber" developed, among many technical devices and substances various toxins, such as ricin, which is but one example. The work of Department 12 "has grown" since the collapse of the Soviet Union. Genetic engineering has brought forth new bioterrorism horrors. And these are to be unleashed in the event of something called "Day X," which signifies, conceptually, the beginning of the next world war—a large-scale war. Soviet military thinkers believe that such a war will tentatively involve the mass use of nuclear as well as biological weapons, concomitant with multiple bioterrorism operations. The KGB thus had its own R&D centers for special toxic matters including bioterrorism toxins and pathogens for use in espionage aims and sabotage (so-called "Fleita" program). In parallel, aerosol-released bioterrorism weapons were often in the possession of Spetsnaz operatives (Soviet military Special Forces).

Connectedly, the manners of the KGB are well illustrated in detail through the Soviet–Bulgarian ricin plot. Georgi Ivanov Markov was born 01.03.1929 in Sofia, Bulgaria and died in London due to induced ricin intoxication. He was executed by DS (Durzhavna Sigornost—Bulgarian State Security) in London on 11.09.1978, thanks to vital assistance knowingly afforded by the KGB. A totally independent journalist, Markov was Bulgaria's most revered dissident and Bulgarian Communism's arch enemy. Bulgarian Communist dictator, Todor Zhivkov, was very well informed about Markov's activities by the DS. In 1977, Zhivkov asked the KGB to help him silence Markov. The Russians did not hesitate. Both President Yuri Andropov and Vladimir Krutchkov, head of KGB, personally approved and ordered General Sergei Golubev (Chief of the Security Service and specialist on "murder") to cooperate with DS. The KGB granted DS access to the resources in the "Chamber."

Golubev received instructions in the KGB headquarter relevant "Chamber," and the next week he flew to Sofia with Ivan Surov. Surov's job was to transmit the Bulgarian Intelligence Service practical know-how in the use of special poisons, which could not be traced after the victim's death. Golubev and Surov discussed with the Bulgarian's intelligence officers the various options of killing Markov. They worked out one plan to use a poison that could be surreptitiously dissolved in tea, coffee, or any liquid that Markov might drink. In 1978, Gen. Golubev traveled to Sofia three or four times to help DS with planning of the secret operation. Three attempts to assassinate Markov followed. The first attempt was made in Munich in the spring of 1978 when Markov was visiting friends and colleagues at Radio Free Europe. Someone put a toxin into Markov's drink at a dinner in his honor. The attempt to kill him failed. The second assassination effort occurred on the Italian island of Sardinia, where Markov was on vacation with his family. The plan also failed for reasons unknown.

Golubev returned to Sofia to work out a new plan to kill Markov. The KGB decided to use a camouflaged weapon. A folding umbrella was adapted with a firing mechanism and silencer to shoot a small pellet at close range, one and a half to two meters. Golubev requested that the KGB Residency in Washington purchase several U.S.-manufactured umbrellas and send them to the Center. The KGB head resident in Washington bought several umbrellas and sent them to the KGB, and an OTU operational technical unit rebuilt the umbrellas. The "Chamber" then adapted the umbrella tip to enable it to shoot the victim with a tiny metal pellet containing ricin. Golubev then took the converted umbrellas to Sofia to instruct the assassin on how to use this weapon. The pellet was supposed to penetrate the clothing and be lodged in the upper skin layer. Consequently, the final, and successful, attempt was staged in London 07.09.1978, on Bulgarian's Communist dictator Todor Zhivkov's sixty-seventh birthday. Before his assassination, Markov received a threatening anonymous phone call: "Not this time," said anonymous caller. "This time you will not become a martyr. You will simply die of natural causes. You will be killed by a poison that the West cannot detect nor treat." The tasked ricin toxin did the job, indeed. On the day of his assassination, Markov worked a double shift at the BBC. After finishing the early morning shift, he went home for rest and lunch. Returning to work by car, he drove to a parking lot on the south side of Waterloo Bridge. It was his habit to take a bus across the half-mile Waterloo Bridge to the BBC head-quarters in the Bush House. After parking his car in a parking lot near the Waterloo Bridge, Markov climbed the stairs to the bus stop. As he neared the queue of people waiting for the bus. he experienced a sudden stinging pain in the back of his right thigh. He turned and saw a man bending to pick up a dropped umbrella. The man who was facing away from Markov, apologized. The assassin then hailed a taxi and departed. Although in pain, Markov boarded the bus to work. But the pain continued.

Markov noticed a small blood spot on his jeans. He told colleagues at the BBC what happened and showed one friend a pimple-like red swelling on his thigh. By evening, he had developed a high fever. He was hospitalized and treated for an undetermined form of blood poisoning. His condition fast worsened. He was not responding to doctor's efforts. The next day he went into shock, and after three days of agony and delirium, he died on 11.09.1978.

An autopsy was performed at Wandsworth Public Mortuary. The doctors found a tiny metal sphere the size of a pinhead in the wound. When they attempted to extract the "pin," a tiny pellet fell on the table. The police took the pellet to the Chemical and Microbiological Warfare Establishment at Porton Down, commonly called the "Germ Warfare Center." There, a team of the England's foremost specialists in forensic medicine, and, reportedly, Dr. Christopher Green of the CIA examined the pellet. The pellet was 1.52 mm in diameter, embedded in his calf, and composed of 90% platinum and 10% iridium. They found that two 0.34-mm holes had been drilled in the pellet, possibly using a high-technology laser at right angles to each other, producing an X-shaped cavity. The holes were empty.

This prevented investigators from establishing the type of substance that had been used, but it was sufficient to determine that Markov had "not died of natural causes." BATS (British Anti-Terrorist Squad), detectives then joined the Scotland Yard investigating team. After weeks of research and experimentation, in January 1979, a Coroner's Inquest in London Gavin Thurston ruled that Georgi Markov had been killed via ricin toxin. Traces of ricin were possibly found later thereupon.

But several years later, two former top KGB officers, Oleg Gordievsky and Oleg Kalugin, publicly admitted Soviet complicity in Markov's murder by means of ricin toxin. The case was dormant until after the arresting of Communist dictator Todor Zhivkov and the fall of the Communist government in Bulgaria in 1989. Although the DS act about the case Markov is destroyed or has been sent to Moscow, there is no doubt that some DS and KGB officers know the true about his death.

In 1991, former chief of Bulgarian Foreign Intelligence Vasil Kotsev, who was identified as the person in charge of the Markov operation, died in a questionable and mysterious automobile accident. A second suspect, General Stoyan Savov, preferred to commit suicide on 09.01.1992 rather than face trial also for destroying the documents. In 1994 the British Parliament asked Russia to help them find 15 past KGB agents who might have been involved in or had knowledge of the murder. The request remains unanswered. The Markov murder case remains officially unsolved. No one has been brought to justice for the murder of Markov, although *prima facie* evidence points fairly clearly at the involvement of Soviet and Bulgarian elements, chiefly the KGB. The Russian KGB officially ceased to exist in November 1991, but its successor organization, the FSB, is functionally extremely similar to the KGB. Even after many details about the related bioterrorism mechanisms were revealed, during the 1990s, and although many alterations took place in Russia, this system did not substantially change.

Iraq

In the past, Iraq conducted bioterrorism in the following cases: In 1988, the Iraqi army deliberately introduced typhoid bacteria into the water supply of the Kurdish city of Sulaimaniyah, bringing about an outbreak. In 1989, outbreaks of cholera were generated as a result of BWA being experimented with on Kurdish populations by Iraq. In 1990, an apparent, severe malaria outbreak that exceptionally occurred in the Kurdish Biharka concentration camp in Iraq has been attributed to Iraqi experimental employment of a BWA. Also, Iraq developed and produced aflatoxin (at least 2200 L) as a long-term debilitating bioterrorism agent intended to be used against the Kurds. It has there-upon been noted that:

The discovery (by UNSCOM, during the 1990s) that Iraq was researching aflatoxin, not a traditional BW candidate, was a cause for some surprise. It is a carcinogen, the effects of which manifest themselves only after many years, and several Western experts have rationalized this Iraqi program only in terms of genocidal goals. If aflatoxin were used against the Kurds, for instance, it would be impossible definitively to prove the use of BW once the symptoms emerged. Another possible explanation is its potential use as an immune suppressant, making victims more susceptible to other agents. However, the aflatoxin declaration may also hide other aspects of Iraq's BW program: according to Iraq's depositions, the production program never encountered any mishap (as other parts of the BW program had) and, to judge from the declared time-frame for the total amount produced, production could never have stopped, even for cleaning of the equipment. This raises the suspicion that Iraq declared an excessive amount of aflatoxin in order to disguise the fact that other, more destructive agents had been produced in greater quantities.

Being a very potent, although typically slow-acting hepatotoxin and nephrotoxin, aflatoxin may have been developed as a BWA by the Iraqis for purposes of long-term terrorism, or some short-term acute impact of yet unknown nature. Iraq was unable to justify the weaponization of aflatoxin from the research data obtained from its own experimentation. One bomb that by Iraq's account should have contained aflatoxin instead tested positive for botulinum toxin and negative for aflatoxin; this indicated another mode of weaponization. And indeed, there is documentary evidence and statements obtained by UNSCOM that Iraq was mixing aflatoxin with riot-control gas. They note that it would not be unthinkable for a leader who has used chemical weapons on part of his population. "It is a great way to keep colonels from becoming generals," said an UNSCOM inspector familiar with the searches. "Saddam Hussein hasn't made any weapon that he hasn't used on his own population, with the exception of Scud missiles." Doubtfully, the entire, tainted past Iraqi–Kurdish interface has been revealed by him since being in prison.

Notably, the Iraqi Intelligence Service provided the BW program with security and participated in bioterrorism research, probably for its own purposes, from the beginning of Iraq's BW effort in the early 1970s until the final days of Saddam Hussein's regime. The Iraqi Intelligence Service had a series of laboratories that conducted bioterrorism work including research into BW agents for assassination purposes until the mid-1990s. The Iraqi Survey Group found that the Iraqi Intelligence service produced ricin and tested it on political prisoners. ISG has not been able to establish the scope and nature of the work at these laboratories or determine whether any of the work was related to military development of a BW agent. But they could certainly suffice to sponsor and support the 2001 anthrax letters' sabotage, together with al-Qaeda, as has previously been suggested. All in all, the option for bioterrorism operations was persistently maintained by Iraq until its collapse in 2003.

Iran

According to Eisenstadt, Iran has probably deployed BWs, which it could deliver via terrorist saboteurs, aerosol tanks mounted on aircraft or ships, or via missiles. Taking care, thus, of the entire spectrum of BWs, Tehran did not ignore their importance in the context of terrorist actions; it equipped itself with micro-warfare means destined to employ bioterrorism agents by on-spot spraying and by contaminating water systems. Iran, as well as Muslim BW possessors like Sudan and Syria, can readily be assisted by some Muslim terror organization, in case they want to carry out bioterrorism acts through nonresidential saboteurs. More concretely, such cooperation between Iran and its terror organization ally—the Hezbollah—has been feared. Other states runing BW programs that may potentially support of sponsor bioterrorism acts include, mainly, Syria, North Korea and Cuba.

Nonstate-sponsored Bioterrorism

Persisting organizations, temporary communes, or sporadic individuals may initiate and conduct bioterrorism acts, without there being any institutionalized assistance from any country. The following section deals with those three types of elements, practically or potentially involved in bioterrorism-related activities. Also, it presents in detail prominent episodes of in-effect bioterrorism.

Al-Qaeda

This terror organization has been, and still is, the most significant one worldwide, in terms of bioterrorism, especially that it was involved, most probably, in the Sept. 2001 anthrax letter attack. In the mid-1990s, while being sheltered in Sudan, its head, Osama bin Laden, financed, in part, the construction of BW (and CW) facilities in Sudan. Later on, members of al-Qaeda were apparently trained in Iraq (by its intelligence apparatus) for BW (and other nonconventional weapons) employment. In 1998, relationship with Iraqi intelligence was established, so as to obtain poisons—appatently toxins—and gases training. After the USS Cole bombing in 2000, two al-Qaeda operatives were sent to Iraq for CBW-related training beginning in Dec. 2000. Iraqi intelligence was "encouraged" after the embassy and USS Cole bombings to provide this training.

Moreover, in August 2002, reports have emerged that Ansar al-Islam, an al-Qaeda affiliate active in Iraqi Kurdistan since September 2001 as a militant group, has been involved in testing various poisons including ricin. According to an ABC News report, the group tested ricin powder as an aerosol on animals such as donkeys and chickens, and perhaps even an unwitting human subject. The experiments were ordered and financed by a senior al-Qaeda official, who was providing money and guidance from elsewhere in the region.

Also, selected al-Qaeda terrorists were guided as to the methods of cultivating germs and preparing toxins to be used as bioterrorism agents and how to convert them into weapons, exploiting easily available equipment and materials. Those who plotted in the caves of Afghanistan have left behind diagrams of American cities and landmarks. Also, manufacturing instructions have been posted on the Internet. One of the simulated operations in Kandahar, Afghanistan, was contaminating a water main of a European city (apparently London) using equipment that could fit inside a backpack. Several al-Qaeda cells have been trained in Afghanistan, where they have learned to use bioterrorism agents, including anthrax, ricin, and botulism toxins. Later, after the fall of the Taliban regime, those groups continued their experiments in the Pankisi Gorge, on the territory of Georgia, bordering Chechnya. Not too far away, in Fallugah, Iraq, an improvised laboratory belonging to Iraqi al-Qaeda-directed rebels was revealed in 2004. It was found to contain materials for making chemical blood agents, as well as a "cookbook" on how to produce a deadly form of anthrax. Two months earlier, notably, the very same Abu Musan al-Zarkawi's derivative group of al-Qaedat ("Tahwid and Jihad"— "Oneness of God and Holy War") tried hard to take care of two women known as the Iraqi anthrax masterminds. It kidnapped two Americans and a British man, threatening to kill them if Iraqi women prisoners were not released. The two Iraqi masterly women were not set free, and the three kidnapped men were then killed.

Another training base was located at Zenica, Bosnia. It is not clear, however, whether any experimentation practically included, beyond toxins, in-effect living germs. Reportedly, bin Laden's associates managed to receive anthrax and plague biological weapons from former Soviet facilities in

Kazakhstan. Records and operations manuals captured in Afghanistan and elsewhere disclose that bin Laden has devoted money and personnel to pursue smallpox, among other biological weapons. Furthermore, uncorroborated testimony in a high-profile Egyptian trial in 1999 indicated that al-Qaeda had equired Ebola virus and Salmonella germs.

al-Qaeda, and particularly its second in command, Ayman al-Zawahiri, a physician, had long been eager to acquire biological agents, particularly anthrax, according to Khalid Shaikh Mohammed, one of Osama bin Laden's top lieutenants. Also, al-Qaeda agents had inquired about renting crop-dusters to spread pathogens, especially anthrax. During interrogations with terror suspects in custody, it has come to light that the al-Qaeda terror group has been actively seeking weapons-grade anthrax. According to an article by Milton Leitenberg, computer hard drives and handwritten notes seized at the home where Mohammed was arrested included an order to buy anthrax, along with other evidence of an interest in acquiring anthrax and other dangerous germs. Until the American invasion of Afghanistan, launched after the Sept. 11, 2001 attacks, al-Qaeda's anthrax program was based in Kandahar, Afghanistan, and was led by two men: Riduan Isamuddin, known as Hambali, and Yazid Sufaat, a Malaysian member of Jemaah Islamiyah, an al-Qaeda-affiliated group. Although Sufaat tried to acquire anthrax, there is no evidence that he was able to procure the appropriate strain used for the 2001 attacks (Ames strain). This does not mean, yet, that al-Qaeda did not obtain that deadly strain through other channels. Hambali had been trying to open a new BW project for al-Qaeda in the Far-East, when he was arrested. Reportedly, anthrax powder was found, eventually, in March 2006 in a house occupied by the Taliban in Afghanistan.

A London-based offshoot was engaged in preparing ricin and botulinum toxins. In January 2003, British authorities arrested six Arab men that intended to produce ricin in their north London apartment, led by Kamel Bourgass, who had been trained in al-Qaeda terror camps in Afghanistan and was specially selected for instruction in making poisons. Accurate recipes and ingredients for poisons including botulinum and ricin (plus cyanide), and the blueprint for a bomb were found in the apartment, in addition to castor beans.

Nonetheless, after the 2001 anthrax letter attack (covered bellow in special subchapter) and the U.S. military operations against al-Qaeda in Afghanistan, on many occasions repeated bioterrorism warnings emerged, stemming from intelligence information and from various announcements made by al-Qaeda. Just as one example, six flights bound for America, including four from Britain, were cancelled after intelligence suggested that al-Qaeda was planning a spectacular attack using a hijacked airliner and weapons of mass destruction, particularly BWs. Along-side with cases of in-effect bioterrorism-oriented activities, like the ricin affair in London, various bioterrorism hoaxes that could not be identified may probably be attributed to al-Qaeda. At any rate, al-Qaeda certainly wants to use biological weapons and widen the scope. The British M15 recently reported, thereby, that al-Qaeda operatives are training in germ warfare, and trying to recruit university students with access to microbiological laboratories, so as to steal virulent pathogens.

Jemaah Islamiah

A Southeast Asian Islamic militant group affiliated with al-Qaeda, this organization does not lag far behind the latter. Connectedly, Dr Rohan Gunaratna, who heads the terror unit at Singapore's Institute of Defence and Strategic Studies, has warned Australia of a new, global generation of Islamist terrorists "armed, trained financed and ideologicised" to use biological weapons. In declaring that part of this new global terror wave would come out of Southeast Asia, he added he found the Jemaah Islamiah group had come extremely close to developing bioterrorism-chemical weapons, recounting an alarming analysis of a Jemaah Islamiah biological-terror rudimentary training manual that was taken from a Philippines safe house in late 2003. His further generalization is notable, saying "It is only a question of time that a group that has these intentions will have the capability to develop them. We are seeing a new generation of terrorists being trained in the use of biotlogical weapons. We rarely saw this in the 1990s but today we are seeing increasingly this kind of training. Groups are being trained to use these agents, though the probability of attack is still low."

Hezbollah

Former CIA director James Wolsey described the Hezbollah as a potential tool for bioterrorism. That threat has been accentuated and is particularly realistic, because the Hezbollah is a radical terror organization, directly supported and encouraged by Iran, which possesses biological weapons. The evident acquisition and successful employment of unmanned drones by the Hezbollah, as well as its access to the sources of the Jordan River, may increase a potential bioterrorism threat posed by this dangerous organization. In 1998 the Hezbollah attempted to obtain biological and chemical weapons through two businessmen situated in Switzerland. Elements of Hezbollah and al-Qaeda joined forces to plan a series of attacks using toxic substances, apparently chemicals and toxins. Groups of al-Qaeda and Hezbollah activists from the Sidon area of Lebanon met in Africa in December 2002, to set up the needed preparations there or in Sidon. The 2006 confrontation between Hezbollah and Israel, demonstrated effective operational capacities of the Hezbollah to employ a variety of Iranian rockets and missiles, some of which are tipped—in Iran—with biological warheads.

Radical Palestinian Terror Organizations

An article appeared on the 13 August 2001 edition of the Lebanon-based Palestinian weekly, *Al-Manar*, stating that there is "serious thinking" among the Palestinians about obtaining BWs. It says regarding BWs that "obtaining its primary components is possible without too much effort, let alone the fact that there are hundreds of experts who are capable of handling them and use them as weapons of deterrence, thus creating a balance of horror. Anyone who is capable, with complete self-control, of turning his body into shrapnel and scattered organs, is also capable of carrying a small device that cannot be traced and throw it in the targeted location." It has been pointed out that Palestinian organizations are inclined to resort to the acquisition and introduction of nonconventional capabilities—in particular biological and chemical—mainly for deterrence purposes. According to that source, many Palestinians believe that biological and chemical weapons are a legitimate and desirable means in the struggle against Israel. Basically, a radical terror organization, like the Hamas, is apt to acquire BWs, although so far it is not known to have obtained them, in that case.

Notably, a novel mode of infection with hepatitis B virus has been suggested, following penetrating human bone fragments due to the explosion of a Palestinian suicide bomber. Connectedly, perhaps, the Tanzim planned to use a suicide-bomber arrested with explosives bearing AIDS-infected blood, the thinking being that anyone who survived would get AIDS. The operation was foiled. Another Palestinian body, the al-Aqsa Martyrs' Brigades (affiliated with the Palestinian Fatah political party) sent an announcement in 2006 to the Ramattan News Agency, stating: "we are pleased to say that we succeeded in developing some 20 different types of biological and chemical weapons, this after a three-year effort", adding that those agents might be employed under certain circumstances.

Aum Shinrikyo Cult

The Aum Shinrikyo Cult ("religion of supreme truth"), a Japan-based apocalyptic religious sect, produced biological agents and tried to use them. The Japanese police discovered that the Aum included among its members skilled scientists and technicians, including some with training in microbiology, who attempted to generate weapons using anthrax, cholera, botulinum toxin, Q-fever, and even Ebola virus. These accounts also suggest that there were four separate attempts to use biological agents, including anthrax once and botulinum toxin three times:

1. In April 1990, the Aum Shinrikyo outfitted an automobile to disseminate botulinum toxin through the engine's exhaust. The car was then driven around Japan's parliament building.
2. In early June 1993, the cult attempted to disrupt the planned wedding of Prince Naruhito, Japan's Crown Prince, by spreading botulinum toxin in downtown Tokyo using a specially equipped automobile.
3. In late June 1993, the cult attempted to spread anthrax in Tokyo using a sprayer system on the roof of an Aum-owned building in eastern Tokyo. The anthrax was disseminated for four days.
4. On March 15, 1995, the Aum planted in the Tokyo subway three briefcases designed to release botulinum toxin. Apparently, the individual responsible for filling the botulinum toxin had qualms about the planned attack and substituted a nontoxic substance. The failure of this attack led the cult to use sarin in its March 20, 1995 subway attack. A helicopter and two UAVs were purchased by the cult and intended to be equiped with sprayers.

Fortunately, the Aum scientists apparently made mistakes in either the way they produced or disseminated the agents, and no one became ill or died from the attacks.

Bhagwan Shri Rajneesh Cult—Typhoid Epidemic

As the summer of 1984 waned, a cult led by the Bhagwan Shri Rajneesh near the town of The Dalles, Oregon, used a biological agent to sicken hundreds in an apparent dress rehearsal to sway the outcome of a local election. Three years earlier, the Bhagwan brought followers with him from India when he immigrated in 1981. The hard-working Rajneeshees were isolationist, with some 150 armed people to keep outsiders away from their ranch. When the Bhagwan decided to enlarge his ranch and his flock, he took over the small town of Antelope, christening the new town Rajneesheepuram.

Oregon's attorney general stated, however, that the municipality was unconstitutional because it did not separate church and state. To outmaneuver the attorney general, the cult's hierarchy hatched a plan to make the Wasco county residents too sick to vote in November 1984, enabling the Rajneeshees to seat their favored candidate on the county court. The cult's nurse was the scientific brain behind attempts to put a bioterrorism plan into action.

Although the cultists considered additional organisms (AIDS and *Salmonella typhi*), the Rajneeshees decided upon *Salmonella typhimurium*, so as to bring about a massive food contamination. The cult bought bactrol disks from a Seattle medical supply company under false pretenses. A trio of cult members worked in a laboratory equipped with an incubator and freeze dryer to brew what they called a "salsa." Several more Rajneeshees were involved in distributing the agent on various occasions. Starting on 29 August 1984, the Rajneeshees began sprinkling their *S. typhimurium* in personal drinking glasses, on doorknobs, and urinal handles; on produce at the local supermarket; and on salad bars in 11 restaurants.

Soon, a steady stream of patients was reporting to local physicians and hospitals, with symptoms ranging from nausea and diarrhea to headache and fever. In total, 751 fell ill. Wasco County commissioners and ordinary citizens were among the victims. Within 4 days, local health-care providers were able to identify the *S. typhimurium* as the source, but over a year passed before there was confirmation that a single strain caused all of the illnesses and the Centers for Disease Control filed its report. No one died in this test to see whether a ballot box could be fixed, but the Bhagwan reportedly observed that one should not worry if a few perished. Law enforcement authorities thought that the Rajneeshees were practicing to poison the water system of The Dalles. Cult members had already put dead rodents and perhaps raw sewage and salmonella salsa into The Dalles' water supply.

Several cult members were involved in the planning and execution of the salmonella attacks, but only two of the Baghwan's chief lieutenants were prosecuted. This pair received multiple concurrent

20 year sentences, among other penalties. According to one analyst who studied the Rajneeshees carefully, the cult did not work its way up the ladder of violence to bioterrorism. Rather, the Rajneeshees appear to have abruptly embarked on their salmonella spree as a means to a specific end.

An epidemiologic analysis was then done. Cohort and case-control investigations were conducted among groups of restaurant patrons and employees to identify exposures associated with illness. All 751 persons with Salmonella gastroenteritis were associated with eating or working at area restaurants. Most patients were identified through passive surveillance; active surveillance was conducted for selected groups. A case was defined either by clinical criteria or by a stool culture yielding *S. typhimurium*. It has been found that the outbreak occurred in two waves, September 9 through 18 and September 19 through October 10. Most cases were associated with 10 restaurants, and epidemiologic studies of customers at 4 restaurants and of employees at all 10 restaurants implicated eating from salad bars as the major risk factor for infection. Eight (80%) of 10 affected restaurants compared with only 3 (11%) of the 28 other restaurants in The Dalles operated salad bars (relative risk, 7.5; 95% confidence interval, 2.4–22.7; $P < 0.001$). The implicated food items on the salad bars differed from one restaurant to another.

The investigation did not identify any water supply, food item, supplier, or distributor common to all affected restaurants, nor were employees exposed to any single common source. In some instances, infected employees may have contributed to the spread of illness by inadvertently contaminating foods. However, no evidence was found linking ill employees to initiation of the outbreak. Errors in food rotation and inadequate refrigeration on ice-chilled salad bars may have facilitated growth of the *S. typhimurium* but could not have caused the outbreak. A subsequent criminal investigation revealed that members of a religious commune had deliberately contaminated the salad bars. An *S. typhimurium* strain found in a laboratory at the commune was indistinguishable from the outbreak strain.

Although the above information pertains to organizational or cultist bioterrorism, the following episodes represent individual bioterrorism.

Shigella Dysenteriae Type 2 Outbreak

Another case of intentional contamination of food with a bacterial pathogen occurred in 1996, involving clinical laboratory workers infected with *S. dysenteriae* type 2. *S. dysenteriae* type 2 is a rare organism, and outbreaks are seldom seen in the general population. After consumption of muffins and donuts anonymously placed in the break room of a Texas laboratory, 12 of 45 laboratory workers developed severe, acute diarrheal illness. Rapid onset of symptoms allowed investigators to retrieve a muffin sample, later cultured and found to contain *S. dysenteriae* type 2, matching those cultured from infected workers. Laboratory reference cultures were found in disarray, and cultures were missing, indicating laboratory cultures had been taken, grown, and used to contaminate foodstuffs. All case patients reported having eaten muffins or doughnuts placed in the staff break room on October 29. Isolates from nine case patients were indistinguishable from *S. dysenteriae* type 2 recovered from an uneaten muffin and from the laboratory's stock strain, a portion of which was missing.

Hepatitis A Outbreak

Another instance of apparent intentional contamination of food with hepatitis A virus was documented in 1965. Twenty-three cases of hepatitis were reported among personnel at a Naval Air Station in 1961. The course of disease among those infected was moderately severe with no deaths. At the time, hepatitis A (infectious hepatitis) and hepatitis B (serum hepatitis) diagnoses were made on clinical and epidemiological grounds. To determine the cause of the infections, an extensive investigation of risk factors was conducted. Dining hall records and food questionnaires identified potato salad as the most likely contaminated food source. Questioning of the sole salad cook revealed that he had experienced symptoms resembling hepatitis, and a background investigation revealed aberrant social behavior. Connectedly, two incidents of inappropriate urination gave investigators a possible route of contamination of the potato salad when coupled with the individuals' symptomology.

Ascaris Suum Outbreak

The last instance of intentional contamination involved four college students who were peculiarly exposed to a massive dose of embryonated *Ascaris suum* eggs (a large ringworm infecting pigs) while attending a Winter Carnival in Canada during February 1970. The most likely source of infection was a meal served to the students during the Winter Carnival.

Anthrax Letters

A colossal event generated by means of a minute amount of anthrax powder, the September 2001 anthrax letter attack, is discussed in detail. The remarkable potentiality of anthrax as a bioterrorism agent in general, and within the context of the letter attack in particular, is demonstrated. Resultant short- and long-term impacts are accentuated, alongside with the severe inability to point at the provenance of the anthrax powder contained in the letters.

The germ *Bacillus anthracis* is the etiological agent of anthrax, a disease primarily of herbivores, but one that humans occasionally acquire through contact with infected animals or with contaminated animal products. The mode of infection may be cutaneous, intestinal, or pulmonary. The latter represents, as well, a distinct form of employing anthrax germs as an inhalable bioterrorism agent, either sprayed (wet aerosol) or powdered (dry aerosol). The efficacy of the aerosol thus generated is shaped by a variety of inherent attributes largely depending on the way the aerosol material has thereby been structured. In general, the aerosol material contains anthrax germs spores—a resilient form of life typifying all species of the genus *Bacillus* sp.—plus various, most vital, additives.

Under optimal meteorological conditions, producing 50% fatalities over a one-square-mile area would require about just 10 g of anthrax spores, in case there is no medical intervention, whatsoever. Additional data show the impact of anthrax in terms of some 20,000 to 80,000 casualties afflicted by 30 kg of this biological agent, as compared with 400 to 6000 casualties afflicted by 300 kg of sarin nerve gas, and 80,000 casualties afflicted by 20 kiloton of a nuclear weapon. Moreover, official U.S. estimates for casualties produced by an airplane, flying upwind of a city, releasing successfully a cloud of anthrax germs, range from 100,000 to three million dead. An individual driving a car around a medium-sized city spewing anthrax out the tailpipe would cause some 70,000 fatalities, and two individuals in two cars in two cities, 140,000 (referring to an unprotected population). These are, of course, traditional theoretical estimates; yet they illustrate the proportional impact of a biological agent, in this case, anthrax—a noncontagious bacterial pathogen. Still, even by 2003, it was held that a little more than two pounds of anthrax spores efficiently spilled into the air over a city the size of New York could be expected to kill more than 120,000 people unless state and federal officials respond much more aggressively than they currently plan to, according to the first comprehensive computer model of such a terrorist act.

The September 2001 anthrax letter attack marked an outstanding, most significant milestone in the course of bioterrorism. It was a quantum leap, scarcely expected in practical terms, albeit with a lot of indicative intelligence preceding the event. Overall, this bioterrorism campaign has been, operationally, complicated, assuming that the spore powder was produced outside the United States. A most comprehensive picture has been presented by the School of Public Health, Department of Epidemiology, University of California. It meticulously covers the technical, epidemiological, medical, and logistical aspects altogether. Seven letters containing anthrax spores were probably mailed, with similar written messages from Trenton, NJ. Five letters were sent on September 18 (postal facilities [probable cross-contamination]), one going to American Media in Boca Raton, Florida (not recovered); a second to the *New York Post* (recovered); a third to Tom Brokaw of NBC News (recovered); a fourth to ABC News (not recovered); and a fifth to Dan Rather of CBS News (not recovered). On October 9, two more letters were sent from Trenton, NJ. (probably cross-contamination) via Brentwood mail processing facility, one to Senator Tom Daschle (recovered), and the other to Senator Patrick Leahy (recovered). Letter(s) cross-contaminated with the Daschle and Leahy letters were sent from Trenton, NJ to Wallingford, CT, with at least one letter probably going to Oxford, CT. The final anthrax case in the outbreak remains a mystery, but possibly arose from contact with the September 18 letters or cross-contamination with the October 9 Leahy letter in Trenton, NJ. To do so, spores from the Leahy letter would need to have adhered to an envelope of another letter destined for the Bronx, New York City. In summary, the 22 cases (one was removed by the CDC) that comprised the American Anthrax Outbreak of 2001 likely had contact with one or more of seven spore-laden envelopes.

Four letters laden with anthrax spores were discovered, all dated by an unknown author as "09-11-01," and all sent from Trenton, NJ. Two letters were postmarked September 18, 2001 in Trenton, one of which was sent to the *New York Post* where it was handled by several staff members, and the other to Tom Brokaw of NBC, opened September 19–25 but not found until October 12, 2001 in case 2's file drawer. The *New York Post* letter, handled but not opened, was found on October 19, 2001. It was dampened before being discovered, turning the spore contents into a granular or clumped state.

The second two letters were postmarked on October 9, 2001 and mailed to the Washington, D.C. offices of Senator Tom Daschle of North Carolina, Majority Leader, and Senator Patrick Leahy of Vermont, Chair of the Judiciary Committee. Both letters went though Washington, D.C.'s Brentwood mail processing facility, which handles all incoming federal government mail. Both letters contained the same anthrax strain and were of the same potency.

The Daschle letter was opened in the sixth floor office at 9:45 a.m. by an aide in the Senator's Hart Senate Office Building suite on October 15, 2001. It was believed to contain about 2 g of powder comprising 200 billion to 2 trillion spores. Based on nasal swabs, all 18 persons who were in the area of Daschle's sixth floor office tested positive for anthrax exposure, as did 7 of 25 (i.e, 28%) in the area of the Senator's fifth floor office (an open staircase connected the two offices). The Leahy letter never arrived at his office. Instead an optical reader misread the handwritten 20510 ZIP code for the Capitol as 20520, which serves the State Department. As a result, the letter was routed to the State Department, where it arrived on October 15, infecting a State Department postal worker (case 20). Shortly thereafter, all mail was isolated and sealed in plastic bags for a later search.

On November 16, 2001, the Leahy letter was found; then after special preparation, it was opened on December 6 in a laboratory setting. It contained about 1 g of anthrax, made fresh no more than 2 years before it was sent. The contents of the enclosed letter were identical to the wording of the Daschle letter. The anthrax spores in the Daschle and Leahy envelopes were uniformly between 1 and 3 ìm in size, and were coated with fine particles of frothy silica glass. More investigation is underway.

Also processed at the Trenton, NJ postal facility was a small number of letters sent to the Southern Connecticut Processing and Distribution Center in Wallingford, CT. Here letters arrived on October 11 that had been cross-contaminated with anthrax spores from the October 9 Daschle or Leahy envelops. Anthrax spores were found on mail-sorting equipment in Wallingford. One letter that went through the Wallingford distribution center was found in Seymour, nearby to Oxford where case 23 resided. Likely case 23 was infected via a similar cross-contaminated letter that came in contact with mail in the distribution center in Wallingford.

Most uncertain is the origin of case 22, although there is a connection between case 22's neighborhood and the Trenton, NJ post office. A printout from the post office showed that an unrelated letter went to a shop around the corner from case 22's home. This unrelated letter was processed 2 minutes after the Leahy letter and 18 minutes before the Daschle letter. Thus the mail sent to case 22 might also have been cross-contaminated with spores from the Leahy or Daschle envelopes. Alternatively, case 22 might have had contact with one or more of the unrecovered September 18th letters following their disposal in Manhattan, similar to case 19 and case 21.

But the anthrax letters affair was not limited to the US. The American embassy in Vilnius, Lithuania, was likewise concurrently targeted. Also, Three businesses in Karachi, Pakistan, were targeted, and received anthrax letters. Anthrax spores were found in a letter sent from Europe to a doctor's surgery in Chile, according to Chilean officials. For the time being, the culmination of bioterrorism worldwide has been this act of distributing mail envelopes containing anthrax spore powder. It reflected noticeable supremacy of a simple act of bioterrorism (irrespective of preparing the anthrax powder in itself, which was very sophisticated), in several senses:

(a) Uncontrollable preparing of the postal envelopes containing the anthrax powder
(b) Uncontrollable, repeated mailings
(c) Undetectable conveying of the mailed envelopes until reaching their various destinies
(d) Untraceable footprints of the perpetrators
(e) Inability to even postulate whether the sabotage was state or nonstate sponsored

Despite or, rather, because of those points of supremacy, the leading agencies responsible for foreseeing or, at the least, deciphering in retrospect such strikes—FBI, CIA, DIA, and the like—were after nearly 2 years still reluctant to grant public access to an unclassified report on lessons learned from the anthrax letter attacks of 2001; the Pentagon has finally released a redacted version of the document. "The anthrax attacks revealed weaknesses in almost every aspect of U.S. bioterrorism-preparedness and response," the report said. "As simple as these attacks were, their impact was far-reaching." The report, authored by David Heyman of the Center for Strategic and International Studies, is based on a day-long forum convened by CSIS under contract to the Defense Threat Reduction Agency in December 2001.

It provides a detailed and informative but hardly unsuspected inventory of shortcomings in emergency preparedness and response. Ironically, the Defense Department's two-year denial of repeated requests for release of the document exemplifies one of the central problems identified in the report: "The failure to communicate a clear message to the public was one of the greatest problems observed during the anthrax attacks . . . [including] failure to provide timely and accurate information." The Department's inability to efficiently process requests for this document suggests that it still has a long way to go to remedy this particular failure. The redacted version of the report was finally released in response to a Freedom of Information Act (FOIA) appeal.

Also, the Pentagon did not contend that the withheld portions of the anthrax report are classified (exemption 1), even though they are said to concern "vulnerabilities and capabilities of the US Government to respond to another... attack." Rather, in an expansive interpretation of the law, it said that release of the redacted portions would make it possible to "circumvent Department of Defense rules and practices...." (exemption 2). See the March 15 transmittal letter from H.J. McIntyre of the DoD FOIA Policy Office here: Mike Denny Senior Force Protection Consultant Guardian Group Inter national (GGI).

In the long run, the impact of the anthrax letter attack still prevails in several respects:

1. Individually, those who survived the infection have not been fully cured.
2. Globally, the short-run impact encouraged terror-oriented entities to persistently explore or increase bioterrorism options.

3. Practically, numerous consequent hoaxes of bioterrorism threats through powder containing post envelopes extremely proved burdensome to wide logistical systems.
4. Environmentally, even as of 2005, rooms contaminated in 2001 are repeatedly disinfected.
5. Publicly, the interface with institutional classified information holders sharpened.
6. Strategically, the provenance of the anthrax powder has not been deciphered, although somewhat traced.

Thus, since the anthrax attacks in 2001, work at the nation's post offices has been disrupted by more than 20,000 incidents of suspicious powder leaking from envelopes and packages. All but a few have turned out to be nothing more than soap, dust, talc, or other nonlethal substances. Sand was the culprit in one incident included in wedding invitations for a beach ceremony. Still, the scares have taken a toll in nerves, lost time, and money. Postal workers have been instructed, if they see something like that to consider it dangerous. The area then is sealed off, and local hazardous materials teams and the Postal Inspection Service are called in. Leaking suspicious powders that turned out to be harmless include powdered Alfredo sauce, ground lentils, pudding mix, and coffee creamer, officials said. Other cases have included leaking samples of detergent, sugar, or baking soda.

In November 2003, a secret cabinet-level "tabletop" exercise, designed to be very stressful to the system was thus conducted, which simulated the simultaneous release of anthrax in different types of aerosols in several American cities. The drill, code named Scarlet Cloud, found that the country was better able to detect an anthrax attack than it was 2 years ago, said officials knowledgeable about the exercise. But they said the exercise also showed that antibiotics in some cities could not be distributed and administered quickly enough and that a widespread attack could kill thousands; particularly, enormous difficulties stopping the spread of contamination through the country and into Canada were observed.

The drill was notable for the top-level attention it drew and the gaps it showed in the effort to protect against bioterrorism. About three dozen senior officials involved in domestic defense, including two cabinet officers—the secretary of homeland security, and the secretary of transportation—as well as the head of the White House's Homeland Security Council, participated in the exercise at the Pentagon's National Defense University.

Moreover, the contents of the former American Media Inc. building in Boca Raton, FL—namely, thousands of boxes—exposed to anthrax in 2001, were set to be decontaminated for a second time to ensure all of the pathogen is eliminated, given the approval of the Environmental Protection Agency and the Palm Beach Country Health Department.

Overall, the impact of the anthrax letter attack was colossal. In a sense, the very fact that the anthrax letter attack has not been deciphered since 2001 is no less meaningful and important than this unprecedented act of bioterrorism itself. In contrast to the wealth of empirical data collected and published with respect to the specific Ames strain of the 2001 anthrax letter attack and the resultant medical cases, a relative paucity of information has been brought out regarding the chemical and physical properties of the substance contained in the mail envelopes, namely the anthrax spore powder. Primarily its provenance has not yet been deciphered. This peculiar powder certainly reflects an outstanding assortment of different disciplines: micro biological, technological, medical, political, and strategic. Connectedly, it still poses, in parallel, an enigmatic, extremely complex intelligence issue that ought to be elucidated, for numerous reasons. Although the anthrax germs used for this act of bioterrorism have been fully identified to be indistinguishable from the strain Ames—a remarkably virulent strain initially isolated in 1981 in Texas but later shared with laboratories outside the United States—it is still not even known whether the anthrax powder contained in the envelopes has been structured in the United States or elsewhere. Various indications point at Al-Qaeda together with Iraq as being the perpetrators.

Overall, dozens of buildings were contaminated with anthrax as a result of the five mailings, which contained, altogether, about 18 gr. of the sabotage spore powder. The decontamination of the Brentwood postal facility took 26 months (and cost US$130 million). The Hamilton, NJ postal facility remained closed for 41 months (its cleanup cost US$65 million). The Environmental Protection Agency spent US$41.7 million to clean up government buildings in Washington, D.C. One FBI document said the total damage exceeded US$1 billion.

Ricin Course

Various traits making ricin the toxin of choice for bioterrorism purposes are discussed. The actual outcome of that appeal, as shown, has for long been relapsing episodes involving ricin, worldwide. Clear tendency emerges of al-Qaeda and affiliated groups, at the least, to persist in deploying ricin, and is doubtfully controllable. Ricin molecules contain a heterodimeric type 2 ribosome-inactivating enzyme (32 kDa), also known as the A chain. It is a very potent cytotoxic RNA N-glycosidase that inactivates eukaryotic ribosomes. It is linked by a disulfide bond to the galactose/N-acetylgalactosamine-binding lectin (34 kDa), also called the B chain. Weakness, fever, cough and pulmonary edema occur 18–24 hours after inhalation exposure, followed by severe respiratory distress and death from hypoxemia in 36–72 hours. Direct administration into the blood system brings about a similar picture, whereas food poisoning is basically slower, certainly dose-dependent. This protein plant toxin may be regarded, foremost, as the prime toxin for bioterrorism, owing to the integral formed by several different characteristics, altogether:

1 High toxicity
2. Atypical symptomatology
3. Effective contraction through respiratory and alimentary tract
4. Effectual administration through blood stream
5. Availability of the raw material (castor beans)
6. Typical dual usability of the raw material
7. Easiness of manufacturing

Ricin's properties have been known since ancient times, and it has a long history of accidental and intentional intoxication. Ricin was studied as a possible weapon in World War I, and the United States, Canada, and the United Kingdom developed it as a field weapon during World War II, also known as Agent W. The World War II effort led to refined ricin in a crystalline form, although it was the amorphous form that was used in high-explosive bombs and shells and in more specialized delivery systems, such as plastic containers and cluster bombs. Attaining effective particle sizes with ricin powder is difficult, and use of the material in water or suspended in glycerol or carbon tetrachloride is more effective. The agent is difficult to detect. It is fairly stable in clear, dry weather, persisting in the soil or environment for up to 3 days.

But the perfect usability of ricin-oriented for sabotage acts, in parallel, has not at all been ignored. The course of ricin oriented sabotage began long before 1978; yet its in-effect emergence took place in that year. It was the successful ricin-based assassination of the Bulgarian anticommunist reporter Georgi Markov that then occurred in London. Two years later, an assassination of CIA agent Boris Korczak occurred in McLean, Virginia, Tyson's Corner, ricin being used as weapon, possibly repeatedly in umbrella configuration.

The attractiveness of ricin did not diminish because it found new grounds in the United States. In 1983, the FBI obtained one ounce of ricin oriented in a 35-mm film canister from an individual in Springfield, Massachusetts, who had manufactured it himself. This is believed to be one of several confiscations of ricin. In 1993, an Arkansas man with survivalist group connections attempted to smuggle

130 g of ricin from Alaska into Canada to use as a weapon. Later, in 1995 two members of the Minnesota Patriots Council were convicted of conspiracy to assassinate a deputy U.S. Marshal and International Revenue Service agents by ricin.

Syria and Iran acquired ricin as a weapon during the 1990s. Also, the Iraqi Survey Group concluded that the Iraqi Intelligence Service produced ricin contemporarily, and tested it on political prisoners. The toxin subsequently became an agent of increasing interest within some Muslim terrorist organizations. Thus, in August 2001, the FSB (Russian Federal Security Service) claimed it had intercepted a recorded conversation between two Chechen field commanders about instructions on the "homemade production of poison" for use against Russian soldiers. Russian authorities reportedly then seized materials, including confiscated papers also containing instructions on how to produce ricin from castor beans. The Russian response did not take place too late, employing the lethal castor molecule. In March 2002 the FSB apparently continued its long tradition of poisoning, while killing Chechen rebel Amir Khattab, by sending him a letter impregnated with ricin.

al-Qaeda got into action. Traces of ricin and instructions on its use were discovered in 2002 in an al-Qaeda house in Afghanistan. The head of an alQaeda affiliate network, Abu Massab al-Zarqawi, was trained in the use of ricin in Afghanistan before he relocated to Iraq in 2002. It was regarded to be an ideal bioterrorism weapon for terrorists. An al-Qaeda suspect arrested in Italy before the 2003 Iraq War told his interrogators that members of the al-Zarqawi network had purchased toxins from Iraq. Ricin, botulinum, and gas-gangrene toxins were the main toxins possessed by Iraq. And, indeed, in August 2002 reports have emerged that Ansar al-Islam, an al-Qaeda affiliate active in Iraqi, has been involved in testing poisons and chemicals including ricin. The toxin powder has been tested as an aerosol on animals such as donkeys and chickens, perhaps even on an unwitting human subject.

The outcome has first surfaced in London, marking the ricin route from Asia onto Europe: London, 5 January 2003. British authorities arrested six men suspected of producing ricin in their north London apartment. All six, including two teenaged asylum seekers and four individuals in their twenties and thirties, are believed to be Arabs from Algeria or other North African countries. On 8 January, a seventh man, age 33, was also arrested in connection with the case. The next day sources in Whitehall indicated that at least one of these seven men had attended an al-Qaeda training camp in Afghanistan, whereas others appear to have received terrorist training in Chechnya and the Pankisi Gorge region of the Newly Independent State of Georgia.

In the apartment where the six original arrestees resided, the authorities found several castor oil beans and equipment that could be used to process those beans. The toxin has not been detected. Five other locales were sub sequently searched in conjunction with this incident, and on 13 January, Scotland Yard officials arrested five more men and a woman in Bournemouth. One day later, another Islamist who was being arrested by Manchester police attacked them with a knife, killing one officer and wounding four others. British antiterrorist investigators soon identified this same 27-year-old Algerian, "Kamel Bourgass" (also known as Nadir Habra), as "a very senior player" in the network thought to be behind the ricin plot.

These events occurred after a series of arrests of other Islamist radicals in Rome, Paris, and London. Because some of these individuals, particularly those in the Rome case, were allegedly planning to carry out terrorist attacks using poisons, the most recent incident in London raised several potentially worrisome questions. One is whether the arrestees actually intended to employ the deadly toxin as an assassination or mass casualty weapon. A second is whether they were linked to components of the al-Qaeda network, such as the Groupe Salafiste pour la Predication et le Combat (GSPC: Salafist Group for Preaching and Fighting) in Algeria, or were instead affiliated with some other Islamist terrorist organization such as the Algerian Groupe Islamique Armee (GIA: Armed Islamic Group). A third is whether certain states that have previously produced and tested ricin as a potential weapon played any role at all in transmitting their technical expertise or unused stocks of ricin to violent anti-Western Islamist groups. Iran, Syria, and Iraq (until occupied, if not later) are known to possess ricin.

Still in Europe, ricin was then discovered in Paris, two months later. Traces of the toxin have been found at a railway station in Paris, according to the French interior ministry. Two vials of the potentially deadly substance were found inside a locker at the Gare de Lyon, according to ministry officials. The locker contained two vials with a powder, a bottle filled with a liquid and two smaller bottles also containing a liquid. The two smaller bottles contained traces of ricin in a mixture that turned out to be a highly toxic. The United States was repeatedly the next station of the ricin course, chronologically, although apparently involving but domestic American perpetrators questing to achieve influence. In October 2003, a metallic container was discovered at a Greenville, SC postal facility with ricin in it. The small container was in an envelope along with a threatening note. Authorities did not believe this was a terrorism-related incident. The note expressed anger against regulations overseeing the trucking industry. But one month later, the target was the White House.

The U.S. Secret Service intercepted a letter addressed to the White House in November 2003 that contained sparkled ricin powder, but it never revealed the incident publicly and delayed telling the FBI and other agencies; the affair was disclosed in February 2004. It was addressed to the U.S. Department of Transportation. The letter—signed by "Fallen Angel" and containing complaints about trucking regulations—was nearly identical to one discovered in October 2003 at a Greenville, SC, mail-sorting facility. But the existence of a similar letter sent to the White House was not disclosed until yesterday, and then only by law enforcement officials who asked not to be identified by name. Until then, the whole thing was absolutely kept under wraps on a national security basis.

Although seemingly—at the least—purely domestic, Secret Service spokeswoman declined to comment on details of the case or why it was kept secret, citing the ongoing investigation. He also declined to comment as to whether workers at the mail facility were tested or underwent decontamination procedures, and said the facility's location was kept secret for security reasons. Officials have previously noted that one mail facility used by the White House is located at Bolling Air Force Base. The letter is believed to have been sent from the Chattanooga area as it passed through a mail facility there. The subsequent and last link in the United States, for now, has been a ricin-containing postal enveloped mailed in Feb. 2004 to the U.S. Senate office of the Majority Leader. Federal investigators have examined about 20,000 pieces of mail in hopes of finding the source of the ricin discovered on Capitol Hill, but so far they have turned up nothing to lead them to a suspect in the case.

One month later, possibly by sheer coincidence, FBI agents searching Miron Tereshchuk's home in March 2004 found firecrackers, chemicals, recipes for ricin, and a postcard with the message "Here is your poison—enjoy," according to documents filed in the Virginia court. Back to Iraq, the same month, the U.S. Army staged raids in Baghdad, uncovering evidence of an attempt to produce ricin, so as to put some in mortar rounds. And again, in the United States, in November 2005, plans for producing ricin, along with bomb materials and diagrams were found in the home of Sergio Maldonado, a 20-year-old man known as a criminal. In a markedly similar event, a jar containing ricin derived form castor beans, along with ricin residue in a bowl, gun silencers, pipe bombs and bomb-making materials, were found in a shed in Nashville, Tennessee. Most probably, the ricin course did not reach an endpoint.

Smallpox Complex

The unique properties and particular importance of smallpox virus are discussed, both as a bioterrorism threat and as a major biohazard in general. It appears to pose, potentially, a colossal menace, which ought to be intensely coped with. The issues of renewed vaccination and ongoing research are then addressed, showing the complexity related to that singular pathogen. The virus causing smallpox appears to be, objectively, the most devastating pathogen ever faced—as far as known—by humanity. Presumably, many billions of people lost their life due to smallpox during human history (an estimated 300- million people worldwide in the twentieth century alone). The virus has been effectively used for bioterrorism purposes. It has successfully been eradicated worldwide, primarily thanks to the fact that it is infective toward man only, hence not having the capacity to endure within any other creature. This plainly means that the absence of this pathogen from human populations signifies for its final elimination, except for persisting in the frozen state in laboratories or, perhaps, in nature. Moreover, the lacking of alternative hosts, apart from man, considerably restricts—both quantitatively and qualitatively—the overall gene pool of this virus and, therefore, its ability to markedly evolve and give rise to novel variants capable of evading human herd immunity, which has extremely been fortified in the past by mass inoculations. Resultantly, the magnitude of susceptible unvaccinated segments of human populations was, at the time, too small to sustain the virus. Consequently, the virus vanished.

Furthermore, the genetic distance between *Variola major*, the virus that generates smallpox, and the monkey-pox virus, which is sometimes regarded as a possible future reproducer of a new variant of human pox, is still appreciable. But the genetic distance from certain viral strains held in some laboratories over the world is zero. And, at the same time, human herd immunity against smallpox is steadily diminishing, since inoculations were stopped (around 1980). The temporal equation thus formed seems to be formidable. Moreover, the sound, natural equilibrium between the spatial distribution of immunized and nonimmunized segments of human populations worldwide has substantially been impaired as a result of vaccinations, particularly since the elimination of the virus (as a natural selection factor) from the wild. Objectively, favoring for a moment an authentic natural perspective, this seems to be, then, a sort of anomaly. Such circumstances may immensely increase the vulnerability of mankind to the impact of an act of bioterrorism involving the smallpox virus.

If not held in some laboratories until now, it would apparently be, then, a non-revivable creature. But in actuality, things are different. The story begins in that there are no clear data as to the overall local attempts to isolate—and, hence, preserve—the virus during the occurrences of natural smallpox epidemics over many countries worldwide throughout the twentieth century, until the last 1972 epidemic. Still, even if assuming the total and complete destruction of this virus worldwide, it is apt to be recreated, based on the knowledge attained on its full genome.

Smallpox (also known by the Latin names *Variola* or *Variola vera*) is a highly contagious disease unique to humans. The causative virus has two variants called *Variola major* and *Variola minor*. *V. major* is the more deadly form, with a typical mortality of 20–40% of those infected. The other type, *V. minor*, only kills 1% of its victims. Many survivors are left blind in one or both eyes from corneal ulcerations, and persistent skin scarring—pockmarks—is nearly universal. Smallpox was responsible for an estimated 300–500 million deaths in the twentieth century. In 1967, for instance, still prevailing worldwide in spite of massive inoculations, the WHO estimated that 15 million people contracted the disease and that 2 million died in that year.

Transmission is by droplets, and infection in the natural disease will be via the lungs. The incubation period for obvious disease is around 12 days. In the initial growth phase, the virus seems to move from cell to cell, but around the twelfth day, lysis of many infected cells occurs and the virus will be found in the bloodstream in large numbers. The initial or prodromal symptoms are essentially similar to other viral diseases such as influenza and the common cold—fevers, muscle pain, stomach aches, etc. The digestive tract is commonly involved, leading to vomiting. Most cases will be prostrated.

The smallpox virus preferentially attacks skin cells, and by days 14–15, smallpox infection becomes obvious. The attack on skin cells causes the characteristic pimples associated with the disease. The pimples tend to erupt first in the mouth, then the arms and the hands, and later the rest of the body. At that point, the pimples, called macules, should still be fairly small. At this stage, the victim is most contagious. By days 15–16 the condition worsens; at this point, the disease can take two vastly different courses. The first form is of classic ordinary smallpox, in which the pimples grow into pauples, and then fill up with pus (turning them into pustules). Ordinary smallpox generally takes one of two basic courses. In *discrete* ordinary smallpox, the pustules stand out on the skin separately—there is a greater chance of surviving this form. In *confluent* ordinary smallpox, the blisters merge together into sheets that begin to detach the outer layers of skin from the underlying flesh—this form is usually fatal. If a victim of ordinary smallpox survives for the course of the disease, the pustules will deflate in time (the duration is variable), and will start to dry up, usually beginning on day 28. Eventually the pustules will completely dry and start to flake off. Once all of the pustules flake off, the patient is considered cured.

In the other form of smallpox, known as hemorrhagic smallpox, an entirely different set of symptoms starts to develop. The skin does not blister, but it remains smooth. Instead, bleeding will occur under the skin, making the skin look charred and black (this is known as black pox). The eyes will also hemorrhage, making the whites of the eyes turn deep red (and, if the victim lives long enough, eventually black). At the same time, bleeding begins in the organs. Death may occur from bleeding (fatal loss of blood or by other causes such as brain hemorrhage), or from loss of fluid. The entry of other infectious organisms, because the skin and the intestine are no longer a barrier, can also lead to multiorgan failure. This form of smallpox occurs in anywhere from 3% to 25% of fatal cases (depending on the virulence of the smallpox strain).

Edward Jenner developed a smallpox vaccine by using cowpox fluid (hence the name vaccination, from the Latin *vacca*, cow); his first inoculation occurred on May 14, 1796. After independent confirmation, this practice of vaccination against smallpox spread quickly in Europe. The first smallpox vaccination in North America occurred on June 2, 1800. National laws requiring vaccination began appearing as early as 1805. The cowpox virus is still the immunogenic tool, dismissing, fortunately, the need to use the smallpox virus itself for vaccine preparation, as is the case with many pathogens. Compulsory vaccinations were increased, and the virus has been wiped out globally.

The last case of wild smallpox occurred on September 11, 1977. One last victim was claimed by the disease in the United Kingdom in September 1978, when Janet Parker, a medical photographer in the University of Birmingham Medical School, contracted the disease and died, and the Professor responsible for the unit killed himself. A research project on smallpox was being conducted in the building at the time, although the exact route by which Ms. Parker became infected has never been fully elucidated. After successful vaccination campaigns, the WHO in 1979 declared the eradication of smallpox, although cultures of the virus were kept by the Centers for Disease Control and Prevention (CD C) in the United States and at the Vector Institute in Koltsovo, Novosibirsk in Siberia, Russia, where a regiment of troops guard it. Under such tight control, smallpox would, it was thought, never be let out again. All other known stocks of smallpox were ostensibly destroyed. Smallpox vaccination was discontinued in most countries in the late 1970s; the risks of vaccination include death (~1 per million), among other serious side effects.

Nonetheless, after the 2001 anthrax attacks took place in the United States, concerns about smallpox have resurfaced as a possible agent for bioterrorism. As a result, there has been increased concern about the availability of vaccine stocks. Moreover, President George W. Bush has ordered all American military personnel to be vaccinated against smallpox and has implemented a voluntary program for vaccinating emergency medical personnel. Vaccination is seriously being reconsidered over many countries. It is also feared that additional stocks of the virus may exist in research collections, the product of the accumulatory nature of microbiologists. Additional collections of the virus almost certainly exist as the result of certain military and biologicol warfare programs, particularly in Russia. Iran, Syria, Israel, China, North Korea, and Cuba have been mentioned as current possessors, as well. The possibility that the virus is currently being held by a terrorist organization has not been excluded.

In light of those circumstances, and considering the extremely undesirable possession of this virus by various countries—hence its expected migration to terror elements, as well—the final and complete destruction of virus stocks held anywhere, and particularly in the CDC and Vector, was ordered in 1993, 1994, 1995, and 1996, but they have not yet been destroyed in those two facilities. Yet the continuation of this actuality has been approved. The World Health Assembly has passed resolutions (WHA52.10) (WHA 55.15) authorizing temporary retention of the existing stocks of variola virus for the purpose of further essential research. The program of research is overseen by the WHO Advisory Committee on Variola Virus Research, composed of members from all WHO regions and advised by some 10 scientific academic experts from such areas as public health, fundamental applied research, and regulatory agencies. Current reports are submitted to the World Health Assembly and are worth detailing due to the uniqueness of the topic at large, as follows.

Articles Summarizing Recent Research Overseen by the WHO Advisory Committee on Variola Virus Research

1. Exploring the potential of variola virus infection of cynomolgus macaques as a model for human smallpox
2. The host response to smallpox: Analysis of the gene expression program in peripheral blood cells in a nonhuman primate model

Abstracts Summarizing Recent Research Overseen by the WHO Advisory Committee on Variola Virus Research—2004

1. Diagnostic Development at the CDC: Update 2004
2. Inferring the Phylogeny of Variola from Genomic SNPs Analysis
3. Variola Morphogenesis effected by an erb-B Tyrosine Kinase Inhibitor: Possible therapeutic functions
4. The WHO Collaborating Center for Smallpox and other Poxviruses at the Centers for Disease Control and Prevention Atlanta: 2004 report on the variola repository

Abstracts Summarizing Recent Research Overseen by the WHO Advisory Committee on Variola Virus Research—2003

1. Analysis of Nucleotide Sequences of Individual Orthopoxvirus Genes
2. Comparative restriction analysis of genomic DNAs of the variola virus strains from the Russian collection
3. Human Combinatorial Antibodies against Orthopoxviruses
4. Update on variola and orthopoxvirus diagnostic development and use
5. Update on search for antivirals against human-pathogenic orthopoxviruses
6. Viability estimation of variola virus isolates from the Russian collection

Abstracts Summarizing Recent Research Overseen by the WHO Advisory Committee on Variola Virus Research—2002

1. Capillary-electrophoresis restriction fragement length polymorphism. A new method for poxvirus fingerprinting
2. Cidofovir Treatment of Variola (Smallpox) in the Hemorrhagic Smallpox Primate Model and the IV Monkeypox Primate Model
3. Genome-wide analysis of the host response to variola infection

4. Lethal infection of primates with variola virus as a model for human smallpox
5. New PCR assays for identification of smallpox virus
6. Variola virus genomics

So far, so reasonable, perhaps. But a dangerous shift might have taken place. American scientists are now awaiting World Health Assembly approval to begin experiments to genetically modify the smallpox virus. Researchers have already been given the go-ahead by a technical committee (WHO Advisory Committee on Variola Virus Research), which accepts the argument that the research could bring new vaccines and treatments for smallpox closer. Still, in the debate during the full assembly of the WHO, whose representatives from 192 member states met from 16 to 25 May 2005, WHO said it will ensure that any research will only be conducted after detailed proposals have been thoroughly examined on a case-by-case basis by the Advisory Committee, paying particular attention to biosafety and biosecurity issues.

Some 200 tons of smallpox virus have been produced by the USSR as a weapon and inherited by Russia. Their fate is unclear. However, details of the development of smallpox as a weapon by the Soviets became available. A report was elicited from General Prof. Peter Burgasov, former Chief Sanitary Physician of the Soviet Army and a senior researcher within the BWP. Admitting that development of BW by the Soviets did take place, in the form of live field tests, he described a "*smallpox incident*" that happened in the 1970s, and was then hashed up: "On Vozrazhdenie Island in the Aral Sea, the strongest recipes of smallpox were tested. Suddenly I was informed that there were mysterious cases of mortalities in Aralsk. A research ship of the Aral fleet came 15 km away from the island (it was forbidden to come any closer than 40 km). The lab technician of this ship took samples of plankton twice a day from the top deck. The smallpox formulation—400 gr. of which was exploded on the island—'got her' and she became infected. After returning home to Aralsk, she infected several people including children. All of them died. I suspected the reason for this and called the Chief of General Staff of Ministry of Defense and requested to forbid the stop of the Alma-Ata—Moscow train in Aralsk. As a result, the epidemic around the country was prevented. I called Andropov, who at that time was Chief of KGB, and informed him of the exclusive recipe of smallpox obtained on Vozrazhdenie Island".

Actually, it was a new lethal strain of smallpox that traveled far and away from the island-based BW testing facility in the Aral Sea, to infect people downwind on a ship. Most of the adults exposed to the strain contracted smallpox despite being immunized. Promptly, remarkably extensive countermeasures, including vaccination, disinfection, and quarantining were conducted.

In March 2003, smallpox scabs were found tucked inside an envelope in a book on Civil War medicine in Santa Fe, New Mexico. The envelope was labeled as containing the scabs and listed the names of the patients that were vaccinated with them. Assuming the contents could be dangerous, the librarian who found them did not open the envelope. This was fortunate, as unlike bacteria (with the exception of those that produce spores), viruses can theoretically survive for many years. The scabs ended up with employees from the National Center for Disease Control, who responded quickly once in-formed of the discovery. The discovery raised concerns that smallpox DNA could be extracted from these and other scabs and used for a bioterrorism attack.

Nevertheless, the chances of successfully doing that seem to be slim, for now. Notably, Ramses V, who lived some 3000 years ago, is the earliest known victim of smallpox, based on an analysis of his mummy. Many virus-like particles were revealed by electron microscopy and identified serologically as smallpox virus in a 400-year-old mummy from Italy. The antigenic structure of the particles was well preserved. The virions in the mummy's skin had lost their viability. Viral antigen was not be detected by EIA or RPHA, and its DNA was not detected by molecular hybridization. Attempts to recover the virus from the frozen bodies of persons who died of smallpox continue in Arctic sites in Siberia, and in Canada.

The *Variola major* virus is very stable and survives in exudates from patients for many months. The virus is unlikely to survive in dried crusts for more than a year. Yet, it can be preserved in sealed ampules at 4°C for many years, and indefinitely by freeze-drying. This leads to the presumption that the virus still may be preserved alive within bodies of victims buried in permafrost. Much more feasible, however, the practical employment of smallpox virus for bioterrorism purposes is remarkably worrisome and reckoned to be a prime threat.

The current, perpetual phase along the smallpox virus course is facilitated, in effect, by an informal Russian-American status quo, one that has virtually been established lately, acknowledging the nontermination of BWs, for the time being. In a sense, the cardinal, unsolved issue of the smallpox virus constitutes an illustrative reflection of that much broader, not as yet untied, tangle. Sheltered by seemingly acceptable justifications of essential ongoing research into the most dreadful pathogen of mankind is thus still being kept in Russia, the United States, and most likely, some other places. It perfectly symbolizes the bivalent potential of further, extremely ominous pathogens held, militarily, by Russia and additional states. In Russia, it is retained, probably, as a stockpiled weapon, alongside with an arsenal of various pathogens and toxins. The argument that full acquaintances with pathogens reckoned as BWA—and, likewise, with their aggressive attributes, in terms of bioterrorism threats—are necessary for achieving effective protection, is a very reasonable one, and may hardly be debated. It is therefore, objectively, a salient dual-purpose factor; particularly as engineered pathogens and bioterrorism menaces are becoming common. Concurrently, and perhaps genuinely, this attitude is applied within the U.S. Army as defensively oriented "*bioprofiling*". At any rate, the U.S. Army Medical Research Institute of Infectious Diseases, at Fort Detrick, has accumulated "credible evidence" that several terrorist groups and nations have obtained, or are trying to obtain, clandestine stocks of smallpox and are actively trying to produce weaponized armaments based on the virus.

Connectedly, an international exercise in dealing with a series of international terrorist attacks involving smallpox virus has shown that the impact would be catastrophic for almost the entire world, and that the lives of millions of people could be lost. This outcome of the "*Atlantic Storm*" session seems all the more alarming given all the measures taken to combat bioterrorism since the 2001 anthrax letters attacks. The fictitious scenario of "*Atlantic Storm*" centered on a wave of attacks with the smallpox virus. The exercise was held at a hotel in Washington, D.C., with some 150 observers present to see how 11 former government officials and leaders of inter-governmental organizations, all with the necessary experience, would deal with such a calamity.

Agroterrorism

The essence and characteristics of agricultural terrorism (agroterrorism) are presented. Reference is here made to infective agents only, meaning pathogens of farm animals and cultivars. Mention is not made here of bioterrorism warfare agents common to man and animals, such as anthrax. Accordingly, various episodes of agroterrorism that took place since WWII are reveiwed.

Agroterrorism is the deliberate introduction of pathogens or chemicals (toxic/ radioactive), either against livestock or crops, for the purpose of causing economic losses, undermining stability and/or generating fear. The direct impacts are economical, logistical, and demographical (up to hunger). Agroterrorism may be conducted in the form of state-sponsored or nonstate-sponsored acts. The out-comes show in the form of epizootics (animal epidemics) or epiphytotics (plant epidemics).

The United States, the USSR, Germany, Iraq, and Iran, foremost, are known to have had programs that included potential agroterrorism pathogens (in Russia and Iran, at least, this inheritance presently persists), as follows:

United states: The viruses causing fowl plague (epizootic avian influenza), rinderpest (cattle plague), hog cholera (swine contagion), and Newcastle disease (poultry contagion), plus late blight of potato fungus, were explored by the United States as candidates for agroterrorism. Weaponized have been the fungal causative agents of wheat rust and rice blast, making the former, explored ones, of no less importance. A wealth of British scientific experience has thereupon been exploited by the US. One salient finding has been in that 3 g of the rice blast fungi per hectare could infect between 50% and 90% of the crops exposed. Other fungal agents evaluated—in that case against drug crops, mainly poppy and coca fields—were *Fusarium oxysporum* and *Pleospora papaveracea*.

Germany: Explored: foot and mouth disease, potato beetle, potato stalk rot, potato tuber decay, wheat fungus, turnip weevils and antler moths.

USSR: Explored: African swine fever virus, rinderpest virus, and the fungi casing wheat stem rust and rice blast. An uncertain part of those pathogens have been weaponized, plus, apparently, cow pox and sheep pox viruses.

Iraq: Explored: sheep pox, goat pox, camel pox, and foot-and-mouth disease viruses; wheat smut and cereal rust fungi. Weaponization of the fungus causing weat smut has been evidenced [30].

Iran: Rinderpest and foot-and-mouth disease viruses, as well as crop fungal pathogens apparently have been explored and possibly weaponized.

Those lists exhibit, basically, the severity of agroterrorism, although principally the spectrum of potential agents is much broader. Thus, mention should be made, in addition, of some further examples. For instance, a 2005 GAO report accentuates the special significance of Asian soybean rust. In an experts meeting "Biosystems and Bioterrorism: Can Arthropods Be Used as Agents of Destruction," the immense importance of arthropods as disease disseminators has been pointed at, with reference being made, among other, to the glassy-winged sharpshooter scare, the Mediterranean fruit fly and the potential for Tsetse and Trypanosomosis reinfestation or establishment in free areas.

Illustratively, the devastating New World screwworm fly, regarded to be the most serious insect pest of cattle in the New World, appeared for the first time in the Old World in Libya, during 1988. It aroused, justifiably, great fear, and the countermeasure conducted was an act of biological warfare in itself, namely the sterile male technique: from December 1990 and until October 1991, sterile male flies at the rates of 3.5 building up to 40 million per week were released so as to suppress the fertile male invaders. The release of sterile flies was terminated 6 months after the last detected case of screwworm myiasis in Libya. Notably, Libya accused the United States of intentionally delivering the initial, reproductive pest, although it was the Mexican-American Commission for Eradication of Screwworms that thereafter carried out the eradication campaign.

Peculiarly, an outstanding agroterrorism-related interface evolved between Cuba and the United States. Cuba has blamed the United States for attacking Cuban crops and livestock on as many as 21 different occasions. According to Raymond Zilinskas, of the few incidents for which information is available, agents include Newcastle Disease (1962), African wine sever (1971, 1979–1980), Tobacco Blue Mold Disease (1979–1980), Sugarcane Rust Disease (1978), and Thrips insect infestation (1997). Only in the case of the Thrips did Cuba make a formal complaint. According to the Cuban account, the United States flew a crop-duster operated by the State Department over Cuba and released the insects. The United States has denied the allegation, and while U.S. agriculture experts discount Cuban claims, the United Nations has undertaken an investigation. Yet, according to Zilinskas, the most likely explanation for all these incidents was nature or accidental human transmittal through commerce. Connectedly, a Florida university professor informed the CIA that a Florida citrus canker outbreak was the result of a Cuban bioterrorism weapons program. Although the CIA could not substantiate the claim, it did investigate the case. During that same time period, Cuba claimed that an outbreak of

Thrips Palmi disease on the island was bioterrorism warfare introduced by the United States. Apparently, no final conclusion can be reached concerning those issues. At any rate, the Cuban file was not the only one within the context of agroterrorism affairs. Since 1915, a variety of agroterrorism-related incidents have taken place, worldwide, and included, mostly, the following events involving animal and plant pathogens/toxins: Richard Ford, a prominent British naturalist, has made the accusation that Germany dropped Colorado Potato Beetles on the United Kingdom during WWII, accounting for their unusual appearance in parts of the United Kingdom. According to Ford the bombs were made of cardboard and contained 50 to 100 beetles. The allegation has not been verified or refuted.

In a Ministry of Forestry report dated June 15, 1950, the East German government accused the United States of scattering Colorado Potato beetles over potato crops in May and June of 1950. The Mau Mau, a nationalist liberation movement, poisoned some 33 steers at a British mission station, using what is believed to be a local toxic plant known as "African milk bush". Ken Alibek, First Deputy Chief of the Russian Biopreparat system, alleged he was informed by a senior Soviet military officer that the Soviet Union attacked the Afghan Mujaheddin with glanders on at least one occasion. According to Alibek, this would have the dual effect of sickening the Mujaheddin and killing their horses, their main mode of transportation. Sometime from 1983 to 1987, a Tamil militant group threatened to use bioterrorism agents against Sinhalese and crops in Sri Lanka. The communiqu' threatened to introduce foreign diseases into the local tea crop and to use Leaf Curl to infect rubber trees.

Queensland's State Premier received a letter threatening to infect wild pigs with foot-and-mouth disease (FMD), which was feared might spread to cattle and sheep, unless prison reforms were implemented within 12 weeks. Ultimately, this incident proved to be a hoax as the perpetrator turned out to be a 37-year-old murderer serving a life sentence in a local jail. In December 1984, Queensland's premier received a similar letter from an unidentified individual. An outstanding pattern emerged regarding the spread of the Mediterranean fruit fly, a major threat to agriculture in California, in 1989. Despite heroic attempts to eradicate this insect, new infestations repeatedly appeared in odd and unexpected places. Concomitantly, the Mayor of Los Angeles received several letters from a group calling itself The Breeders, which claimed to be spreading the insect to protest California's agricultural practices. In 2003, Israel has been blamed for spreading foot-and-mouth disease in the Palestinian Authority territory.

It so happened that the majority of antihuman bioterrorism agents are basically and currently pathogens of animals, making them zoonotic. The sense lying in that phenomenon is in that, naturally, those pathogens rarely infect humans; hence human herd immunity against them is marginal, bringing about considerable vulnerability. Some of those zoonotic pathogens are important as both antihuman and anti-animal agents, like Rift Valley fever, epiornithic avian influenza (*"fowl-plague"*), glanders, anthrax, and brucellosis. They are potentially usable for both agro-and bioterrorism. But another class of pathogens includes specifically livestock attackers. The FMD virus is seemingly their best representative. It is, indeed a formidable agroterrorism agent.

It was again, thus, a viral epidemic—rather an epizootic—this time belonging to the category of livestock attacking agents, which exhibited the aggressiveness of an agroterrorism-patterned course, in that case—the FMD virus. Although very rarely infective toward humans, it is extremely contagious and virulent for mammalian farm animals. It is therefore a prime candidate for agricultural bioterrorism and a very effective one.

Great Britain was the arena, 2001. Despite a single outbreak of FMD in cattle on the Isle of Wight, Hampshire in 1981, there had been no outbreaks of FMD in Great Britain since 1968, until 2001. On 20 February 2001 an outbreak of FMD caused by the O1 Pan Asia strain of virus was confirmed in pigs in an abattoir in Essex. The source of the infection was traced to a pig unit in northeast England where disease was believed to have been introduced at the beginning of February. The provenance of the causative agent could not be identified. Deliberate introduction has not been ruled out. Sheep on a neighboring holding became infected by airborne spread from the pig unit. These sheep were subsequently moved through markets in Northumberland and Cumbria between 13 and 22 February 2001. Disease was then disseminated to many other parts of Great Britain and Northern Ireland as a result of movements through markets and dealers before the existence of disease in the country was recognized. Notably, between 20 February and 30 September 2001, a total of 2025 apparently resultant FMD outbreaks were confirmed in Great Britain; a further 4 were confirmed in Northern Ireland. Over 4 million animals were killed as part of the FMD control program. The epidemic was essentially sheep based, other classes of livestock becoming infected through direct contact with infected sheep or through the movements of people, vehicles, and fomites.

The impact of the epidemic was colossal. The overall economic costs in the food and farming sectors of the U.K. economy totaled an estimated £5 billion, roughly $10 billion. This figure compares with an annual gross output of the entire U.K. agricultural sector of £25 billion. The U.K. economy suffered other economic costs associated with the outbreak of FMD. Outside the agricultural sector costs, the United Kingdom endured additional losses to the leisure and tourism sector of the economy. The U.K. Department of Environmental Food and Rural Affairs estimated that the leisure and tourism sector of the economy lost £5–6 billion pounds as a result of the outbreak of FMD in 2001.

Finally, an image of a list of livestock diseases found in a cave in Afghanistan was used as evidence that terrorists are considering attacks on agriculture. It has been accentuated, in connection, that there are many operatives that were planning such acts.

Narcoterrorism

The nature and specific features of narcoterrorism are discussed. Various connotations of narcoterrorism, which are compatible or concerned with biosabotage-related activities, are presented. The main terrorist organizations involved in narcoterrorism worldwide are outlined.

Primarily, narcoterrorism is a term coined by former President Belaunde Terry of Peru in 1983, when describing terrorist-type attacks against his nation's antinarcotics police. In the original context, narcoterrorism is understood to mean the attempts of narcotics—actually, recreational drugs—traffickers to influence the policies of government, the enforcement of the law, and the administration of justice by the systematic threat or use of violence. Pablo Escobar's ruthless dealings with the Colombian government is probably the best known and best documented example of narcoterrorism.

The term has become a subject of controversy, and it is being increasingly used for known terrorist organizations that engage in drug trafficking activity to fund their operations and gain recruits and expertise. Such organizations include, mainly, FARC, ELN, and AUC in Colombia, Hezbollah in Lebanon, and al-Qaeda through-out the Middle East, Europe, and Central Asia. Although al-Qaeda is often said to finance its activities through drug traf ficking, the 9/11 Commission Report notes that "While the drug trade was a source of income for the Taliban, it did not serve the same purpose for al Qaeda, and there is no reliable evidence that Bin Laden was involved in or made his money through drug trafficking."

Although financial considerations seem to be the leading ones, narcoterrorism is often marked, substantially, by a constant attempt to sustain and enlarge the proportion of drug consumers in a given target population, hence weakening the latter physically, mentally, and economically. In that sense, it is indeed a sort of terrorism. But beyond the direct effects of narcoterrorism, it is very meaningful, although secondarily, in that it greatly facilitates the ongoing spread of blood-transmitted pathogens, such as AIDS and hepatitis, having their own significant and demographic attritional impact.

Moreover, usually the drugs consumed by narcomans are in fact psychotropic plant toxins: heroin, cocaine, opium, hashish, marijuana, and so on. Narcoterrorism is often based on massive cultivars of the related plants that are currently being overseen by the concerned terror organization, namely self-production of the involved hallucinogenic phytotoxins thereafter consumed by narcomans. In addition, the terrorists engaged in producing those phytotoxins accumulate the know-how and experience needed, basically, for the manufacturing of typical plant toxins, such as ricin, aconitine, and other potent ones. Chemical refinement is often essential. Also, the financial, technical, and logistical infrastructures involved in drug trading may be appreciably supportive of narcoterrorism, bioterrorism, and agroterrorism altogether. Like agroterrorism, narcoterrorism may be regarded, thus, as an additional variant of bioterrorism, although rather of a different sphere.

Most (more than half, certainly) of drug consumption worldwide is fueled by directed narcoterrorism. Some terrorist groups, like Colombia's FARC, collect taxes from people who cultivate or process illicit drugs on lands that it controls; others, including Hezbollah and Colombia's AUC, traffic in drugs themselves. Moreover, some terrorist groups are supported by states funded by the drug trade; Afghanistan's former Taliban rulers, for instance, earned an estimated $40 million to $50 million per year from taxes related to opium. The drug trade is also a significant part of the economies of Syria—which has funded terrorist organizations such as Hezbollah, the Popular Front for the Liberation of Palestine-General Command, and Palestinian Islamic Jihad—and Lebanon, a haven for numerous terrorist groups including Hezbollah and Hamas.

The drug trade is extremely lucrative. Heroin, cocaine, and marijuana are uncomplicated and cheap to produce, but because they are illegal and therefore risky to supply, they can earn more than their weight in gold on the vast international black market. The United Nations estimated that the illicit drug business generates about $400 billion per year. Also, because the drug trade is secretive, terrorists can amass large sums of cash without being detected by authorities. The terror organizations involved in narcoterrorism at large are mostly the following ones:

1. The Revolutionary Armed Forces of Colombia (FARC), a Colombian leftist group, which raises funds by taxing coca farmers in the Switzerland-sized zone of the country it controls. Experts say FARC may force peasant farmers to grow the coca used to make cocaine. It also makes money by protecting cocaine laboratories and clandestine airstrips and by trafficking in drugs locally.
2. The National Liberation Army (ELN), another Colombian leftist group, taxes growers of marijuana and opium poppies and protects drug-lab operations. But it generates far less of its funding from drugs than does FARC.
3. The United Self-Defense Forces of Colombia (AUC), which includes several right-wing paramilitary groups, says it gets 70% of its income from processing and exporting cocaine. It claims to be leaving the drug business, but experts doubt that all of its members will comply.
4. Remnants of Shining Path, a Peruvian leftist group, finance some operations by "protecting" cocaine smugglers in jungle areas under its control and by taxing the coca trade.
5. Some members of the Liberation Tigers of Tamil Eelam, a Sri Lankan separatist group, traffic in heroin, and the group reportedly has close ties to drug-trafficking networks in nearby Burma.
6. Hezbollah smuggles Latin American cocaine to Europe and the Middle East and has smuggled opiates out of Lebanon's Bekaa Valley, although poppy cultivation there is declining.
7. The Kurdistan Workers' Party (PKK), a Marxist separatist group based in Turkey, taxes ethnic Kurdish drug traffickers, and individual PKK cells traffic in heroin.
8. The Real IRA, an Irish Republican Army (IRA) splinter group that opposes the peace process in Northern Ireland, is suspected of trafficking drugs, although the extent of its involvement is unclear.

9. Basque Fatherland and Liberty (ETA), a separatist group in Spain, is reportedly involved in drug trafficking.
10. al-Qaeda does not appear to have direct links to the drug trade. But its former protector in Afghanistan, the Taliban, supported itself in part through opium poppy production and trafficking.

Chaotic countries constitute warm nests for narcoterrorism. Drug traffickers and terrorists tend to thrive in failed states with ineffective governments that have been destabilized by war and internal conflict, experts say. For example, Colombia—a large, fragmented country in the throes of a decades-long conflict over power and resources—produces 80% of the world's cocaine and 70% of the U.S. heroin supply. Lebanon has been plagued by drug traffickers and terrorist groups since its own harrowing 15-year civil war began in 1975. In Afghanistan, the 1990 retreat by occupying Soviet troops left the econom ically devastated country vulnerable to control by warlords and Islamist extremists. Furthermore, by promoting violence, tax evasion, and lawlessness, terrorists and drug traffickers make it harder for a weakened state to form a stable central government. All in all, the magnitude of narcoterrorism is a remarkable one, and coping with it is difficult and complicated. Narcoterrorism is, in a sense, a long-term attritional mode of terrorism. It is unlikely to diminish, and the main way to effectively struggle against it is expediently to remove the drug producing cultivars themselves. Significant achievements were thus reached by mass employment of fungi that specifically attack those cultivars: cocaine plantations in Columbia and opium plantations in Uzbekistan—a sensible mode of biological warfare by itself.

Paradoxically—yet sensibly, by all means—vast narcoterrorism cultivars were eliminated by agroterrorism-like warfare launched in the last decade, including the effective use of specific fungi capable of destroying poppy fields in Uzbekistan and coca fields in Columbia.

Novel Agents

Novel biological agents constitute a category of enormous interest, in many senses. It is apt to chiefly be pronounced in terms of paradigmatic combat power multipliers on the one hand, and plain bioterrorism parameters, on the other hand. Reference is made, however, to the inability of terrorist organizations to develop or acquire novel bioterrorism agents, unless extraneously assisted. A combat power multiplier is defined, primarily, as a warfare element sufficient enough to balance a quantitative inferiority of troops. This concept bears, however, a broader meaning in the context of strategy and military affaires. In these areas, the power multipliers have greater and more complex implications, starting with terror attacks and ending in an overall geopolitical power balance at its highest level, such as international pacts as we saw in the rivalry between NATO and the Warsaw pact.

The future battle field is absorbing, tentatively, a variety of multifunctional technologies. So, the sheer importance of these power multipliers is less in balancing the quantity disadvantage and more as a pragmatic method to decrease the number of the fighting corps (order of battle). Connectedly, a unique range of action is dedicated to biological, chemical, and radiological guerilla warfare technologies, both terrorism-oriented and military-oriented. This section will discuss these technologies and their ramifications at the macrolevel, within the biological sphere, synthetic biology being, thereby, the chief platform.

Anti-Organism Power Multipliers

Anti-organism power multipliers are based on technologies designed to harm humans, farm animals, or cultivars, whether during offensive, defensive, or calm situations. Although the new generation of these power multipliers is characterized by nonlethal (or sublethal) weaponry, some of them are distinctively lethal. This new generation include:

1. Novel toxins
2. Bacteria and viruses in a supremely engineered condition

Toxins are being upgraded as power multipliers. This being the case, through the following biotechnological featuring:

1. Molecular design, avoiding or decreasing the body ability to activate an immunological response
2. Molecular design that reinforces their toxicity
3. Embedding coded genes (regarding protein toxins) in noncontagious bacteria and turning these into "production lines"
4. Embedding coded genes in contagious bacteria and viruses and making these even more harmful

The range of toxins designed to perform as power multipliers is vast. Here are two examples, representing both ends of the spectrum: The Pepper spray and the group of agents called "Prions."

The Oleoresin Capsicum (OC) called "the Pepper spray" can be naturally found in hot chilies. The OC has been recently found as more efficient than the common police incapacitating agents, because it causes a faster and longer lasting reaction. The spray can be used for on-spot or wider purposes. Simultaneously, the "Pepper gel" was also developed. This gel is launched from its container by air-pressure; when contact occurs, the gel clings to any surface (if it touches the face, it may cause temporary blindness). The gel formula contains 10% of OC mixed with the gel. The gel is not flammable.

Prions, on the other hand, are extremely destructive protein molecules. They are the cause of "Mad Cow Disease" (Creutzfeldt–Jacob Disease). The prions are infectious molecules, which means their penetration to the body brings about normally functioning proteins that turn into abnormal proteins like themselves. The infection-like condition they cause is developing slowly but deadly. They are host-specific. The research of prions, chemically and biologically, is in progressive process and some see them as one of the future measures designed to target a specific civil population for long-term influence. Some prions harm a variety of farm animals.

Supremely Engineered Bacteria and Viruses

Genetic engineering is intruding this field, in two main ways:

1. The probability of finding gene fragments of highly virulent extinct pathogens is more likely than finding the complete genome and succeeding to revive it. At any rate, an intervention of genetic engineering is necessary to reconstruct and assemble the genome so it can imitate the natural pathogen as a living-reproducing system. In that manner, the polio virus has been recently produced, out of the blue, in laboratories. Similarly, the devastating 1918 "Swine Flu" virus has lately been reconstructed and resurrected.
2. The ability of the defender to immunize its population even against the most virulent variants forces the offender to engineer them so immunity will turn out as ineffective.

Genetic engineering is covering far more than those two just mentioned, by creating different and sophisticated power multipliers. The current front in genetic research is promising great achievements for the medical treatments of humans, animals, and plants disease by what is referred to as gene therapy. But, a military aspect of this research also exists. This aspect permits a new form of bioterrorism warfare to take place—genetic warfare. An unavoidable outcome is the discussion on how to use these methods of genetic treatment as a weapon: how to deploy these weapons of genetic warfare and how it is possible to expose the deployment of these weapons.

In his futuristic-realistic article, Mark Willis predicts the appearance of the biological genetic-engineered warfare agents according to the following criteria:

1. Synthetic viruses
2. Cellular pathogens bearing unusual virulence
3. Cell-like synthetic entities that cannot reproduce, as vectors of biochemical warfare agents

4. Dormant and secret pathogens
5. Pathogens specific to farm animals and agricultural vegetation
6. Pathogens specific to ethnic groups
7. Long-lasting or delayed-effect biological warfare agents
8. Ethnic pathogens that can cause autoimmune diseases such as infertility

In practice, at the last decade, we saw the use of specific fungus able to destroy poppy fields in Uzbekistan and coca fields in Columbia. In future perspective, there is no doubt that this is just the tip of the iceberg.

Anti-Inanimate Object Power Multipliers

Anti-inanimate object power multipliers are derived from technologies aimed to harm, disrupt, or jam weapon systems or other valuable assets. They can be implemented during times of offense, defense, and calm. In this context, power multipliers designed to contaminate water or food sources will not be regarded as an anti-inanimate object power multiplier because water and food are used, in that case, to attack humans, serving as vehicles. To our discussion, mention is made, then, of bacteria that can be fed from key materials, naturally or genetically engineered. That includes:

1. Plastic, like polyurethane (for example, digesting and removing the special cover enables specific aircrafts to reduce their radar signatures, and by that allowing their detection)
2. Rubber, steel, and paint used in strategic and logistic facilities
3. Asphalt used in runways
4. Crude oil and petrol

Bioengineering Availability

This ethical–technological entanglement has begat a discussion, both locally and globally, concerning increasing or reducing bioengineering availability of the power multipliers being discussed. That, while the freedom of information principle, universal communication interfaces, and the natural curiosity of different scientific circles are taking their place and diverting the reality toward a constant increasing technology availability at large. The fact that a lot of these novel agents are defined as nonlethal (ethical, so to speak) and antiriot countermeasures is contributing to this trend. This trend is also encouraged by the involvement of a university's laboratories in the military R&D process. Those universities, especially in Western countries, mostly get the publication they want.

The latest developments in the fields of political and strategic thinking regarding the use of existing or developing weapon systems (including nonlethal biological weapons) and the ramifications over the operational doctrine in the context of the contemporary trends in the international relations are very significant. This last publication maintains that the alleged revolution of the military-technology affairs has to be considered in light of discussions on military use of nonlethal weapons in existing and future conflicts. The issue is presented from a political-strategic point of view, criticizing the revolution in military affairs as a starting point in the discussion on the use of nonlethal weapons during conflicts. These issues are presented to politicians and strategic analysts asked to formulate a technology-based policy that may be used in future political/social conflicts. The danger of neglecting other important dimensions in politics and strategy, emphasizing the "force to force" aspect, are considered.

Most of the scientific and technological developments mentioned here are openly reported and documented in the United States, which is probably the world leader on these subjects. Russia is, probably, not far behind, but seems to lessen the publishing of this domain. The Russian BWs are very advanced, and Russia also puts a lot of effort in biological espionage, trying to get its hands on relevant knowledge and technological means.

At large, the global research for upgrading biological power multipliers is striving to develop:

1. New measures: both new categories and new means included in already known categories.
2. Measures that although they are known, the enemy will not be able to detect, identify, and handle. That may happen due to objective-inherent technological limitations (in such case, then, measures that have to be activated from a far, with no offender presence) or by using a known technological weakness the enemy suffers from.
3. Measures that will complicate the enemy's ability—military demogrophical, or economical—significantly and even decisive, although known by the enemy.
4. Specific measures designed against a given rival, affecting his military forces, population, or assets uniquely.

The range covered by these new agents is amazing by both its extent and its intensity, starting with incapacitating agents like Pepper spray and ending, hypothetically for now, with ethnical weapons, targeting specific races only. Not in vain, these two examples represent, even if superficially, derivatives of two powerful, inexhaustible technologies—molecular biology and genetic engineering. So, the Pepper spray is becoming a more favorable substitute to the regular tear-gases, being a molecular copy of the biological extract in the hot Mexican chile. So, the biological-ethnic weapons—whose mechanism is using specific genetic elements in the target race or nationality—are conceivably prone to be the unavoidable outcome of highly complex genetic mechanisms, being deciphered by man.

Toxins can be produced in three alternative methods:

1. Extracting it from a natural source (the classic mode)
2. Chemically synthesizing the biological molecule, after its full and accurate identification
3. Producing it by a gene able to code for it (when it is a protein molecule)

The range of scenarios, where the novel agents discussed can be used is vast, in any parameter:

1. Activation by state or terror organization, if only by an individual (that can also be sent by state)
2. Activation in a concealed or open manner
3. Activation in order to achieve an affect in the short, medium, or long range
4. Activation during a military conflict or during an international nonmilitary conflict
5. Activation against humans, animals, plants, or still objects
6. Activation at times of offense, defense, or at calm

Any combination of the parameters or the subparameters is possible.

Today and in the near future it is not expected that the availability of sophisticated biologically engineered power multipliers will proliferate. It will probably be an asset of few supremely qualified laboratories. However, with time they will become more and more accessible, presumably. With no connection to the BW agents that the Iraqi government has produced in its time (undoubtedly, industrial amounts), it is appropriate to mention two agents reflecting an unusual way of thinking suiting aspects aforementioned, although on an embryonic level:

1. Camel poxvirus—a pathogen that can attack humans, but not those who live next to camels and so are naturally immune. The Iraqis have also used this virus as a model to the small pox virus.
2. The fungal toxin aflatoxin, which generates terrible diseases, but only on the long term (was apparently destined to be used against the Kurds in Iraq).

In Russia, or elsewhere, chimeras of VEE-smallpox virus, Ebola-smallpox virus, and snake-toxin-gene-bearing influenza virus have possibly been developed successfully, but this has not been verified or refuted. Furthermore, it was recently argued that advances in nanotechnology could be used in the development of new types of biological (and chemical) weapons, based on the dual-use application of nanotechnology in the fields of biotechnology and medicine, which can be used for offensive purposes. Such a potential military application of nanotechnolgoy could undermine existing international laws that ban biological weapons.

To sum, the technological absorbability (of a country) is indeed the cardinal factor, but it is not sufficient for these frontline technologies to be adopted (even more so—for their upgrading) by one. But mention is made of the option that hostile countries or organizations can get their hands on standardized, instantly usable, weapons. The discussed novel agents are very sophisticated, and so transferring, maintaining, and operating them may be very complicated. However, it is possible that hostile elements will get extraneous assistance at these aspects as well. Particularly, a great deal of these weapons includes, so-called, nonlethal and anti-inanimate agents, hence more obtainable. Referring to the increasing threat of novel bioagents, Steven Block, former president of the Biophysical Society, was quite pessimistic: "The biological weapons threat is multiplying and will do so regardless of the countermeasures we try to take. You can't stop it, any more than you can stop the progress of mankind. You just have to hope that your collective brainpower can muster more resources than your adversaries."

Exploitability of Biotechnology and Biomedicine

The vast space inevitably formed by biotechnology and biomedicine, in terms of dual usability, is briefly presented. Its affinity to bioterrorism-oriented activities is shown, with regard to both pathogens and toxins. Two prominent toxins—botulinum and ricin—are thereby visited, to accentuate the scarcely observable border-line lying in between legitimacy and illegitimacy.

Apparently, the dual usability marking the fields of biotechnology and biomedicine, namely their capacity to serve for desirable and undesirable purposes at the same time, is the most extreme one, comparing with almost any other scientific domain. A relatively simple instance of this: the undisputable need to thoroughly understand the mechanisms underlying the above-described alternating profile of drug resistance of *Vibrio cholerae* potentially enables, in parallel, the creation of a multistable pathogen. The shift is fairly slight, if any.

Fundamentally, all categories of biomedicine targeted at infectious diseases— antibacterial and antiviral drugs, vaccines, and antisera—as well as gene therapy are apt to be exploited for improper development, parallel to their impressive, invaluable advancements. Moreover, regretfully, a principle of "*amplified reversibility*" underlies the undesired, yet inevitable, usability of biomedicine and bioengineering resources for the purpose of bioterrorism. That is to say, although most pathogens and toxins have found a way to become harmless and beneficial, thanks to the scientific comprehension gained from their usefulness in various respects, that very paved course may readily be reciprocal; in particular their road back to pathogenicity and virulence—often appreciably amplified, artificially—may take place in the form of accidental leakage or bioterrorism acts.

In pragmatic terms, two dimensions of exploitability can be observed: One is the general modularity of equipment and materials that can equally be employed for innocent or bioterrorism-oriented activities. The other one is the various untainted activities currently engaging specific pathogens and toxins that are reckoned, at the same time, as potential agents for bioterrorism; hence, they are prone to undergo, in principle, a turnover at the level of intentions and practice of their possessors. Thus, the harvest of a seed virus propagated for subsequent production of a vaccine by attenuation may equally be kept as is, before attenuation takes place, serving as a weapon. In actuality, the two courses are not in contrast with each other; hence, they may expediently be applied in parallel, in whatever proportions the possessor chooses, so as to attain effective camouflage.

The principle is fairly plain, even an old one. In 1939, the active ingredient of curare—an ancient plant toxin weapon still in use by Indians—was isolated for the first time. In 1943, it was introduced successfully into anesthesiology. Curare provided adequate muscle relaxation without the depressant effect of deep anesthesia induced by ether or chloroform. Over the last 20 years, physicians have used curare to ease the stiffened muscles caused by polio and to treat such diverse conditions as lockjaw, epilepsy, and cholea (a nervous disorder characterized by uncontrollable muscle movements). Eventually, more effective treatments were found for these illnesses, but the active ingredient of curare, d-tubocurarine, led to the skeletal muscle relaxant Intocostrin, which has been used in surgery ever since. Synthetic analogs of d-tubocurarine are used tens of thousands of times per day in the operating room.

Tubocurarines reflect, yet, but one, relatively marginal example of the dual exploitability of biotechnology and biomedicine. Ricin toxin and botulinum toxin are more actual agents, as shown. Global castor seed production for civilian purposes is around 1 million tons per year. The beans are widely used for the production of castor oil, making their control impossible, practically. The castor oil manufacturer may readily use the remains of the beans for obtaining ricin. Moreover, ricin in itself is typically a dual-use substance. Because of its cytotoxic potency, modified ricin is being used for the selective killing of unwanted cells and for the toxigenic ablation of cell lineages in transgenic organisms. Ricin is the most commonly used toxin in conjugates for selective cell killing, so-called targeted toxins. Beneficial uses of ricin include, potentially the treatment of cancer and AIDS. Recently, there is, indeed, increasing interest in the medicinal applications of ricin as immunotoxin, which have been successfully applied in several human diseases. In addition, the mole-cule of ricin in itself is the precursor for the preparation of toxoid and anti-serum.

Ricin can be targeted to specific cells, such as cancer cells, by conjugating the RTA subunit to antibodies or growth factors that preferentially bind the unwanted cells. These immunotoxins have worked very well for *in vitro* applications, e.g., bone marrow transplants. Although they have not worked very well in many *in vivo* situations, progress in this area of research shows promise for the future. In bone marrow transplant procedures, RTA-immunotoxins have been used successfully to destroy T lymphocytes in bone marrow taken from histocompatible donors. This reduces rejection of the donor bone marrow, a problem called "*graft-vs-host disease*" (GVHD). In steroid-resistant, acute GVDH situations, RTA-immunotoxins helped alleviate the condition. Also, in autologous bone marrow transplantation, a sample of the patients own bone marrow is treated with anti-T-cell immunotoxins to destroy malignant T cells in T-cell leukemias and lymphomas:

For the *in vivo* treatment of solid tumors, considerable problems can arise due to poor access of the immunotoxin to the tumor mass, lack of immunotoxin specificity, and further disadvantages. Still, research efforts to expand and develop immunotoxins and therapies for clinical use in cancer and AIDS are continuing with strategies using recombinant DNA technology. On the whole, the following examples of recent studies may be noted: Oncologic applications: Immunotoxin treatment of brain tumors; cytotoxins directed at Interleukin-4 receptors as therapy for human brain tumors; bispecific monoclonal antibodies for the targeting of type I ribosome-inactivating proteins against hematological malignancies; tyrosine kinase inhibitors against EGF receptor-positive malignancies; targeting tumor vasculature using VEGF-toxin conjugates; and gene therapy with immunotoxins. Alternative applications: effects of selective immunotoxic lesions on learning and memory; targeting toxins to neural antigens and receptors; *in vivo* testing of anti-HIV immunotoxins. All in all promising, apparently, but yet legitimating the access to purified ricin. Botulinum toxin constitutes another notable case. The most poisonous molecule ever identified, compared with any other natural or synthetic molecule, could not gain, apparently, a title better then "A Bug with Beauty and Weapon."

The germ *Clostridium botulinum*, a gram-positive, anaerobic spore-forming bacterium, is distinguished by its significant clinical applications as well as its potential to be used as a producer of a singular bioterror agent. Growing cells secrete botulinum neurotoxin, a multitype protein bearing exceptional toxicity. Although botulinum toxin is the causative agent of deadly neuroparalytic botulism, it also permits a remarkably effective treatment for involuntary muscle disorders such as torticollus, dystonia blepharospasm, strabismus, hemifacial spasm, certain types of spasticity in children, and other ailments. It is also used for "off label" indications such as migraine headaches. Furthermore, this extraordinarily potent toxin is also used in cosmetology for the treatment of glabellar lines and is well-known as the active component of the anti-aging medications Botox and Dysport. In addition, recent reports show that botulinum neurotoxin can be used as a tool for pharmaceutical drug delivery. However, botulinum toxin remains the deadliest of all toxins and is a potent agent of bioterrorism. Among seven serotypes, *C. botulinum* type A is responsible for the highest mortality rate in botulism, and thus it has the greatest potential to act as a bioterrorism weapon. Genome sequencing of *C. botulinum* type A Hall strain (ATCC 3502) has been completed. It may readily serve to dually engineer the related molecule in terms of toxicity, antigenicity, and stability.

The availability of medicinal Botox is not likely to contribute to a terrorist attack as the vials contain dilute toxin: approximately 0.3% of the lethal inhalational dose estimate and 0.005% of the lethal oral dose estimate. Yet if available right before being diluted, it would certainly be an attractive object. Obviously, the toxin is needed for producing a toxoid and an antiserum. Finally, the next two examples may tentatively illustrate an entire scope of the exploitability of biomedicine and biotechnology through its two edges, namely the rudimentary one as against the sophisticated one. The former can be demonstrated, then, by crude fermentation of various fungi for the manufacturing of antibiotics or mycotoxins (a dual-use biotechnology largely adopted by the then USSR), whereas the latter one is the usage—for now experimental—recently made of viruses as drug delivery systems, owing to their unique capacity to inwardly parasitize host cells. This biomedical horizon appears to be fascinating, and a far reaching one, in both a desirable and an undesirable fashion.

Preventive and Countermeasure

Having been recognized as a prime threat with global potentiality, different approaches and schools configured to fight bioterrorism are here discussed, rather exhibiting the absence of adequate preparedness. Moreover, various factors, some inherent, may hinder the effectual establishment of future preparedness and are considered. Much progress has though been achieved and is reviewed, particularly in the United States. An endeavor is taking place in Europe and Russia. All over, the efforts are doctrinal, scientific, and logistical, both preventive and reactive.

Aiming to defy any sort of assistance lent by (or from) states to terrorists within the entire context of biological, chemical, or nuclear weapons, the UN Security Council formulated in 2004 a resolution saying that "... All States shall refrain from providing any form of support to non-state actors that attempt to develop, acquire, manufacture, possess, transport, transfer or use nuclear, chemical or biological weapons and their means of delivery. All States, in accordance with their national procedures, shall adopt and enforce appropriate effective laws which prohibit any non-state actor to manufacture, acquire, possess, develop, transport, transfer or use nuclear, chemical or biological weapons and their means of delivery, in particular for terrorist purposes, as well as attempts to engage in any of the foregoing activities, participate in them as an accomplice, assist or finance them ...". Globally, apart from many national frameworks, various international initiatives have been founded, aimed at the prevention of, and coping with, possible bioterrorism scenarios. In 2006, the U.N. General Assembly released its new counterterrorism strategy. It recommends development of a "*biological incidents*" database by the United Nations and its member countries, in order to fight the threat of bioterrorism.

In Europe, much progress was achieved during 2004-2006, owing to the New Dedence Agenda (NDA) (later on renamed as Security and Defence Angenda—SDA) —a regular professional discussion forum involving NATO, the EU, and the World Health Organization plus national ministries, industry figures, and journalists, to debate safety and defense issues. It aims to raise awareness in Europe of the bioterrorism threat and to define a set of recommendations for EU policy makers to prevent and protect against attacks.

The 2004 NDA conference outlined that security awareness at epidemiology research laboratories across the industrialized world is lagging behind the growing threat of bioterrorism. Tighter cooperation is needed among laboratories, international customs, and transport authorities, and NATO could provide important logistical and communications support in the event of a bioterror attack in Europe. Notably, Roger Roffey, research director of the Swedish Defense Ministry's Department of International and Security Affairs, accentuated that "The risk of bioterrorism is on the rise, and one of the deficiencies we all face concerns the control of bioterrorism agents within laboratories and their transfer beyond, especially at labs across the former Soviet Union. We should expect bioterrorists to go beyond an attack by aerosol delivery into product-tampering of crops and animals, into our very food and water supplies. We need new multilateral initiatives to improve biosecurity facilities." The 2005 NDA conference was an example of excellent EU-U.S. collaboration in the context of bioterrorism. If there was one conclusion that could be drawn from the conference, it was that such teamwork had to be duplicated in the actual fight against bioterrorism. Not that the event lacked ideas, as these were ever present. But there were few signs of real cooperation, and the specter of different "*threat perceptions*" was forever hovering in the background. This line strengthened in the 2006 SDA conference.

The Interpol and the European Homeland Security Association pay much attention to bioterrorism threats. Interpol President Jackie Selebi recently observed that "Major panic, temporary paralysis of government functions and private businesses and even civil disorder are all likely outcomes of a bioterrorism attack. In fact, bioterrorism appears particularly well suited to the small, well-informed groups. A bioterrorist's lab could well be the size of a household kitchen and the weapon built there could be smaller than a toaster, and the range of options available to terrorists will continue to grow." Furthermore, he warned of bioterror attacks on livestock or the food chain. Interpol Secretary General Ronald Noble added that "There is no criminal threat with greater potential danger to all countries, regions and people in the world than the threat of bioterrorism. There is no crime area where police have as little training than in preventing—or responding to—bioterrorist attacks. Terrorists do want to use biological weapons. The threat is worthy of immediate preparation".

French Interior Minister Dominique de Villepin called for creation of a UN-affiliated organization to track potential biowarfare agents and keep them away from terrorists. He did not propose giving inspection powers to such an agency, but said that biotechnology companies, laboratories, hospitals, and universities need to better monitor themselves on issues of hiring, pathogen work, and access to sensitive areas. Connectedly, in Britain, MI5 officials recently warned British laboratories that Islamist terrorists—chiefly al-Qaeda, through recruited university students—may try to steal deadly pathogens. Scientists and lab staff handing biological agents such as samples of avian flu, tuberculosis, rabies and polio, have been told their security measures will be vetted by police. In consequence, police is supposed to conduct background checks on scientists and others who work with restricted materials at universities, hospitals and pharmaceutical firms. Government officials are intended to inspect such laboratories, and regular audits are planned of agent inventories. The idea is that it will be up to scientists to prove they have good reason for using the materials in their work, according to a senior of the British National Institute for Biological Standards and Controls.

During 2006, cooperation between prominent European states and Russia considerably strengthened. Thus, in Kyiv, Russia, the highly qualified Interpol Workshop on Preventing Bioterrorism took place. Also, a fairly thorough "Strategic Study on Bioterrorism" produced by 20 high level bio-experts from the Russian Federation and other European countries, was released by the Center for Strategic and

International Studies. In Israel, much concern was raised that regular microbiological laboratories—particularly those located in the Palestinian-occupied territories—may be used as minifactories for producing bioterrorism agents. It has therefore been decided that the National Security Council—in coordination with the General Security Service, Ministry of Health, academic institutions, and industrial bodies—will oversee such laboratories. The Israeli Parliament building and facilities are expected to be reviewed for potential vulnerabilities to biological (and chemical) terrorism. Air conditioning and other ducts are expected to be examined to determine any entry point for airborne agents.

In some Muslim states, professional forums intended to fight bioterrorism have been formed. In Iran, parallel to its ongoing, progressing BW program—which includes, among other things, guerilla means for applying bioterrorism warfare— The First Conference on [the] Campaign Against Bioterrorism was held in Tehran. The conference, which was a joint project of the Iranian Red Crescent Society (IRCS) and the infectious diseases department of the Tehran Medical Science University examined the health risks posed by bioterrorism and attempts to develop an action plan for use by relief workers in the event of a bioterror event. Over 300 IRCS relief instructors attended the event along with IRCS managers and students from the University.

In Saudi Arabia, where there are still elements in support of al-Qaeda, the Center of Studies and Research at Naif Arab University for Security Sciences in Saudi Arabia held a seminar on bioterrorism. Experts participating in the seminar were from Saudi Arabia, Jordan, Bahrain, Comoros, Sudan, Syria, Palestine, Qatar, Iraq, Kuwait, Lebanon, and Egypt.

Beyond comparison, however, is the effort against bioterrorism made by the United States. The preventive and countermeasures taken by the United States against bioterrorism are indeed the most impressive ones, in terms of concept, thoroughness, and scope. They are nourished by fundamentals that preceded the 2001 anthrax attack, which means, dually, that on the one hand the need for pre-emptive preparedness was soberly recognized in advance, and on the other hand, that the saboteurs succeeded to carry out their attack plan despite the defensive preparedness already established, then, by the United States.

In principle, a variety of ways in which the U.S. agencies were implementing President George W. Bush's April 2004 Biodefense for the 21st Century initiative, organized around the four "pillars" of awareness, prevention, detection, and response. Project Bioshield Presidential law reflects the genuine national American incentive to get prepared toward the bioterrorism threat. In this fashion, lately (2004), the President of the United States signed a new law to implement a $7.8-billion (estimated) project aimed to develop advanced vaccines. This law permits the government to use, in case of national emergency, medications and treatment not yet approved by the FDA. President Bush said this step will help the country to be better prepared in case of a terror attack. Also, said Bush: "It sends a message about our direction in the war on terror. We refuse to remain idle while modern technology might be turned against us." The President also added: "We will rally the great promise of American science and innovation to confront the greatest danger of our time."

The U.S. Homeland Security Subcommittee on Prevention of Nuclear and Bioterrorism Attack handles the bioterrorism threat. It pointed out that the United States must seek the proper balance between agility of response and countermeasure stockpiling in defending against bioterrorism. Moreover, the United States is pursuing multiple avenues of defense against a possible terrorist attack using bioengineered pathogens. Top leaders such as the Homeland Security Secretary have stepped up calls for greater use of terrorist threat information in setting a hierarchy of planning and spending priorities. Witnesses warned the Government Reform National Security, Emerging Threats and International Relations Subcommittee, though, about limits to what can be known about potential engineered threats. They stressed the need for maintaining a broad, flexible array of counter-measures. Homeland Security and the Health and Human Services Department have developed a strategy to address the potential for a bioengineered attack, a document that highlights monitoring of scientific research around the world, as well as broad countermeasure development to give the United States flexibility when confronting an unknown pathogen. Complementarily, two annexes of the new U.S. National Response Plan are particularly relevant to bioterrorism: Emergency Support Function 8 (Public Health and Medical Services) and the Biological Incident Annex. These annexes describe specialized application of the NRP to the delivery of public health and medical services and biological incidents.

Within that colossal program, the Bush administration's fiscal 2006 budget plans for civilian bioterrorism defense measures total at least $5.1 billion, according to a new nongovernmental analysis. The amount brings the total requested since 2001 to at least $27.7 billion. The budget request includes increases for protecting national food and water supplies and a significant decrease for funding state and local public health departments, compared with requested spending last year.

Further budgetary and organizational details are worth mentioning, then, as presented in that publication. The fiscal 2006 budgeting, an aggregate of spending across numerous agencies, reflects as much as a $2.5 billion drop from what was sought for fiscal 2005, but the decrease results mostly from the absence of a one-time appropriation last year for drug and vaccine purchases through 2008 as part of the Project Bioshield law. "Civilian biodefense spending, not including the Bioshield bill, has reached a consistent level of about $5 billion from fiscal 2003 to fiscal 2006," the article says. The fiscal 2006 total in the study does not include Defense Department budgeting for civilian bioterrorism defenses, as do previous years' figures, because the Pentagon "was unable to furnish numbers for the requisite programs," the study says.

Military bioterrorism defense spending for civilians in the previous two fiscal years averaged about $200 million. The analysis says, though, that those figures do not truly account for all Pentagon funding for civilian bioterrorism defense measures. "Some DOD research has direct civilian benefit, but because the majority of these funds are primarily military in application, these lines were excluded from calculation of total DOD expenditures," it says.

As in previous years, the largest amount of money—$4.1 billion according to the article—was budgeted for the Health and Human Services Department, which funds the National Institutes of Health, the Food and Drug Administration, and the Centers for Disease Control and Prevention. The article describes a planned $130 million cut to CDC funding for state and local public health departments, bringing the total CDC budget request down to $797 million. Another substantial cut is a $119 million reduction from the National Institute of Allergy and Infectious Diseases' budget for research facility construction, down to $30 million, and intended to "offset the increase in research funding," the analysis says. The Homeland Security Department's $362 million budget is roughly the same as for fiscal 2005—except for the $2.5 billion drop reflecting the advanced purchase for fiscal 2005 under the Bioshield law.

The Agriculture Department was budgeted $354 million, a 26% increase, for bioterrorism defense activities, the State Department $71.8 million, and the National Science Foundation $31.3 million, particularly, in accordance with Homeland Security Presidential Directive 9 (HSPD-9), Defense of United States agriculture and food, January 30, 2004. Finally, the Environmental Protection Agency received an 87% increase to $185 million, primarily for decontamination capabilities, to protect water and food supplies, and for training, the study says.

Apart from doctrinal and laboratory studies conducted by those agencies, field studies are being carried out as well. Scientists from several agencies released two tracer gases in a 2-km^2 area of midtown Manhattan. In a series of experiments, they are tracking how harmful particles might disperse through street canyons, subway tunnels, and buildings. Dubbed the "Urban Dispersion Project," this

Department of Homeland Security-sponsored effort aims to produce a computer model of airflow patterns that could help state and local officials better respond to an emergency or to a bioterrorism act. The studies are intended to conclude in 2007.

Overall, a possible counterproductive outcome has been assessed, naturally, as some scientists are concerned that the increase in the number of researchers working in the United States to counter bioterrorism elevates, potentially, the risk of an attack and the accidental release of biological agents. More than 300 institutions and 12,000 individuals have access to weaponizable biological agents, said Richard Ebright, a Rutgers University molecular biologist and critic of the expansion in biodefense since the anthrax attacks of 2001. Biodefense watchdog, the Sunshine Project, claims that 97% of principal investigators who received grants from the U.S. National Institute for Allergy and Infectious Diseases from 2001 to 2005 to study six biological agents had not previously conducted similar work. The explosion of "NIAID newbies" increases the likelihood of accidents, said Edward Hammond, U.S. director for the Sunshine Project. Jeanne Guillemin, a senior fellow at the Security Studies Program at the Massachusetts Institute of Technology, has the view that increasing access to pathogens heightens the chances that rogue scientists could use them in an attack. "What [NIAID Director Anthony Fauci] and others haven't thought through is the particular kind of expertise, from basic bench work to aerosolization, that comes with defensive biological weapons programs".

Furthermore, the extreme, objective complexity of implementing bioterrorism-defense measures aroused, unavoidably, critics saying that despite substantial funding on bioterrorism defenses since the Sept. 11 terror attacks, the country remains substantially unprepared for a mass-casualty bioterrorism attack. A variety of concrete steps and moves has been conducted, however, as follows.

Nonetheless, a large bioterrorism research network has been established in the United States. The U.S. National Institute of Allergy and Infectious Diseases supports 11 academic institutions throughout the United States, which operate as Regional Centers of Excellence for Biodefense and Emerging Infectious Diseases Research. The new network is working diligently to uncover new knowledge and create preventive, therapeutic, and diagnostic tools that will leave us far less vulnerable to bioterrorism, and is regarded as a key element of a U.S. strategic plan to counter bioterrorism and emerging infectious diseases. Each Center for Excellence leads a group of local universities to conduct research on next-generation treatments for anthrax, smallpox, plague, and other diseases. The consortiums encourage bioterrorism research, train personnel, maintain support resources, push for research on the development of new countermeasures, open facilities to researchers from academia and the business world, and provide support for first responders. Within that framework, an 83,154-square foot Biosafety Level 3 laboratory is to be constructed as part of George Mason University National Center for Biodefense and Infectious Diseases. Personnel at the facility will conduct research on development of techniques and products to combat bioterrorism and treat natural infectious disease outbreaks. Researchers will focus on bioterror threats identified by the U.S. government, such as anthrax, tularemia, and plague, along with diseases such as SARS, West Nile virus, and influenza. In addition, Army Medical Research and Materiel Commander Eric Schoomaker focused on the coming benefits of interagency cooperation at the planned National Interagency Biodefense Campus at Fort Detrick, MD. The Defense, Health and Human Services and Homeland Security departments are participating in the campus project.

At the same time, the multiplicity of pathogen holding research facilities is disadvantageous in that they are vulnerable to technical intelligence assaults, thefts and sabotage acts which may serve bioterrorism. This applies, in principle, to a variety of biotechnological resources at large, and thereby propelled, for example, the Congressional Seminar on Preventing Terrorist Exploitation of the Biotechnology Revolution, (June 5, 2006). Connectedly, perhaps, an FBI secrecy initiative formed with key bio-facilities such as the Public Health Research Institute (PHRI) in Newark, New Jersey, so as to refrain from "publicly disclose which specific select agent pathogens and/or strains are stored at PHRI."

In practical terms, early detection systems of various pathogens gained high priority. BioWatch—a Department of Homeland Security's effort to collect air samples form dozens of cities around the country to detect biological agents—biosensors have been deployed in more than 30 urban areas (at a cost of $79 million for 2006). Air is thus monitored air 24 hours a day and samples are collected daily and taken to labs that are part of the Centers for Disease Control and Prevention Laboratory Response Network. The results are provided within 12 to 36 hours.

Connectedly, the U.S. Postal Service has installed more than 1000 biological agents—anthrax plus two undisclosed agents—detectors at 271 mail processing facilities since the 2001 anthrax mailings. Moreover, President Bush has staked out the right of the U.S. government to open citizens' mail without first obtaining a warrant. A further methodology, mass spectrometry based "finger print" data base, has been developed by the Food and Drug Administration (FDA) National Center of Toxicological Research (NCTR), for immediate differentiation between biological contaminants, toxins and other, nontoxic substances. Although the concerned device cannot distinguish between living and dead cells, it is highly advantageous in terms of instant findings. Also, nanotechnology could significantly increase the speed of detection of an act of bioterrorism or a natural outbreak. Using a diagnostic test, researchers can measure the frequency change of a nearinfrared laser while it scatters a virus' DNA or RNA. The change in frequency is distinct.

Beyond, the most advanced biodetectors are the Triangulation Identification for Genetic Evaluation of Risks—the first multi-purpose diagnostic system that can work with samples of various materials. It can simultaneously identify all pathogens in a soil, water, air or blood samples within four hours, and roughly five such devices are now being used in the US by the US Army and Agriculture Department. In connection, a comprehensive national surveillance network—Project Tripwire— aimed at detecting diseases in wildlife that may be linked to bioterrorism, is being developed by the Wildlife Center of Virginia. Coping with specific pathogens is complicated, naturally, though the very fact that a certain pathogen is being referred to removes a lot of vagueness. Illustratively, the optional adoption of a pre-attack line of defense, as against a post-attack one, is indeed an intriguing one. Researchers from United States and Canada said post-attack anthrax immunization and antibiotic therapy is more effective than pre-attack vaccination. Still, this is doubtfully the correct strategy concerning smallpox, for instance, particularly considering the irrelevance of antibiotic drugs.

Currently, cities and counties throughout the United States are creating stockpiles of anthrax countermeasures that mirror the drugs available in the Strategic National Stockpile. The distributed stockpiles are necessary because it would take too long to distribute countermeasures from the National Stockpile. The drugs, given to cities to prepare for a terrorist attack, are meant to immediately treat first responders in the event of an anthrax attack without having to wait for drugs from the National Stockpile. The 2001 anthrax letters sabotage was at any rate a cardinal turning point. Using those attacks as a case study, a group of U.S. researchers have developed a risk-based decision-making system that they believe will allow governments to make better judgments following a bioterrorism attack. In "Bayes, Bugs and Bioterrorists: Lesson Learned from the Anthrax Attacks," Kimberly Thompson, Robert Armstrong, and Donald Thompson argue that governments must develop "decision trees," or methods for evaluating several courses of action, following a bioterrorism attack. They claim this would improve the evaluation of costs, risks, and benefits and would create more effective policy development.

"Using this type of approach, the government can better characterize the costs, risks and benefits of different policy options and ensure the integration of policy development," the report states.

"Additionally, confirmed use and refinement of decision trees during exercises will provide analysis of the long-term consequences of decisions made during an event and give policymakers insights to improve initial decisions." The study, dated April 2005 and published by the National Defense University's Center for Technology and National Security Policy, says poor planning prior to the fall 2001 bioterrorism attacks in which anthrax was sent to U.S. Senate office buildings through the mail led to improper allocation of resources after the attack. The report estimates the direct costs to the Postal Service could exceed $3 billion, with additional expenditures of over $1 billion for unnecessary countermeasures.

Despite the attack, coordination between U.S. agencies has made development of a comprehensive response plan difficult. To remedy the problem, the report urges establishing a decision tree so that multiple paths of action can be evaluated at once, making individual agency's responsibility more clear. "With this approach, analysts can quickly communicate with decision makers about the implications of combinations of options," the report says. "We emphasize that this approach of focusing on decisions provides a means to cross interdisciplinary and other boundaries... and consequently it provides a useful organization and com munication tool to promote effective management." The report adds that decisions should be separated into different categories, including who should be immunized, what response should be, how to allocate Strategic National Stockpile resources, how to contain biological agents, and how much information should be made public. The Health and Human Services Department should head the effort to form the decision tree, drawing on the expertise of other agencies when necessary.

The 2001 anthrax attacks clearly demonstrated the need for a better decision-making process, the report says. Lack of investment in the public health infrastructure, a poor understanding of the disease caused by anthrax, inadequate training of first responders, and poor communication are just a few of the problems that plagued the response to the attack. The report argues that a decision tree would have vastly improved response, allowing for a better understanding of who should be vaccinated, how relevant agencies should have responded, a better plan for containment, and improved information management. The report is careful to say that it is not critical of the 2001 response. However, researchers believe a decision tree would have prevented panic and yielded a more appropriate response. Researchers hope decision trees can guide policy discussions as a comprehensive response plan is formulated. "Given our recent experience with anthrax, the specific decision trees for anthrax are offered, as an analytical tool to aid future policy decisions," the report says. "Indeed, the lessons learned from the 2001 attack should facilitate the use of these trees."

Plague has been visited as well, when a wide-scale drill took place in the United States in November 2003. The drill was an effort to follow up on weaknesses in federal emergency response plans identified in a simulated pneumonic plague bioterrorism attack. That exercise, called Top Off 2, was organized by the Department of Homeland Security and involved 8000 local, state, and federal officials. It simulated a pneumonic plague attack on Chicago (and a radiological attack on Seattle).

As for smallpox, the United States intends to acquire up to 80 million doses of the modified virus Ankara smallpox vaccine, as part of its defense against the threat of smallpox virus being used for bioterrorism purposes. It would be useful for people who could suffer reactions to the existing vaccine. That includes patients with suppressed immune systems or those with the skin condition eczema. The vaccine contract could be worth more than $1 billion. President George W. Bush has ordered all American military personnel to be vaccinated against smallpox and has implemented a voluntary program for vaccinating emergency medical personnel. Stockpiling and vaccination is seriously being reconsidered over many countries. Japan is a recent example; after announcing in 2001 that it would begin stockpiling enough vaccine for 3 million people, a governmental panel of experts recommended—in July 2005—

the stockpiling of smallpox vaccine for 56 million people in preparation for a possible bioterrorism attack. Russia, with its efficient oral—plus aerosol—vaccines, does not lag far behind. Lately, an international exercise—the "Atlantic Storm Scenario" in dealing with a series of international terrorist attacks involving smallpox virus has shown that the impact would be catastrophic for almost the entire world, and that the lives of millions of people could be lost. This outcome of the "Atlantic Storm" session seems all the more alarming given all the measures taken to combat bioterrorism since 11 September 2001. The Atlantic Storm Scenario has been preceded by "Exercise Global Mercury," which was the first worldwide simulation project modeling a smallpox bioterrorism attack.

Considering influenza virus to be the most powerful potential bioterrorism weapon, Madjid et al. proposed several steps to address the threat of influenza as a terrorist weapon, including the following:

1. The Centers for Disease Control and Prevention should classify influenza virus as a "critical agent" for bioterrorism.
2. Immunization should be expanded, possibly by requiring it for all medical personnel.
3. Laboratories that work with influenza virus should strengthen their security.
4. Antiviral drugs should be stockpiled, and vaccine-making capacity should be increased.
5. The government should consider a gene-sequencing and vaccine development program.
6. Surveillance efforts should be increased and should include incentives for reporting of clinical cases.
7. The fitting of ventilation systems with virus detection and inactivation.

A super-flu virus, particularly a pandemic derivative of the current H5N1 avian flu, would presumably kill 200,000 and up to 1.9 million Americans, plus may millions sickened, according to recent estimates. A government's plan to fight such contagion designates not just who cares for the diseased, but who will keep the country running amid the chaos. Specific countermeasures include stockpiling of both the anti-flu drug Tamiflu as well as avian flu vaccine. Still, the protean nature of influenza type A virus at large may be defying. Experts in Hong Kong observed that the human H5N1 strain that surfaced in northern Vietnam during 2005 had proved to be resistant to Tamiflu. Also, the present antigenic quality of the H5N1 may undesirably alter. Also, the present intact strain of avian flu, as isolated from its human victims, and although not yet a contagious pathogen, is a putative bioterrorism agent itself, due to its respiratory infectivity, lethality, and panic-causing nature.

In general, then, ideally—although seemingly impractically—a complete genetic inventory of all pathogenic strains found worldwide could provide the proper basis for initial, rather essential, inquiry into bioterrorism acts. It may facilitate, as well, controlling the registration of culture collection so as to hamper theft of dangerous pathogens. Thus oriented, the United States is making an effort to fully catalog and selectively to obtain prioritized pathogenic strains such as those then included in the Soviet BW program. Within that context, Kazakhstan, Azerbaijan, Ukraine, and Georgia are appreciably cooperative.

Consequently, more than 60 pathogens—including anthrax and plague strains— from the former Soviet Union's Azerbaijan-based biological weapons program plus epidemiological system arrived at Dover Air Force Base in Delaware. In Azerbaijan—largely a Muslim country—several facilities—including field-test site—were engaged in the then USSR BW development program plus epidemic control. The samples were transferred as part of the Cooperative Threat Reduction program with Azerbaijan, aimed at getting the U.S. help to improve security for pathogens.

Moving to Russia, a different picture emerges with regard to a country fully acknowledging the essentiality of anti-bioterrorism moves, while still possessing an inventory of BWs and an active BW program. The anti-bioterrorism outline and legislative base that were established in Russia—so as to deny possible access by terrorist states and terrorist groups to dual-use biotechnologies, plus materials—

have been described by Vorobiev. He thereupon pointed at potential international cooperative efforts to be implemented, accordingly. Eventually, in 2001, a commitment was achieved between Russian and U.S. Presidents. Vladimir V. Putin and George W. Bush, to pursue cooperation to counter the threat of bioterrorism, including a focus on health-related measures.

American assistance to Russia within the "Reduce the Common (WMD) Threats" program fared much. In the bioterrorism sphere, a chief course of that program for conversion has been the anti-bioterrorism one. The Novosibirsk-based Biopreparat-affiliated Vector microbiological center has been a pioneering facility, within that context. A long time before others, Vector's Director, Academician Sandakhchiev, started to cooperate with international institutions, and already in the early 1990s focused on issues related to monitoring and prevention of bioterrorism. In addition, there are plenty of microbiological laboratories all over Russia eager—for financial, professional, or even ideological reasons—to save forbidden strains, toxins, equipment, and information. On the other hand, with time the Americans became more attentive to Russian arguments about development of anti-terror measures.

Consequently, The Russian-U.S. BioIndustry Initiative (BII) began in 2002, constituting the newest proliferation threat reduction program. It aims to counter bioterrorism through targeted reconfiguration of large-scale, formerly Soviet BW research, development, and production facilities for civilian purposes, by creating Russian-U.S. research partnerships. Collaboration has then been established in 2003 between the International Science and Technology Center (ISTC), Moscow, and the Boston-based Center for Integration of Medicine and Innovative Technology (CIMIT), to implement the BII. Conversion is thus intended to take place through formation of systems in Russia to link scientists, physicians, and engineers to solve medical and scientific problems, and to identify innovative technologies and commerciali zation opportunities. Also, the U.S. Defense Department has been increasingly engaged in efforts to secure from proliferation dozens of former Soviet pathogen collection and research facilities included within the "*anti-plague system*," widespread across 11 former Soviet states (excluding Russia). Apparently, many of those facilities lack sufficient safety and security and their scientists on average are poorly paid. The concerned, so called Anti-Plague Institutes, are thus being turned into controllable "central reference laboratories".

PROJECTIONS AND PROGNOSIS

Built-in limitations, which interfere with comprehending and foreseeing the course of bioterrorism, are outlined and discussed, together with objective constrains that restrict the scope of countering it. Nonetheless, the conjunction of methodological intelligence monitoring, systematic biosecurity globali zation, and creative scientific research may furnish a crucial tool for effectively fighting bioterrorism.

The very supremacy of mankind, in terms of know-how and technology, may possibly make it prone, paradoxically, to self-destruction, in various manners. Bioterrorism is one main way to materialize that undesirable predisposition. Apparently, an outstanding conjunction marked the recent decade, bringing about the prominence of bioterrorism as a colossal issue, including:

1. Internet-contained unclassified and declassified information.
2. The outcomes of the birth of the formerly Soviet republics—particularly the Muslim and semi-Muslim ones—with their Soviet BW inheritance, namely highly qualified, equipped facilities, culture collections, and many unemployed experts, plus partial Islamic orientation.
3. The accelerated augmentation of international terrorism, at large.
4. The rise and persistence of al-Qaeda with its radical philosophy and unlimited financial resources.
5. The global strengthening of Islam and its fundamentalistic inclination.
6. Extremely meaningful breakthroughs made in life sciences and apparatus engineering.
7. The increasing emergence and reemergence of infectious diseases worldwide.

Altogether, the ongoing integration of those various, interacting factors will probably shape, both conceptually and practically, the future of bioterrorism, one way or another. If a new breed of anarchistic multinational terrorists—not necessarily connected with al-Qaeda—is currently sprouting up, as at times claimed, the outcome may be unforeseeably catastrophic. The outlining—let alone structuring—of a defensive alignment that would fully address the bioterrorism threat is, objectively, an impossible mission. Even while referring, primarily, to natural (nonengineered) pathogens and toxins, and assuming a consensus prioritizing anthrax, smallpox, plague, influenza, ricin, 'and botulinum, one can hardly face the two main resultant questions:

(a) How to be best prepared toward each of those agents?

(b) Should other potential bioterrorism agents be totally ignored, and if not— what ought to be the respecting mode of preparedness?

And, beyond, of course—what about potential engineered pathogens and toxins? Is it unfeasible, for instance, to form an anthrax germ resistant to the antibiotic Ciproflaxin? Overall, the immeasurable complexity thus formed seems to be insoluble even if budgetary aspects are ignored. Although frustrating, those issues can and should in part be practically administrated by bioterrorism-strategic planners, provided they are fully aware of and acknowledging the concurrent constraints and limitations.

Increasing success of acts of so-called conventional terrorism is not regarded to decrease the potentiality and potency of bioterrorism (or other WMD-terrorism). Recurrent operations of conventional sabotage—even if fully effective—may intensify a perpetrator's daring quest for escalation and resonance through varitype means and modes of terrorism. Perhaps the most significant feature of bioterrorism, the ratio between the low probability of threat realization on the one hand, as against the high impact generated in case of threat realization on the other hand, is an extremely problematic factor for the defender. Let alone, that bioterrorism act that took place—the enthrax letters—in effect looks, in part, successful. In a sense, the very fact that the anthrax letter attack—apparently the most significant bioterrorism act ever conducted—has not been deciphered since 2001 is no less meaningful and important than this unprecedented act of bioterrorism itself.

Apparently, the prime and ultimate apparatus to cope with the bioterrorism threat is effective monitoring by intelligence sources, at least in that if adequately structured it would expediently shape the real and concrete needs and deeds of defense, in whatever sense. Therefore, intelligence ought to be supremely prioritized. All defensive measures have to actually form as derivatives of the intelligence picture, which may certainly be dynamic, though, in itself. The defense planner would not like that dynamics, in case the latter is not a plainly evolving one, but this is an inherent disadvantage. Conversely, yet, or rather complementarily, the defense planner may rely on his own considerations, as long as they can objectively be figured out. The significance of intelligence has been accentuated by the U.S. House of Representatives Homeland Security Subcommittee on Prevention of Nuclear and Biological Attack Chairman John Linder, who called for better coordination between intelligence and disease-fighting agencies. "Science, tools, reagents and technology may be ubiquitous. Scientists, however, are not," Linder said. "We have to do a better job of keeping track of those individuals with skill sets that are attractive to potential terrorists."

In conjunction, it has been accentuated that a harmonized international regime that enhances biosecurity is essential for reducing the risk of bioterrorism. Presumably, like other security regimes, this will entail mutually reinforcing strands, which need to include enactment of legally binding control of access to dangerous pathogens, transparency for sanctioned biodefense programs, technology transfer, and assistance to developing countries to jointly advance biosafety and biosecurity, global awareness of the dual-use dilemma and the potential misuse of science by terrorists, and development of a global ethic of compliance. To work, this effort must be undertaken collectively, using the international and regional institutions that already have a role to play in providing safety and security. To those two essential elements—methodological intelligence monitoring and systematic international endeavor—should be added the dimension of creative scientific research. Apparently, the prospects for attaining a breakthrough in upgrading preparedness lie in the integral formed, then, by those three different spheres (beyond the self-evident readiness achieved by means of doctrine-structuring and medical stockpiling). The scientific sphere seems to bear enormous potential. Specific immunoglobulins may constitute a good example of a not yet adequately developed defensive tool, which potentially can be very efficient against pathogens and protein toxins, both for instant prophylaxis and treatment for as well as detection. This tool may be valid against both recognized and future engineered agents, provided that biotechnological processes will allow for at once production of fully specific immuno globulins against a given agent.

Seemingly, to the least, this direction is worth elaborating on. Unlike vaccines and antibiotics, which are largely prioritized, antisera are less noticed, apparently unjustifiably. Antisera could constitute an optimal means for treatment, provided that instant and specific ethiological diagnosis is available. Studies and case reports evaluating convalescent plasma as therapy (or prophylaxis) of infectious diseases showed to be fairly promising. In the event of a bioterrorism attack, the usefulness of active immunization may be limited. Vaccine efficacy often requires time, multiple doses, and a competent immune system. Prophylactic immunization might provide an effective defense against bioterrorism agents but has the disadvantage that many individuals would have to be vaccinated to protect against an attack that might never occur. In this situation, even a small number of vaccine-related side effects would be unacceptable. In addition, vaccines do not induce protective immunity in all recipients, especially immunocompromised individuals. Such inadequacies should carefully be considered. Yet in contrast, passive immunization involves the administration of preformed antibody to provide a state of immediate immunity. The two modes of immunization are used together in certain circumstances, such as rabies prophylaxis following possible exposure, where a passive antibody provides immediate protection and a vaccine elicits a protective immune response.

A protective antibody suitable for passive immunization could be used in concert with vaccines and drugs to provide a multilayered defense against attacks with biological agents. It should be possible to create a strategic reserve of immunoglobulins against the major biological warfare agents that can be rapidly administered to exposed individuals in the event of an attack. The availability of a strategic reserve of specific antibody preparations would have a significant deterrent value, as aggressors would be aware that the lethality of their weapon could potentially be counteracted by prompt administration of antibody to susceptible individuals. As antibody can be administered intramuscularly, immunoglobulin preparations could be packaged in self-injectable, disposable, single-use containers. Self-administration of antidote would avoid taxing the health-care system with the need for intravenous administration. Given the stability of immunoglobulin preparations, it should be possible to store antibody for many years. Developing, producing, and stockpiling antibody reagents for defense against bioterrorism agents is a sensible strategy that needs to be considered as steps are taken to prepare against the threat of bioterrorism. On the whole, so it seems, the practicality of antisera should rather equalize that of vaccines and drugs, if not beyond. Connectedly, it has been highlighted that, in the U.S. National Institute of Allergy and Infectious Diseases work on boosting the human innate immune system, a strategy is formed that could lead to countermeasures that would be useful against a wide variety of different agents.

Such strategy may become vital, owing to the considerably diminishing usefulness of antibiotics against bacterial pathogens, as predicted by Prof George Poste, Director of the Biodesign Institute at Arizona State University and an advisor to the U.S. President: "Frankly, most governments are asleep at the switch"; he predicts that from 2010 to 2015 will be a "window of vulnerability" when the toll of the super-bug will reach its peak as a result of naturally augmenting antibiotic resistance. Antibiotics may therefore be appreciably replaced by other protective agents, such as antibodles, receptor decoys, dominant-negative inhibitors of translocation, small-molecule inhibitors, and substrate analogues.

A new horizon may be gained through the Neugene antisense technology. Neugene antisense "*rapid response therapeutics*" are synthetic compounds that mirror a critical portion of a disease-causing organism's genetic code and bind to specific portions of the target genetic sequence. Like a key in a lock, Neugene antisense compounds are designed to match up perfectly with a specific gene sequence, blocking the function of the target gene. Resultant antisense preparations have been able to block the cellular mechanisms used by the causative agents of anthrax, Ebola and Marburg, during pathogenesis. Another variant has been reported to block ricin toxin as well.

Relying on a similar principle, a novel drug has lately been developed that could expectedly be used to treat people exposed to anthrax bacteria specifically engineered to overcome antibiotics, due to an increasing concern that therapeutics developed for bioterrorism agents may be rendered ineffective if the microbial target is altered intentionally. This problem could be overcome, however, by designing inhibitors that block host proteins used by pathogens or their toxins to cause disease.

Thus, although the bioterrorism threat stemming from nonengineered pathogens and toxins is more or less characterized, in terms of expected impacts (although not in terms of likelihood, timing, and locality), the vagueness marking the threat posed by engineered pathogens and toxins is intriguing. Synthetic biology may be a key arena. Security experts fear that scientists building synthetic biochemical compounds could create a pathogen with no natural countermeasures, hence the possibility of making an unprecedented deadly bioterrorism weapon. Synthetic biologists are combining existing chemical components of DNA or RNA taken from cells and viruses to form compounds that do not occur naturally. Scientists hope to use this technology to produce computers, medicines, and energy sources. The field is attracting attention from investors and prominent biologists; yet some biologists and security experts warn that these new compounds could be used to develop a biological weapon. "There are certainly a lot of national security implications with synthetic biology."

Concerns were played down that a new agent could exterminate the human race but warned that the threat of new, engineered pathogens remains serious [368]. Scientists are already exploring ways to self-police synthetic biological research, including requiring reports of sales of materials that could be used to create a tailored biological-weapon. "There are now tens of thousands of people, worldwide, who could engineer drug-resistant anthrax," said Professor Kenneth Alibek, who as a consultant to the U.S. government has received numerous briefings on U.S. and Soviet biological weapon programs.

A testimony prepared to the House of Representatives Homeland Security Subcommittee on Prevention of Nuclear and Biological Attack may well illustrate the issue of bioengineered agents. Addressing it, National Institute of Allergy and Infectious Diseases Director Anthony Fauci contented that agents could be made more virulent through "resistance to one or more antibiotic or antiviral drugs, increased infectiousness or pathogenicity or, in the somewhat longer term, a new virulent pathogen made by combining genes from more than one organism. As the power of biological science and technology continues to grow, it will become increasingly possible that we will face an attack with a pathogen that has been deliberately engineered for increased virulence." Fauci added, however, that creating an agent whose transmissibility could be sustained on such a scale, even as authorities worked to counter it, would be a daunting task. "Would you end up with a microbe that functionally will ... essentially wipe out everyone from the face of the Earth? ... It would be very, very difficult to do that," he said. Centers for Disease Control and Prevention Director Julie Gerberding said a deadly agent could be engineered with relative ease that could spread throughout the world if left unchecked, but that the outbreak would be unlikely to defeat countries' detection and response systems. "The technical obstacles are really trivial," Gerberding said. "What's difficult is the distribution of agents in ways that would bypass our capacity to recognize and intervene effectively."

Today, the CDC's list of pathogens that must be reviewed comprises more than 60 agents. Each of them may completely be explored, so as to become fully manageable. But the catch is in that the existent pathogens are recognized—hence controllable—yet currently available for the potential attacker. whereas the unknown future engineered pathogens will scarcely be available, yet hardly controllable. The dichotomic menace thus emerging is an extremely challenging one. Possibly, as mentioned, immunoglobulins, polyvalent inhibitors, and other opproaches, may furnish a solution. All in all, the threat of bioterrorism is indeed a challenging one and bears, potentially, overwhelming, somewhat enigmatic impacts. Henry Crumpton, the US State Department Coordinator for Counter-Terrorism, described a biological attack on West "simply a matter of time", adding that such an attack could pose an even greater menace to security than a nuclear strike. U.N. Secretary General KofiAnnan, in the General Assembly, laid emphasis on the hazardous conjunction of bioterrorism and biotechnology:

"The international community must give a higher priority to developing new strategies against bioterrorism. Biotechnology has value in the fight against disease, but scientific advances could also "bring incalculable harm if put to destructive use by those who seek to develop designer drugs and pathogens. Soon, tens of thousands of laboratories worldwide will be operating in a multibillion-dollar industry," Annan said, according to the Associated Press. "Even students working in small laboratories will be able to carry out gene manipulation. U.N. nations should consider organizing of forum of governmental officials and science and public health experts to develop a strategy "to ensure that biotechnology's advances are used for the public good and that the benefits are shared equitably around the world." Finally, perhaps most plainly forwarded by the head of the Interpol, Ronald Noble, the bioterrorism treat has been featured as a global, severe, unprecedented menace: "The world is ill prepared for the looming threat of a bioterrorism attack. The danger of an al-Qaeda attack has not diminished since the 9/11 strikes on the US. The potential cost of a bioterrorism attack left no room for complacency. When you talk about bioterrorism, that's one crime we can't try to solve after it happens because the harm will be too great. How could we ever forgive ourselves if millions or hundreds... or tens of thousands of people were killed simply because our priorities did not include bioterrorism?" Noble acknowledged that governments and security agencies were better organized against the threat than ever before, but "none of us can let our guards down and assume that the problem has been addressed". Were al-Qaeda to launch a "spectacular bioterrorism attack which could cause contagious disease to be spread, no entity in the world is prepared for it," he said. "Not the US, not Europe, not Asia, not Africa." He may possibly be right.

12

Proteomics

The completion of the Human Genome Project represented a significant milestone in the journey toward understanding the genetic basis of disease. By dissecting the genetic blueprint of an organism, we can begin to understand the gene-derived cellular milieu and how subtle biochemical balances maintained within this milieu are regulated by the switching on or off of one or more genes, thus the regulation of protein expression. Proteomics represents a means by which proteins of interest can be analyzed en masse and specifically in the context of whatever possible cellular/biological/pharmacological process is being examined. However, this is, by no means, the limit of the proteomic pathway. For example, simply looking for changes in protein expression between normal and disease states, or as a consequence of a particular drug treatment, does not allow one to know whether the changes observed were the cause, or simply the result, of the particular perturbation. Instead, proteomics provides the starting point for the emerging field of "*functional proteomics*," where changes observed in a particular system are linked to the functional consequences of the change, thus building a comprehensive global picture of cellular function and the interactivity of proteins within it. Proteomics is generating considerable interest and investment in the pharmaceutical and biotechnology industries for its potential for identifying drug targets for the development of lead compounds, validating drug targets, examining protein and drug pharmacokinetics, identifying disease biomarkers, as well as developing diagnostic tools. Thus, this particular chapter will have a specific focus not only on the proteomic technologies available, but also on the application of proteomics in areas particularly relevant in the field of biomolecular pharmacology.

Historical View

A somewhat surprising finding from the genome project was the relative paucity of human genes (<30,000) and—even considering splice variants—the predicted proteins coded would fall well short of the anticipated 1-1.5 million proteins needed to account for the complexity of human life. Thus it is immediately apparent that the axiom of "one gene, one protein" is not true in all cases. For example, several isoforms of one protein, each often having quite distinct functions, can result from the alternate splicing of a single gene. In addition, following translation from mRNA, many proteins frequently undergo modifications that either add or remove various prosthetic groups (e.g., phosphorylation/dephosphorylation, glycosylation, alkylation, and amidation), which can have profound effects on protein function. The presence of a gene in a sequenced genome does not guarantee that it will be expressed, and there is a poor correlation between mRNA levels and the abundance of protein product within a cell. The regulation of protein expression and posttranslational modification provides the link between the genome and the phenome, resulting in health or disease, and underpins the importance of the emerging field of proteomics in applying genomic science to human disease. Unlike the genome, which is essentially static throughout the life of an organism, the protein complement of a cell is always changing under the influence of a host of physiological and pathological stimuli.

Thus a proteome might best be thought of as a snap-shot of the cellular protein expression profile at any given time. The field of proteomics, then, refers to the systematic, comprehensive, and often large-scale analysis of both the type and the level of proteins expressed in a specific—often very complex—tissue/ cell extract, or the identification of specific protein sets involved in a particular pathway/interaction. Proteomics, or proteome analysis, is a series of sophisticated technologies that allow proteins, their interacting partners, and protein systems to be analyzed on a scale previously only seen in the genomic arena. Proteomics can be used not only for advancing fundamental understanding of cellular function but also for identifying drug targets, screening potential lead compounds, and identifying biomarkers for a host of diseases, including neurological disorders, heart diseases, infectious diseases, and various cancers. Because the vast majority of drugs are targeted at proteins and because most disease states are manifest at the protein level, attention is becoming increasingly focused on investigating the protein complement of the genome, referred to as the proteome.

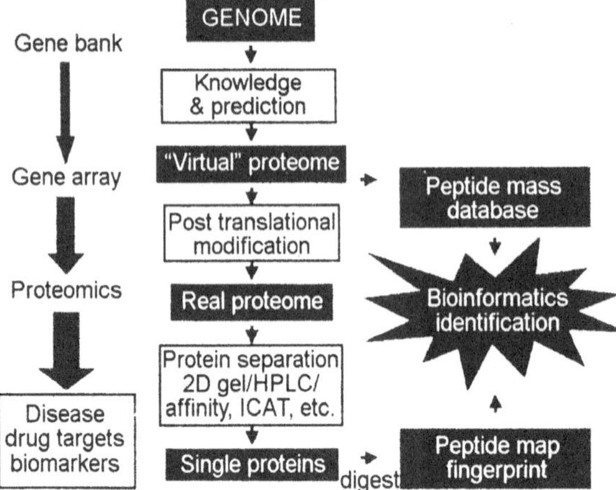

Fig. 12.1. Schematic diagram showing the relationships between proteomics, genomics, and the generation of biological knowledge.

Worldwide genome research has led to the development of new strategies, reliance on high throughput, high-sensitivity protein separation, protein sequencing, and data analysis. It is now possible to identify individual protein components of complex mixtures in an automated system without resorting to the difficult and laborious biochemical isolation of individual proteins. All that is required is to separate the protein components [two-dimensional gel electrophoresis/high-performance liquid chromatography (HPLC)/affinity probes, etc.], analyze the pattern of protein expression, and isolate the protein(s) of interest; after proteolytic digestion, identification is readily achieved by mass spectrometric analysis and comparison with protein/genome databases.

Access to this technology is now crucial in all areas of biological research. The complete decoding of human genome means that all proteins present in a cell/tissue extract can theoretically be identified by proteome analysis. Thus an established proteome profile for a control tissue can be compared with profiles obtained from a similar experimental sample. For example, normal or disease-free tissue or blood samples can be compared with profiles obtained from similar samples taken from diseased patients. Likewise, samples from control and experimental animal tissues or cell lines can be similarly analyzed. Differences in the proteome profile will not only allow the precise identification of the proteins involved in the disease process, but will also show which specific proteins are being "turned on" or "turned off," as well as identify posttranslational modifications. Such information has enormous value in unraveling the complex pathways involved in disease processes. Because the vast majority of drugs are targeted at proteins and because most disease states are manifested at the protein level, attention is becoming increasingly focused on investigating the protein complement of the genome, referred to as the proteome. Unlike the genome, which is essentially static throughout the life of an organism, the protein complement of a cell is always changing under the influence of a host of physiological and pathological stimuli. Thus a proteome might best be thought of as a snapshot of the cellular protein expression profile at any given time. The field of proteomics, then, refers to the systematic, comprehensive, and often large-scale analysis of both the type and the level of proteins expressed in a specific—often very complex—biological system. The tremendous interest in this technology within the biotechnology, pharmaceutical, and academic communities derives from the ability to characterize novel protein–protein interactions (ligand/receptor, etc.) and to identify novel drug targets and new therapeutic agents.

Proteomic Technologies

Proteomic analysis requires a series of sophisticated technologies, which, when linked together, allows proteins (and their interacting partners) and/ or protein systems to be analyzed on a scale previously only seen in the genomic arena. Given the vast number of proteins that are expressed by any one cell (approximately 10–20,000), a proteomic analysis requires technologies and methodologies that are able to not only resolve, but also analyze, large numbers of proteins with a reasonable degree of throughput. For some years, the "classical" approach to proteomics used two-dimensional electrophoresis (2-DE), coupled with protein sequencing by Edman degradation chemistries and simple mass spectrometry (MS), to facilitate protein resolution (2-DE) and identification, respectively. In more recent years, techniques such as chromatographic separation [particularly reversed-phase HPLC (RP-HPLC) and ion exchange HPLC] and affinity probing/baits, coupled with sophisticated high-resolution mass spectrometry, have been used with success to expand the scope and power of proteomic research. Regardless of the particular technology used, most proteomic studies can be divided into three distinct steps, namely: preparation, separation, and identification.

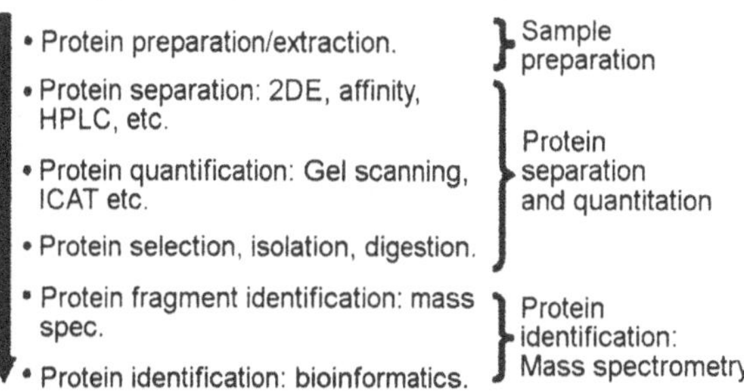

Fig. 12.2. Diagram illustrating the key proteomic technologies and the direction of flow from one technology to the next.

Sample Preparation

One of the most crucial considerations in proteomic analysis is sample preparation because this will ultimately dictate the number and type of proteins that can be processed. The first priority is to establish the precise protein system to be studied [e.g., will this be a comprehensive and exhaustive catalogue of every expressed protein within a tissue or cellular extract, or is only a small subset of a cellular proteome (e.g., only phosphoproteins or membrane-bound proteins) sufficient for analysis?]. Whether a full or partial proteome, or even a limited number of specific proteins is required for analysis, it is crucial that the extraction technique provide maximal protein recovery while preserving the integrity of the protein complex to be examined. Furthermore, the method of preparation must be totally compatible with the separation methods to be used. This is particularly important for separation technologies that are reliant on protein–protein interactions or drug/ligand/antibody, etc. interactions. Poor recovery of proteins is clearly a disadvantage, especially in the analysis of low- abundance proteins, whereas poor recovery of particular types of proteins (e.g., hydrophobic or basic proteins) can skew the interpretation of an overall protein expression profile. Furthermore, because the proteome is a time-dependent entity, any extraction procedure should be designed so as to preserve the protein profile at the time of protein complex formation. Most proteomic analyses are performed on cellular systems and, as such, require an initial lysis step to liberate the contents for separation and analysis. Because the disruption method used will very much depend not only on the particular cell under investigation but also on whether analysis of the full or partial proteome is required, this aspect of proteomic analysis may require a number of rounds of experimentation to develop an optimal extraction protocol. Unfortunately, many of the more interesting proteins expressed in a cell are some of the least abundant and are often obscured by a swamping excess of cytoskeletal/structural proteins, heat-shock proteins, other chaperones, and other much more abundant proteins. To overcome this problem, there are a number of enrichment procedures that can be used to concentrate low-abundance proteins prior to analysis. Of growing interest to the proteomic community is the application of laser dissection microscopy as a means of obtaining pure cell populations. This technology allows the selective removal of visualized cells excised from tissue sections for subsequent proteomic analysis.

Protein Separation and Quantitation

The majority of proteomic studies focusing on tissue and cellular extracts have been performed using 2-DE for the separation of proteins, the so-called "*classical proteomics*." One of the major strengths of 2-DE is its unparalleled resolving power, with a typical gel able to resolve somewhere around 1000–2000 proteins. Moreover, the expression pattern displayed on a 2-D gel is amenable to quantitation, thereby allowing the up-regulation or down-regulation, de novo synthesis, or disappearance of a protein to be determined. This technique is essentially a combination of isoelectric focusing (IEF) and conventional sodium dodecyl sulfate polyacrylamide gel electrophoresis (SD S-PAGE), and separates mixtures of proteins, first, by their overall charge or isoelectric point, and, second, by their molecular weight. Similarly, changes in either the charge and/or molecular weight of proteins can be readily observed on 2-DE gel as a physical translocation from one region of the gel to another. This is a particular strength when examining posttranslational processing changes such as phosphorylation, occurring as a consequence of a particular treatment/disease process.

Quantitation of proteins stained in a gel in the past has been reliant on simple scanning of gel images followed by the crude quantitation of spot staining intensity. With the development of sensitive fluorescent dyes (with differing excitation and emission wavelengths), together with massive improvements in imaging technologies, particularly the development of high-resolution software, differential 2-DE fluorescent analysis, Fluorescence Difference Gel Electrophoresis (DIGE), allows a quite exquisite and sensitive quantitation of proteins separated by 2-DE. This technology allows the mixing of two or even three samples, each having its own selective fluorophor. The mixture is then run on a single 2-DE gel and the images are captured at different excitation and emission wavelengths. By overlapping the images, it is easy to visualize protein differences between the samples. Furthermore, this technology (DIGE) overcomes the problems/inconsistencies of gel-to-gel variation.

Although highly resolutive, 2-DE has a number of not insignificant inherent limitations. By analyzing the codon bias of proteins (a method of predicting the abundance of a protein in a cell) in a yeast extract, Gygi et al. showed that most spots typically seen in whole cell "proteomes" are from highly abundant proteins, cytoskeletal proteins, etc., whereas low- abundance proteins such as signaling molecules, kinases, transcription factors, etc. (often the most interesting proteins) are poorly represented. Of course, one way to overcome this limitation is to load more samples onto a gel, although this can produce artifacts such as streaking and smearing—often obscuring important information. Moreover, detecting low-abundance proteins with even the most sensitive detection methods often requires very high loads (milligram quantities) of total protein.

Commercial isoelectric focusing strips that have high resolving power over a narrow pH range ("zoom" gels) and have the added advantage of accepting much higher protein loads than broad pH range strips are now available; thus, to a certain degree, this problem can be overcome. However, another limitation of 2-DE is the limited "window" over which proteins can be resolved. Proteins whose molecular weights fall outside the resolving power of SDS-PAGE ($> \sim 150$ and $< \sim 10$kDa) and those that are particularly hydrophobic are poorly represented in 2-D profiles. Similarly, alkaline proteins are traditionally difficult to resolve on 2-D gels.

2-DE is, by no means, the only method used in proteomic research; indeed, much effort has gone into identifying alternate strategies for protein separation given the obvious limitations of 2-DE. Examples of other, largely column-based, chromatographic separation techniques used, either alone and/or in combination, include: ion exchange, size exclusion, and reversed-phase chromatography. One interesting development that has gained considerable momentum for what is termed "shotgun" or "bottom-up" proteomics is multidimensional protein identification technology (MudPIT). This technique uses the combined resolving power of RP-HPLC and ion exchange, with the separated peaks identified by tandem mass spectrometry. Briefly, a soluble protein mixture is digested with trypsin and the resultant digest is subject to fractionation on a cation exchanger; RP-HPLC is then used to resolve the resultant peptide digest peaks. Each peak is then subject to tandem mass spectrometry on-line for precise protein identification. This technology is also amenable to reasonably accurate quantification using isotope-coded affinity tagging (ICAT) technology. This technique involves the selective labeling of cysteine residues in a protein with isotope-coded affinity tags. The reagent has three constituent groups: first, a biotin group, which binds to an avidin affinity support (purification); second, a linker, which has the isotope tag; and third, a reactive group, which links to the cysteine thiol group. Very simply, one linker will have no deuterium and the second linker will have eight deuteriums; thus the peptide digest fragments can be run together (e.g., control vs. treated) and the ratio between the peptides can be determined by mass spectrometry, which will easily distinguish between the two isotope tags; the resulting MS/MS spectrum will allow identification of the peptide fragment.

Other separation tools include capillary IEF, capillary zone electrophoresis, and affinity enrichment. These alternate chromatographic and immunological techniques have some advantages over 2-DE in that the separated protein is in a soluble (and sometimes nondenatured) state, allowing a higher yield and facilitating subsequent (in-line) biological assays, thereby readily adding a "functional" component to the proteomic study.

Protein beads, chips, and/or other affinity-based supports represent an important emerging technology for the separation of proteins from complex mixtures and/or for the examination of specific protein–protein interactions. For example, protein chips consist of arrays of small spots on a solid support (e.g., aluminum, glass, etc. plate), with each spot containing a protein capture moiety or bait, either chemical (e.g., hydrophobic/hydrophilic surface) or biochemical (e.g., antibodies, receptors, domain fragments, and peptides), designed to trap proteins of interest. Other supports such as magnetic beads and derivatized solid supports, etc. can also be used to "fish out" proteins of interest. Crude cellular extracts, or partially purified protein fractions can be applied to the solid support following which noninteracting material is washed off, leaving only those proteins that interact with the immobilized bait. Solid-phase supports have considerable potential for use in diagnostic kits and high-throughput analyses. One disadvantage of many protein supports is that due to conformational changes and the nonphysiological environment employed, the interactions formed between the bait and target proteins may not necessarily reflect true in vivo interactions. Ultimately, the separation method used, as with the extraction procedure, will depend largely on the analysis required. Having resolved an extract into its individual components, a detection procedure is employed, and the selected proteins (of interest) are then isolated and subjected to identification by mass spectrometry.

Protein Identification: Mass Spectrometry

At the heart of any proteomics facility is high-quality mass spectrometry. Prior to the advent of biological MS in the early 1990s, analysis of spots from 2-DE gels and/or HPLC/conventional chromatography etc. relied on time-consuming and relatively insensitive procedures such as amino acid analysis, immunological detection, or sequencing via Edman degradation chemistry. The development of methods for "*soft ionization*" for mass spectrometers allowed the handling of large biomacromolecules, and subsequent developments facilitated the sensitive and rapid analysis of large numbers of proteins. MS of peptides/proteins is achieved by first ionizing the analytes, using either one of two different methods, then detecting and determining the ion mass. A matrix-assisted laser desorption ionization (MALDI) ion source uses a high-energy laser to ionize peptides or small proteins from a solid sample, whereas an electrospray ion source operates by generating ions from a charged nebula of aqueous sample (e.g., HPLC Eluate).

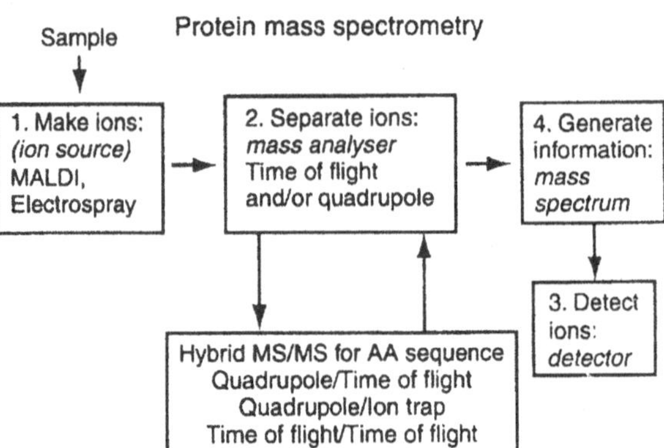

Fig. 12.3. Flow diagram outlining the basic principles involved in the mass spectrometric analysis of protein and peptides.

MALDI time-of-flight (TOF) instruments measure the precise molecular mass of the peptide analyte by reference to its time of flight to a detector at the end of an extended flight tube, whereas electrospray instruments employ multiple quadrupole electromagnetic mass filters. Both types of instruments are able to produce limited sequence information (minimally approximately five to six residues, often much more) by analyzing protein degradation products. MALDI-TOF can be used to glean sequence information by making use of the phenomenon of postsource decay (PSD), whereby a small population of proteins is sequentially fragmented into constituent amino acid residues from which N-terminal sequence can be inferred. However, collision-induced decay (CID) is used in a similar fashion on electrospray instruments fitted with tandem quadrupole filters. A stream of gas is introduced between the two quadrupoles to collide with analytes and induce fragmentation; the masses of the fragments are then analyzed in the second quadrupole (CID) and sequence is inferred in a similar fashion as for PSD.

The strength of MS in proteomic research becomes apparent when a protein to be studied is first digested by using one or more proteolytic enzymes that can cleave proteins at specific residues, producing a characteristic and unique fingerprint of tens to hundreds of constituent peptides. A MALDI-TOF-MS can then be used to rapidly analyze these peptides to produce a peptide mass fingerprint (PMF). The PMF for a protein is essentially specific for that protein and is used as a search query against a database of PMF-like entries generated as theoretical digests of protein sequences. Limited sequence information for several peptides from a protein digest can be used in conjunction with PMF data to increase the likelihood of finding a matching protein during database searching.

Sensitivity and accuracy are two of the most important aspects of MS as it applies to proteomics; the more sensitive is the MS employed, the less likely one would need to include an enrichment procedure prior to separating proteins. Recent advances in biological mass spectrometry have considerable utility in this aspect of proteomic research. Among the new generation of mass spectrometers are the QTOF instruments, which combine the advantages of both MALDI-TOF and electrospray platforms, where ions from a front-end multiple quadrupole ion source are fed into a TOF reflectron flight tube. These instruments offer greater resolution and sensitivity over conventional triple quadrupole instruments, thus allowing both improved sensitivity and greater sequencing capacity in a single instrument. Adding the capacity to hold ions in an electromagnetic "*ion trap*" means that mass spectrometers with this added capability offer even greater sensitivity and enhanced resolution and capacity. The minimum accuracy that one might expect from either a MALDI-TOF and/or electrospray mass spectrometer is a single mass unit (i.e., the ability to distinguish peptide masses that differ by a single hydrogen atom). The more accurate an instrument is, then the better are one's chances of obtaining reliable identification with PMF database matching. Finally, TOF–TOF hybrid mass spectrometers are proving enormous value in ultra high-throughput proteomics. Although lacking in absolute sequencing sensitivity, these instruments can scan through and identify extremely large numbers of peptide fragments in one very rapid analysis. One of the largest bottlenecks in proteomic research is the separation stage, especially if a 2-DE component is employed. One way to overcome this problem is to combine the separation and identification stages, such as is the case with Ciphergen's surface-enhanced laser desorption ionization (SELDI) technology. This approach uses a protein chip containing entrapped proteins as the sample stage for direct MALDI analysis. By eliminating an otherwise lengthy separation step, SELDI and similar technologies have the potential to provide extremely high throughput to routine proteomic analyses.

Pharmaceutical Applications of Proteomics

The significance of proteomics in the pharmaceutical and biotechnology industries is as follows:

1. Proteins are the commercial endpoints of most esearch works in the biological/biomedical sciences.
2. Proteins carry out nearly all controlled biological functions.
3. Protein–protein interactions control most cellular processes.
4. Most diseases are treated at the protein level.
5. Proteins are extremely valuable products for the pharmaceutical, food, environmental, and related biotechnological industries.
6. Proteomics represents the key to understanding nonlinear biological processes.

Proteomics should not be viewed simply as a methodical cataloguing of any and all proteins expressed by a given cell/tissue/extract, etc. at a given time. Instead, proteomics represents a means by which proteins of interest can be analyzed en masse and specifically in the context of whatever cellular processes were active (or not) at the time of preparation. However, this is, by no means, the end of the proteomic pathway. For example, simply looking for changes in protein expression between normal and disease states does not allow one to know whether the changes observed were the cause of the disease or simply the result. Instead, proteomics provides the starting point for the emerging field of "*functional proteomics*," where changes observed in a particular system are linked to functional consequences of change, thus building a comprehensive global picture of cellular function and interactivity of proteins within it. Proteomics is generating considerable interest and investment in the pharmaceutical and biotechnology industries for its potential for identifying not only drug targets for the development of lead compounds but also disease biomarkers, as well as for developing diagnostic tools. The identification of a particular disease can be facilitated by detecting and/or quantitating one or more proteins (or by-products) specific to that disease, referred to as biomarkers.

For the purposes of this particular chapter, there will be specific focus on areas where proteomics is starting to generate valuable information for biomolecular pharmacologists. This includes the following:

1. Proteomic screening, biomarker discovery, and diagnostics (discovery of molecular markers for diagnosis and monitoring disease; molecular dissection of genetic or pharmacological perturbation subtype individuals to predict response to therapy)
2. Drug target identification and validation by proteomics (discovery of novel, biologically active molecules and validation of drug targets)
3. Pharmacokinetic proteomics (ADME analysis, formulation, stability studies, and pharmacokinetics).

Classically, proteomics has been applied to examine gross changes in the cellular expression of proteins as a consequence of a disease process and/ or a particular drug treatment and/or protein expression differences in experimental animal models. This approach has indeed yielded a lot of very valuable information and has certainly provided valuable insights into the proteins involved. For example, the field of neuroscience is particularly well suited to analysis with proteomic techniques, given the complexity of neuronal signaling and the diversity of cellular responses. An area where there has been a particular focus is neurological disorders such as schizophrenia and Alzheimer's disease—just two of the many representative areas of neuroscience research. The potential for these techniques to help unravel the underlying pathology of complex neurological and neuropsychiatric conditions is considerable. The careful cataloguing of postmortem tissues and appropriate storage in tissue banks have allowed the systematic analysis of protein expression changes as a consequence of a particular disease process and, when matched to gene array data, provide even further insights into the disease process. Similar approaches have been used in screening changes in various cancers and cardiovascular diseases. However, all these studies have limitations and, as mentioned earlier, the challenge is always to delineate the differences in protein expression between cause and effect. The development of more sophisticated technologies, robotics, and improved bioinformatics has allowed researchers to take a far more targeted approach, and the areas of functional and focused proteomics are both creating a greater impact and are providing far more useful information, especially in the pharmaceutical sciences.

Proteomic Screening, Biomarker Discovery, and Diagnostics

Perhaps the area in proteomics that is generating most excitement at the moment is applications focusing on biomarker discovery. The development of protein chips, high-throughput mass spectrometry, and sensitive quantitation (ICAT, DIGE, etc.) has provided a very potent series of enabling technologies for biomarker discovery. Very simply, a tissue extract, blood sample, urine, cerebrospinal fluid (CSF), or any other fluid can be passed over a chip, or subject to other chromatography-based capture device (single-dimension HPLC, MudPIT, Affinity, 2-DE, etc.). The retained and/or separated peptides/proteins are then both quantified and identified by either single or tandem mass spectrometry. Any protein or peptide differences manifest as a consequence of a particular disease, then that particular protein has the potential to be a biomarker or used for diagnostics. One of the pioneering technologies in this area and one that has generated much interest and discussion is SELDI-based screening. This technology was developed by Ciphergen and has been successful along with other chip-based technologies for biomarker screening. The concept is simple in that a chip that has been coated with either a specific affinity tag or other chromatographic support is exposed to a defined tissue extract or biological fluid of interest. After washing, the chip is then fed directly into a purpose-built mass spectrometer. The mass spectrometer then calculates and defines the mass of every adhering component and plots the masses in a format similar to a gel. Then by comparing the mass profiles of samples taken from control/healthy/nondrug-treated patients with samples taken from treated/sick patients, it is possible to rapidly identify any protein changes. These proteins can be subsequently identified by MS/MS technologies. This technique has provided leads in the quest for valid biomarkers, particularly in the cancer area where early diagnosis is crucial to some of the cancers including liver, pancreas, lung, etc. Of course, the technology is not restricted to oncology, but has also been applied in other areas such as urology, renal diseases, diabetes, etc.

Of course, SELDI technology is only one of the many technologies that can be used for biomarker screening. Other companies have introduced competing technologies and, of course, there are other chip technologies (e.g., hydrogel) that can also be applied. Most proteomic technologies can be adapted to biomarker screening. Many of the markers identified are clearly surrogate and often are very much the consequence of the disease rather than having any causal component. For example, protein fragments that occur in cancer patient screens could come from highly abundant proteins that are being degraded as a consequence of protease up-regulation, specifically in the case of various cancers, by matrix metalloproteases. These high-throughput screening technologies are not limited to simply biomarker discovery, but can be used to predict responses to therapies and to monitor the consequences of drug therapies. Recently, improved analytical and bioinformatics tools have driven attention on pattern recognition approaches rather than single-marker tests for prognostic forecasting. It is expected that predicting metastasization based on tumoral protein patterns will soon be a reality. However, currently available technologies either limit the number of proteins that can be analyzed simultaneously, or they are expensive, difficult, and time-consuming. Moreover, the tools adapted for expression proteomics might not be the same as those for prognostic studies that require investigation of protein function over time.

Drug Target Identification and Validation by Proteomics

One of the areas where proteomics has made the biggest impact in the pharmaceutical/biotechnology industries is in drug target identification and validation. One of the many challenges the pharmaceutical industry faces is the specificity of candidate drugs and the precise nature of molecular targets being affected. Functional proteomics provides a very useful approach to examining drug specificity and drug target identification.

The most common approach and one that has been very successful is where a drug, or indeed a molecular library of candidate drugs, is tethered to a solid support or chip. An appropriate extract from cells (untreated and/or stimulated), tissue extracts/fluids taken from control or treated animals, diseased or normal biopsies or postmortem tissue extracts, etc. is then washed over the chip/solid support and any interacting proteins or peptides will then adhere to the drug bait. The complex can then be washed (with varying degrees of stringency to make a crude assessment of binding affinity) and then the adhering proteins can be eluted. The eluate, often only containing a few proteins, can then be submitted to proteomic analysis and all the binding partners identified. This technique can also be applied to identify both protein complexes and the mechanism by which these complexes are formed, by simply attaching specific proteins of interest to the solid support and then any drug that can either perturb or prevent complex formation can be analyzed following separation and mass spectrometric identification. Other strategies to identify potential targets involve the covalent cross- linking of a drug to its protein target; the covalent complex can then be isolated and the binding protein(s) can be identified following enzyme digestion and mass spectrometric identification.

One of the biggest issues currently facing both the biotechnology and pharmaceutical industries is drug target validation. Proteomics has been very successfully applied to the validation of specific drug targets. Applying these techniques, of course, requires knowledge of the potential targets and, in particular, the biological pathway to be perturbed or enhanced, specifically knowledge of the precise proteins involved. A broad-based approach is to simply look at gross protein changes as a consequence of a specific drug treatment, and then focus on expression differences for specific proteins involved (e.g., a signaling cascade and/or transcriptional or secretory event linked to a receptor drug target). Thus the downside of such an approach is that, very often, the proteins of interest are of low abundance and are masked by high-abundance (structural, chaperone, or other) proteins present in the particular extract; this is a particular problem when looking at plasma/serum where over 95% of the total protein comprises only four or five protein types—thus the linear and dynamic range for protein detection is much reduced. A far more attractive approach is to use proteomics to evaluate specific protein–protein interactions and the effect a particular drug might have on this interaction, and/or to examine the consequence of a particular drug treatment on an array of representative proteins that have been selectively isolated from the tissue/plasma milieu. Of course, in this context, proteomics embraces specific enabling technologies such as yeast two hybrid and fluorescent quenching technologies such as BRET, FRET, etc. to examine particular protein–protein or protein–drug interacting pathways.

Pharmacokinetic Proteomics

With massive advances in mass spectrometry over the last 5 years, both in terms of sensitivity and throughput, more and more applications have been identified and developed for the analysis of proteins and peptides in biological matrices with the result that some of the more traditional methods are being slowly discarded. One area—although perhaps still very much in its infancy—is the application of proteomics for fine in vivo pharmacokinetic analysis of proteins and peptides. Mass spectrometry has been very much the tool of choice for the analysis of pharmacokinetic profiles for nonproteinaceous drugs and other small-molecule blood-borne constituents; however, with the advent of more discriminating and sensitive technologies, specifically sophisticated "*ion trap*" -based mass spectrometry, it is now possible to measure and monitor specific peptides and proteins accurately in complex biological matrices including blood. However, there are still issues to overcome given the speed and throughput allowed by these technologies; it could be argued that some of the more classical technologies [enzyme-linked immunosorbent assay (ELISA), radio-immunoassays, etc.] will be replaced by high-sensitivity mass spectrometry-based techniques for the pharmacokinetic analysis of protein-based and peptide-based therapeutics. Certainly, in vitro proteomics has been used extensively to monitor peptide and protein stability in complex biological matrices such as plasma and other fluids and tissue extracts, where the peptide of interest is incubated with the biological extract, aliquots are removed at predefined time points, and the integrity of the protein/peptide is assessed by HPLC and mass spectrometry. Indeed, for the design and analysis of stable peptide analogues, proteomic-based approaches are now the method of choice to monitor protein and peptide stability and availability. The major advantage a mass spectrometric approach offers over some of the more traditional, largely immunologically based technologies is that mass spectrometry gives an absolute identification of the protein and/or peptide, whereas an immunological technique only measure the epitope(s); thus by using mass spectrometry, any changes to the core structure of the protein or peptide are immediately apparent. Furthermore, monitoring structural changes provides a valuable insight into metabolic pathways, and, of course, with peptides and proteins, it is important to bear in mind that subtly modified forms may still retain biological activity. Finally, mass spectrometric/ proteomic approaches have aided enormously in the area of peptide and protein formulation, where it is easy to rapidly monitor the structural integrity of a protein under a variety of different storage conditions, diluents, etc.

In summary, proteomics is a series of sophisticated enabling technologies, which allows, for the first time, proteins (and their interacting partners) and/or protein systems to be analyzed on a scale previously only seen in the genomic arena. However, proteomics should not be thought of as supplanting genomics; rather, the two should be seen as complementary disciplines/approaches. Proteomics provides a potential means by which the vast information obtained from ventures such as the Human Genome Project can be annotated, better understood, and applied to the prevention and cure of diseases. In the field of molecular pharmacology, proteomics, although in its relative infancy, is starting to have an impact. There are examples in the literature where proteomics is being used to monitor disease progression, identify novel drug targets, validate existing targets, and identify and characterize novel disease biomarkers, and, finally, proteomics is starting to establish a role in the analysis of fine pharmacokinetics. It must be remembered that this is an emerging field and that the technology is now only starting to move from the development phase into real applications. Clearly, the technologies will continue to be improved and refined; thus the role of proteomics in the pharmacological sciences will become increasingly important as we move toward a greater understanding of integrated biological systems using the information gained from the various proteomic genomic and other molecular technologies.

13

Gastroretentive Systems

Oral controlled release (CR) dosage forms (DF) have been extensively used to improve therapy of many important medications. However, in the case of narrow absorption window drugs, this pharmaceutical approach cannot be utilized, as it requires sufficient colonic absorption of the drug (which contradicts the definition of narrow absorption window agents). On the other hand, incorporation of the drug into a CR-delivery system, which releases its payload in the stomach over a prolonged time period, can lead to significant therapeutic advantages owing to various pharmacokinetic (PK) and pharmacodynamic aspects. Gastroretentive dosage forms (GRDFs) are a drug delivery formulation that are designed to be retained in the stomach for a prolonged time and release there their active materials and thereby enable sustained and prolonged input of the drug to the upper part of the gastrointestinal (GI) tract. This technology has generated enormous attention over the last few decades owing to its potential application to improve the oral delivery of some important drugs for which prolonged retention in the upper GI tract can greatly improve their oral bioavailability and/or their therapeutic outcome.

This article reviews some of the latest developments in GRDF technology from a pharmaceutical point of view. It also highlights the PK and/or pharmacodynamic rationale for the development of GRDFs for certain drugs that are either absorbed in the upper GI tract or have local activity there.

The main approaches examined thus far to extend gastric residence time (GRT) of a delivery system have been low-density GRDFs to induce buoyancy above the gastric fluid, high-density GRDFs to retain the DF in the body of the stomach, concomitant administration of drugs that slow the motility of the GI tract, and bioadhesion to the gastric mucosa. Another approach, which in our view is the most promising, is expandable GRDFs. These GRDFs are easily swallowed and reach a significantly larger size in the stomach owing to swelling or unfolding processes that prolong their GRT. After drug release, their dimensions are minimized with subsequent evacuation from the stomach. Our experience has shown that gastroretentivity is significantly enhanced by the combination of substantial dimensions together with considerable rigidity of the DF. This combination enables the GRDF to withstand peristalsis and mechanical contractility of the stomach. Positive results were obtained in preclinical and clinical studies evaluating GRT of expandable GRDFs. Narrow absorption window drugs compounded in such systems have improved PK and pharmacodynamic properties absorption properties.

GI Physiology

It is worth briefly reviewing the role of the stomach in terms of anatomical structure and physiological function to understand its implication in the development of GRDFs. The stomach is composed of the following parts: the fundus, lying above the opening of the esophagus into the stomach; the body; the central part; and the antrum. The pylorus is an anatomical sphincter situated between the most terminal antrum and the duodenum. The motility of the stomach differs remarkably between the fasted and the fed state. The motoric activity in the fasting state, termed "inter-digestive myoelectric motor complex (IMMC)," is a 2 hr cycle of peristaltic activity that is generated in the stomach and progresses toward the ileocecal junction. It aims to clear the stomach and the small intestine of indigested residues, swallowed saliva, and sloughed epithelial cells. The IMMC is composed of four phases: the first phase lasts for 45–60 min with a few or no contractions. The second phase consists of intermittent irregular sweeping contractions and involves bile secretion and lasts until the intense peristaltic contractions of the third phase start. The peristaltic waves of the third phase, also called the "*housekeeper phase*," last for 5–15 min and decrease gradually in the 4th phase to prepare the stomach for the next cycle. Following meals, food is stored•in the upper part of the stomach, and approximately 5–10 min after food ingestion, the stomach motor activity starts and persists as long as the food exists in the stomach (2–4 hr). The peristaltic contractions of the proximal stomach slowly compress the food toward the pyloric sphincter, and the stomach contents are evacuated.

The pyloric sphincter causes an appreciable constriction of the lumen at the gastroduodenal junction. The width and height of the pyloric ring and the diameters of the pyloric aperture, sphincteric cylinder, and duodenal bulb were measured by radiography during the motor quiescent phase of the IMMC. The mean width of the ring was 4.7 mm, and the mean height 11.1 mm; the depth was approximately the same on the greater and lesser curvature sides. The mean inner margin of the opening by which the lumen of the stomach communicates with that of the duodenum in the motor quiescent phase is 8.7 mm. The mean diameter of the sphincteric cylinder is 57.1 mm, and the mean diameter of the duodenal bulb is 35.8 mm. The circular musculature of the pyloric sphincteric cylinder is complex structure consisting of various loops arranged into a system of rings. The right canalis loop is the muscular part of the pyloric ring. The left canalis loop is located at the oral end of the cylinder. The two loops meet and interlace on the lesser curvature in a muscle torus or knot, from which they diverge to encircle the greater curvature. The loops are connected by intervening circular as well as by overlying longitudinal fibers; many of the latter dip into the right canalis loop. Generally, the residence time of food in the stomach depends upon its nutritive and physical properties, but many other factors are involved in gastric transit performance of DFs including age, gender, posture, osmolarity, and pH of food, mental stress, and disease state. Liquids are emptied rapidly from the stomach, while non-fatty solids and semisolids are emptied slower. Solid or semisolid fats empty much more slowly than aqueous liquids owing to a nervous mechanism inhibiting gastric peristalsis and floating over gastric liquids. Indigestible solids and DFs are not retained in the stomach for over 2 hr when administered in the fasting state owing to the IMMC, while their gastric retention time (GRT) in the fed state depends mostly on the DF size as well as the composition and the caloric value of food.

In general, large DFs have longer GRT in the fed state in comparison to the fasting state and are retained for further digestion and evacuation toward the end of the fed state, or by the subsequent "*housekeeper wave*." As the GRT of DFs is a function of the length of the digestive process, theoretically, continuous feeding can prolong their GRT for more than 24 hr. The transit time in the duodenum is very short and ranges from 5 to 10 min. Unlike the gastric transit, the transit in the small intestine is remarkably constant irrespective of the fed or the fasted state or the type of the DF and lies between 2–4 hr in most populations.

Approaches for GRDF Development

Increasing the GRT of DFs can be achieved in several ways. Naturally, food high in calorie value or containing fats and some amino acids can slow gastric emptying and intestinal transit. Certain drugs such as metoclopramide are known to decrease the gastric motility and thus increase the GRT of drugs that are administered concomitantly. However, it is not acceptable to add a second drug to improve bioavailability. Recently, some sophisticated technologies have been developed to increase the GRT of drug formulations utilizing different features of the stomach anatomy and physiology. Some of these technologies have been adapted by pharmaceutical companies to improve the bioavailability and therapeutic utilization of existing drugs, although it is more likely that the success of these technologies is more valuable in the development of new drugs.

Expandable DFs

Expandable DFs are oral delivery devices that increase their size considerably after ingestion; the extended dimensions are aimed to be retained in the stomach and consequently increase their GRT. These DFs are planned to release their drug content in the stomach and be subsequently evacuated owing to the decrease of their dimension and rigidity. Different expandable DFs have been developed over the last three decades. Originally, these DFs were developed by Laby for veterinary use. The design of expandable DFs usually takes into consideration some basic configurations: a small configuration having a suitable size for convenient oral intake, expanded form that is achieved in the stomach and which should have an appropriate size that inhibits its gastric emptying through the pyloric sphincter, and finally a small form achieved after active drug release that allows their evacuation.

The expanded device should be rigid enough to remain intact and survive the gastric mechanical forces. Besides, the rate of drug release should be appropriate to achieve optimal absorption of the drug from its absorption window. The first designed GRDF for human use was suggested by Johnson and Rowe on the basis of expansion in the stomach and it was composed of thiolated gelatin, a cross-linking agent, and a drug. Once the device reaches the stomach and is exposed to gastric fluids, the thiolated gelatin hydrates, swells, and cross-links to form a matrix too large to pass through the pylorus. Additives like a nondigestible hydrophilic colloidal material can be added to increase the swelling ratio.

Swelling DFs

The techniques applied for achieving expanding properties for GRDFs are usually swelling or unfolding. Swelling devices are, in most cases, based on a hydrophilic polymer prepared from a combination of polyethylene oxide and hydroxypropyl methyl cellulose that form a hydrogel, which can achieve both CR and swelling properties. Mamajek and Moyer have designed a GRDF consisting of a nonhydratable membrane envelope that is drug and fluid permeable; a drug reservoir, an expanding agent, and a swellable resin are enveloped and the whole device expands owing to osmotic pressure. Another swelling device developed by Urquhart and Theeuwes exhibits high swelling properties exhibiting 2–50 fold volume increase, which retains device evacuation from the stomach not only because of its large dimension but also because of maintaining the stomach in the fed mode by means of mechanical sensation. By incorporating the active drug into wax-walled tiny pills, a CR of the drug is achieved.

Some of the swelling devices reported in the literature have shown extended gastric retentive properties when studied in dogs. However, the transit characteristics of these formulations in man were very similar to those reported previously for other single unit matrix systems. Recently developed GRDFs by Chen et al. involve the use of a superporous composite that combines a high swelling rate with a 100-fold increase of the initial volume and a substantial mechanical strength. These DFs have shown good gastroretentive properties in fed dogs, but they yet have to be tested in humans.

Unfolding DFs

Unfolding GRDFs are usually planned to extend from their initial small configuration to their unfolded large size in the stomach after oral intake. Owing to the mechanical properties of the device, the gastric liquids induce its opening or expanding. Unlike the swelling devices, the unfolding GRDFs are manufactured in their maximal size and are folded into their minimal geometry to enable convenient intake, thus also have to include "*obstructing means*" that increase their rigidity and thus inhibit their evacuation from the stomach. The effect of size, shape, erodibility, and mechanical shape of the unfolded devices was conducted by Caldwell et al. The geometric configurations of the developed devices were continuous stick, ring, tetrahedron, planar disc, planar multilobe, and string. All the devices had the following properties: sufficient resistance to forces applied by the stomach to prevent their rapid passage through the pylorus, their presence in the stomach still allows the free passage of food in the stomach and desired in vivo circumference larger than 5 cm, to ensure gastroretentivity. Studies in beagle dogs have shown that gastroretentivity, assessed as the number of devices retained in the fasting stomach at 24 hr, can remarkably be influenced by the geometry of the unfolded DFs and by the type of test species and increases remarkably as a result of enhanced mechanical properties and decreased polymer erosion.

Recently developed unfolding GRDFs in our lab have a rectangular shape and are composed of rigid components with large dimensions to enhance gastroretentivity. The device is composed of a thin drug–polymer matrix that is surrounded by rigid polymeric strips, all covered from both sides in a sandwich form, by identical membranes, which connect and maintain them intact. Each separate component is designed to evacuate from the stomach rapidly, while the combination of them all in this platform yields prolonged GRT. The GRDFs were retained in the stomach of dogs and humans for prolonged and comparable time spans of at least 6 to 10 hr. In both species nondisintegrating tablets and equivalent DFs, which are identical to the GRDF but lack the rigid frame, had short GRT (up to 2 hr), thus showing the unique gastroretentive properties of these GRDFs.

Floating Formulations

Floating microcapsules were first described by Sheth and Tossounian as forms that can float on the gastric contents owing to their lower bulk density. Usually, floating formulations are prepared from hydrophilic matrices that either have a density lower than one or their density drops below one after immersion in the gastric fluids owing to swelling. Cellulose ether polymers are often used as the floating matrices, and low-density fatty acids can be incorporated as well to decrease hydrating rate and increase buoyancy. More sophisticated devices were developed later and involved the use of various film-coating techniques, incorporation of a floating chamber that is filled with harmless gas, or a liquid that gasifies at body temperature. These forms are often called "hydrodynamically balanced systems" (HBS) as they can maintain low density and keep floating even after hydrating. When a floating form is administered with food, the device remains buoyant on the surface of the gastric contents in the upper part of the stomach and moves down toward the pyloric sphincter while the meal empties. The reported GRT of such floating devices varies from 4 to 10 hr. The active drug is progressively released from the formulation matrix and thus introduced to the proximal intestine where it can be absorbed.

Various techniques have been proposed as floating devices, and their performances have been mostly assessed by in vitro methods to evaluate their floating and drug release properties. Sato et al. have prepared riboflavin-containing microballoons that showed an improved gastroretentivity and bioavailability in vivo in human. Yet, the authors have observed that there was poor correlation between the floating properties and the drug release kinetics. They suggested that to optimize the in vivo performance of this DF, the floating properties should be improved in such a way that will not negatively affect the drug releasing properties. However, this mean of GRDF suffers from very high variability in its in vivo performance in human studies and is very much affected by changes in posture and gastric fluid volume.

Bioadhesive Formulations

Bioadhesive or mucoadhesive formulations were originally developed for increasing GRT and controlling drug delivery of all kinds of drugs. The technique involves coating of microcapsules with bioadhesive polymer, which enables them to adhere to intestinal mucosa and remain for longer time period in the GI while the active drug is released from the device matrix. The cationic chitosan polymers are pharmaceutically acceptable to be used in the preparation of bioadhesive formulations owing to their known ability to bind well to gastric mucosa. Taking into consideration the quick turnover of intestinal mucus and the reasonably constant transit time of food and drug in the intestine being independent of size, shape, density or fed state, it is hard to find published data that demonstrate that bioadhesion can actually increase the transit time in the intestine. Thus, the extended transit of such formulations has yet to be confirmed by direct measurement using labeling methods or scintigraphy rather than using circumstantial methods, such as gastroretentivity, as demonstrated in area under the plasma level vs. time curve.

High-Density Systems

In this approach, a device having higher density than the gastric fluids sinks in the bottom of the stomach and its GRT might increase owing to the fact that it may remain for longer times in the lower part of the stomach. Rechgaard et al. demonstrated that for sinking in the gastric fluids, such a device should have at least a density of 1.4 g/ml. Either by using a single unit heavy tablet or multiunit dose in the form of pellets, almost identical GI transit times were observed. However, limited success has been reported so far for high-density devices as GRDFs.

Drug Candidates for GRDFs

Many researchers have been fascinated lately by the development of GRDFs, although it is obvious that this technique can provide a good solution for only a limited number of drugs that are already used in the clinic. This is because most drug candidates that would benefit from GRDF could not reach the market in the absence of such a reliable GRDF. In the searching process for GRDF candidates, several questions may be taken into consideration. The stability and solubility of a given compound in gastric juice is of great importance. According to the biopharmaceutical classification of drugs in terms of their solubility and intestinal permeability introduced by the Food and Drug Administration (FDA) in 1995, drugs are categorized in four classes. Only class I compounds are defined as those with high solubility and high permeability, and are predicted to be well absorbed when given orally, while all other compounds (classes II–IV) suffer from low solubility, low permeability, or both and display variable absorption in different regions of the human GI tract and as a consequence, their oral bioavailabilities can be affected by the limited "*absorption window.*"

This region-specific absorption can be related to differential drug solubility and stability at different regions of the intestine owing to changes in environmental pH and degradation by enzymes present in the lumen of the intestine or interaction with endogenous components such as bile or active transport mechanisms for drugs involving carriers and pump systems. It seems very important to understand why a drug may display a site-specific or narrow absorption window to be able to improve its bioavailability. Pre- formulation studies may provide crucial characteristics of drug's physical and chemical properties. Other in vitro studies for detecting drug permeability using caco-2-cultured cells or in vitro rat intestine segments (USSING chambers) for determining drug absorption rate can provide helpful information, although extrapolation to humans may be uncertain.

The dosing regimen is another important issue that should be evaluated before incorporating a drug into GRDF. Some drugs may exhibit a long half-life, and their dose regimen is once daily. In contrast, other drugs may have a short PK half-life, but still are given once daily owing to a prolonged pharmacodynamic half-life. In both cases, the development of a GRDF may be considered unnecessary unless a new application like local treatment of the GI wall or targeting the intestine mucosa is aimed. GRDF is the formulation of choice when the drug is mainly absorbed in the upper GI tract, and a reduction of plasma level fluctuations is required to minimize concentration-dependant adverse drug reactions. When a drug is mainly absorbed in the upper part of the GI tract and the unabsorbed fraction, which arrives to the colon, may cause serious local side effects, the GRDF is an excellent solution to reduce the appearance of such drugs in the colon. A good example for such compounds is antibiotics. Certain drugs that have been suggested before to benefit from a GRDF are listed in Table 1, some of them have been successfully incorporated in experimental GRDF and have been reported to be examined in humans, and a few of them have also reached clinical phase II.

METHODS TO ASSESS GASTRORETENTIVITY OF GRDFs

Unlike other formulations, the kinetics of transit of the GRDF along the GI tract, and especially in determining its GRT are very important. It requires, in most cases, an imaging technique that can locate the GRDF in vivo. The following methods have been utilized so far to assess gastroretentivity.

Magnetic Resonance Imaging

Magnetic resonance imaging (MRI) is a noninvasive technique that is not associated with radioactivity and allows observation of the total anatomical structure in relatively high resolution. The visualization of the GI tract by MRI has to be further improved by the administration of contrast media. For solid DFs, the incorporation of a superparamagnetic compound such as ferrous oxide enables their visualization by MRI. The technique is safe and allows obtaining many pictures from the same subject.

Radiology (X-Ray)

In this technique, a radio-opaque material has to be incorporated in the DF, and its location is tracked by X-ray pictures. The technique is used to evaluate gastroretentivity of GRDFs and the disintegration rate of DFs in vivo, and also to determine the esophageal transit. Although it is considered cheap and a simple method to use, its major disadvantage is the safety issue owing to repeated exposure to X-ray that increase the risk for the volunteers.

γ-Scintigraphy

Gamma scintigraphy relies on the administration of a DF containing a small amount of radioisotope, e.g., ^{152}Sm, which is a gamma ray emitter with a relatively short half-life. The isotope has to be incorporated into the GRDF in advance. Then, a short time prior to the study, the formulation has to be irradiated in a neutron source that causes it to emit γ rays. The emitted ray can be imaged using a "*gamma camera*"—a form of a scintillation counter, combined with a computer to process the image, and thereby the DF can be tracked in the GI tract. This technique is elegant and provides proper assessment of gastroretentivity in humans.

Gastroscopy

Gastroscopy is commonly used for the diagnosis and monitoring of the GI tract. This technique utilizes a fiberoptic or video system and can be easily applied for monitoring and locating GRDFs in the stomach. However, it is too inconvenient to conduct the procedure frequently in the same experiment for one subject. In human, the procedure can be applied with or without slight anesthesia while it requires complete anesthesia in dogs.

ASSESSMENT OF GRDF PERFORMANCE IN VIVO

The most common laboratory animals used for absorption analysis are rats, while dogs are the more commonly used animals for evaluation of oral CR-DFs. Prior to clinical evaluation, canine studies are usually carried out, for direct evaluation of gastroretentivity, for PK/pharmacodynamic proof-of-concept, or both. Despite some basic differences between the digestive tracts of humans and dogs, overall there are enough similarities to make the dog a useful screening tool. The two major differences between human and dog stomach activity are the gastric emptying time after eating and the pH in the fasting state: the gastric emptying time of food in the fed state is significantly longer in dogs than in humans. In the dog, an 8-mm tablet can be retained in the stomach for more than 8 hr following a small meal, and IMMC is abolished for about 8 hr. To prevent overestimation of the GRDF performance, the outcome of canine studies is considered as a preliminary screening prior to human studies.

Unlike the human stomach, which can reach a pH 2 at fasting state, the fasting dog's stomach pH is 5.5–6.9. Changing gastric pH of a dog may be unnecessary in evaluating nongastroretentive CR-DFs owing to their inherently short GRT. However, assessment of GRDFs may demand intervention: using gastric acidification by pentagastrin intramuscular injection, gastric-acidifying tablets, e.g., glutamic acid hydrochloride, acidulin, or direct administration of acidic buffer. Hence, dogs can be considered a good model for initial gastroretentive evaluation of a new device. On the other hand, pigs cannot be considered a proper model as they normally have a longer gastric retention of pellets and ordinary tablets than human. The most important conclusion from all previous studies is that the best model for human is human.

PK and Pharmacodynamic Aspects of GRDF

It has been established that the selection of a proper drug delivery system should comply with the PK and pharmacodynamic properties of the drug to ensure which input strategy would be most beneficial for achieving significant therapeutic advantages. It seems very important to clarify a variety of PK and pharmacodynamic aspects to establish the rational selection of GRDF as the best mode of administration for certain drugs.

PK Aspects of GRDF

Absorption window

An important PK aspect to be investigated when considering a GRDF candidate is the absorption of the drug along the GI tract and verifying that there is an absorption window at the upper GI tract. Various experimental techniques are available to determine intestinal absorption properties and permeability at different regions of the GI tract. In general, appropriate candidates for CR-GRDF are molecules that are characterized by better absorption properties at the upper parts of the GI tract.

Active transport mechanism

When the absorption is mediated by active transporters that are capacity limited, sustained presentation of the drug to the transporting enzymes may increase the efficacy of the transport and thus improves bioavailability.

Enhanced bioavailability

Once a narrow absorption window is defined for a compound, the possibility of improving bioavailability by continuous administration of the compound to the specific site at the upper GI tract should be tested. For example, although alendronate, levodopa, and riboflavin are three drugs that are absorbed directly from the stomach, it was found that gastric retention of the alendronate in rats, produced by experimental/ surgical means, did not improve its bioavailability, while the bioavailability of levodopa and riboflavin was significantly enhanced when incorporated in a GRDF compared to non-GRDF CR polymeric formulations. In vivo studies remain necessary to determine the proper release profile of the drug from the DF that will provide enhanced bioavailability as different processes, related to absorption and transit of the drug in the GI tract, act concomitantly and influence drug absorption.

Enhanced first-pass metabolism

By increasing the GRT, a CR GRDF provides a slow and sustained input of drug to the absorption site and enhances absorption by active transporters on one hand. On the other hand, the same process may also enhance the efficiency of the presystemic metabolism by the metabolic enzymes cytochrome

P450 (in particular CYP3A4 that is dominant in the gastric wall). This is an important aspect that should be taken into consideration as it means that increasing the absorption efficacy will not necessarily lead to enhanced bioavailability. While CYP450 is found in the upper part of the intestine and its amount is reduced toward the colon, the P-glycoprotein (P-gp) levels increase longitudinally along the intestine and it exists in highest levels in the colon. If a drug is a P-gp substrate and does not undergo oxidative metabolism (e.g., digoxin), a CR-GRDF may improve significantly its absorption.

Elimination half-life

When drugs, with relatively short biological half-life, are introduced into a CR-GRDF, sustained and slow input is obtained, and a flip-flop PK is observed. This can enable reduced dosing frequency and consequently an improved patient compliance and therapy.

Local therapy

The continuous input of active drugs obtained from a CR-GRDF can be utilized for attaining local therapeutic concentrations for the local treatment of the stomach and the small intestine.

Examples for GRDF selection owing to PK considerations

L-Dopa is a prodrug of dopamine and is known as the drug of choice for the treatment of Parkinson's disease. L-Dopa has a narrow absorption window and is actively absorbed from the upper part of the small intestine. The large fluctuations in L-Dopa plasma concentration cause severe side effects. Hence, there is a PK rationale to elevate the extent of absorption while minimizing the maximum plasma concentration (C_{max}) obtained, following oral administration of a sustained release (SR) formulation of L-Dopa. A recently developed unfolding GRDF formulation of L-Dopa showed, in a Beagle dogs model, a remarkable extension in the length of the absorption phase in comparison to non-GRDF, which led to flatter plasma.

These results are important in the development of a GRDF to achieve a delicate interplay in PK factors, prolonged absorption, and sustained blood levels for a compound that has a narrow absorption window owing to active transport and a steep pharmacodynamic profile and is suspected to first-pass metabolism. Based on these results, a new expandable GRDF of L-dopa, with different rigid polymeric matrices, was evaluated in healthy volunteers compared to SR formulation.

Although the tested GRDF formulations showed extended GRT (up to 8 hr), the areas under the plasma concentration vs. time plot were very similar owing to some lag time in drug release observed, following the administration of the GRDF, which may be corrected, according to the author's suggestions, by incorporating an immediate release fraction of the drug into the device. The data clarifies that the GRDF enhances the absorption phase of L-Dopa.

Riboflavin is another narrow absorption window compound that lacks adverse effects and does not affect the gastric motility. It is often used as a model drug to assess the PK aspects of newly developed CR-GRDF in animal and human subjects. When comparing the plasma concentrations of riboflavin following its administration as a CR-GRDF, oral solution or a CR formulation it can be clearly observed the significant increase of the duration of plasma levels obtained by the GRDF.

Pharmacodynamic Aspects of GRDF

For most of the drugs, a better delivery system would significantly minimize the fluctuations in blood levels and consequently improve the therapeutic benefit of the drug as well as reduce its concentration-dependent adverse effect. This feature is of special importance for drugs with relatively narrow therapeutic index and narrow absorption window (e.g. L-Dopa). While the continuous and sustained mode of administration attained by CR-DFs is mostly attributed to the PK advantages, there are certain pharmacodynamic aspects that have to be considered.

Selectivity of receptor activation

The effect of drugs that activate different types of receptors at different concentrations can be best controlled with minimization of fluctuations and attaining flatter drug plasma levels.

Minimized rebound activity

When a given drug intervenes with natural physiological processes, it is more likely to provoke a rebound effect. This can be successfully avoided by its slow input into the blood circulation, which will minimize the counter activity and increase the drug efficacy. This has been demonstrated for furosemide. Furosemide is a widely used loop diuretic indicated for the treatment of different pathological conditions such as congestive heart failure, hepatic cirrhosis, and chronic renal failure. It has a narrow absorption window and mainly absorbed from the stomach and the upper part of the small intestine. Following administration of furosemide, the natriuretic effect rapidly disperses and is concealed before the next administration. This problematic aspect in furosemide therapy is mostly attributed to the natural homeostatic compensatory mechanisms. Lately, it has been demonstrated that the diuretic and natriuretic effects of furosemide can be significantly improved, following a continuous input (intravenous infusion) compared to immediate release DFs. Beside the narrow absorption window, this pharmacodynamic feature of the drug provides another rationale for the development of a GRDF for furosemide.

When furosemide was incorporated in a GRDF by Klausner et al., the device was delayed in the stomach up to 5 hr as detected by X-ray, and its drug delivery and absorption profile were shown to be slow and extended as described in the urinary excretion rate vs. time plot. This slow and extended input of furosemide resulted in improved and extended diuretic effect as described in the diuresis vs. time plot.

Enhancing beta-lactam activity

Some drugs, such as beta-lactam antibiotics, have a nonconcentration-dependent pharmacodynamics, and their clinical response is not associated with peak concentration, but, rather, with the duration of time over a critical therapeutic concentration. SR formulations of these drugs could provide prolonged time of plasma levels over the critical concentration and enhance their efficacy.

Minimized adverse activity in the colon

As beta-lactam antibiotics have a narrow absorption window lying in the upper part of the small intestine, a GRDF can be more beneficial as it can minimize the appearance of these compounds in the colon and thus prevent any undesirable activities in the colon including the development of microorganism's resistance. which is an important pharmacodynamic aspect.

Pharmacodynamic rationale for the development of metformin GRDF

Metformin is mainly absorbed in the upper part of the GI tract with high tendency to adsorb to the intestinal epithelium owing to its ionized nature at physiological pH, and thus its absorption patterns are affected (mainly paracellular), and it causes remarkable GI side effect. This fact, together with the finding that metformin active sites are mainly found in the GI tract and the liver, makes metformin a good candidate for GRDF. The blood concentrations of metformin following administration of metformin in different DFs and the glucose-lowering effect of each formulation is described above. The figure describes two modes of rapid administration, oral solution (PO bolus) or fast-releasing formulation (CR-tablets I) in comparison to a CR GRDF (CR-tablets II) and equivalent input by duodenal infusion.

Although initially there seemed to be both a PK and a PD rationale to develop metformin GRDF, when such formulations were evaluated in a rat model, there were no significant differences in the pharmacodynamic effect regardless of the input rate of the drug. This interesting finding is contributed, most probably, to the affinity of the positively charged drug to the GI wall, thus yielding a slow rate of drug absorption, even following the administration of drug to the upper GI region, and also to "first-pass PD effect" of metformin. The development of GRDFs can be advantageous for the administration of some important drugs and significantly improves their therapeutic outcome. Gastroretentivity of a DF can be achieved by the development of devices that can significantly expand their volume by unfolding or swelling, adhere to intestinal mucosa, or have the suitable density to sink or float over the gastric fluids. Before the incorporation of a certain drug into GRDF, some important criteria should be taken into consideration to assess the possible benefits that this mode of administration will contribute to the therapeutic outcome. The in vivo gastroretentivity reported for different types of GRDF has to be closely evaluated to distinguish between the cases where the retentivity is contributed by the GRDF itself or by extended GRT owing to other factors, mainly high-calorie meal.

14

DOSAGE FORMS

The administration of medications to pediatric patients is in many ways difficult because health care providers and parents are faced with many challenges not experienced, or experienced to a lesser degree, than when medications are prescribed for and taken by adults. First, less information is available about the use of most medications for pediatric patients. In fact only about 20% of drugs marketed in the United States have labeling for pediatric use. Milap Nahata, in a 1999 article on pediatric drug formulations, stated that "only five of the 80 drugs most commonly used in newborns, and infants are approved for pediatric use." Second, many drugs that are used for some pediatric patients are not in appropriate dosage forms for use by children. This includes even some medications approved for use in pediatric patients. These issues have resulted in many questions that need to be answered about drug administration to pediatric patients. For example, is the drug approved for use in pediatric patients and in what age groups? If not approved, is there scientific information that enables us to determine whether the drug is safe and effective for pediatric patients of various ages? If the drug is available commercially for pediatric use, what dose should be administered and how frequently? What route should be used for administration, and what dosage form selected? If the drug is not available in an appropriate dosage form for childhood use, can it be prepared extemporaneously? Is there stability studies, palatability tests, clinical data in children, etc. that pertain to the extemporaneous formulation? How should the drug be monitored for effectiveness as well as for adverse effects? Information determined in adult medication studies may not be applicable to pediatric patients because of pharmacokinetic and pharmacodynamic differences as well as differences in disease states for which a particular drug might be used. Many questions about the use of particular drugs in various age groups of pediatric patients can only be answered through well-designed, randomized controlled studies in pediatric patients who need certain medications for particular health problems.

In 1997, the Food and Drug Administration (FDA) proposed new regulations for how pharmaceutical manufacturers would access safety and efficacy of certain new drugs that could have pediatric indications. Thereafter, the FDA and the American Association of Pharmaceutical Scientists (AAPS) held a conference with academicians, pharmaceutical industry representatives, and U.S. Pharmacopeia (USP) representatives to discuss these proposed FDA regulations.

The FDA Modernization Act (FDAMA) of 1997 contains within it financial incentives for the development and marketing of drugs that could be used for pediatric patients. Some of these incentives include an extension of 6 months on market exclusivity and waiving fees for supplemental applications needed for receiving the approval of drugs for pediatric use that are already approved for adult use. In addition, the FDA published a list of drugs approved in adults for which additional pediatric data may produce health benefits for pediatric patients. For drugs on this list, FDA may ask a pharmaceutical manufacturer why it has not sought approval of a particular drug for pediatric use. So far there has not been much advancement in this area. This may be due to the wait for final approval of FDAMA.

Various medical and pharmacy organizations have worked hard throughout the years in their efforts to better educate children, parents, educators, and health care providers about the medications and their appropriate use. Indeed, individuals who help care for children may not be adequately trained to educate children about medications that they need to use. Therefore in June 2000, the USP started the development of three target initiatives: principles for educating children about their medications, guidelines for developing and evaluating information for children, and developing specific curricular information in a modular format. The USP position about educating children about medications may be found on their website. The following information pieces have been developed by the USP:

1. Guide to Developing and Evaluating Medicine Education Programs and Materials for Children and Adolescents (joint publication of the American Health Association and USP)
2. A Kid's Guide to Asking Questions about Medicines
3. Teaching Kids about Medicines
4. Talking to Children about Their Medicines (pamphlet developed jointly by Pfizer and USP to be disseminated to pediatricians and children's families)
5. An Annotated Bibliography of Research and Programs Relating to Children and Medications

The USP has started working with the National Center for Health Education in New York to develop educational materials that can help school systems nationwide to know more about medications that students may need to take. The USP also adopted the following resolution to address the work that needs to be done in the area of health education: "Facilitate and contribute to the development of a rational school medicines policy, including guidelines for student, faculty, and staff medicine education, for acquisition, transport, storage, administration, use, and disposal of medicines; for protection of privacy; and for record-keeping in primary and secondary schools. Initiatives should be undertaken in collaboration with appropriate partners."

The USP has been working with the National Institute of Child Health and Human Development (NICHD) to develop a list of drugs for which more pediatric information is needed to insure proper use in children. The USP is also evaluating similarities and differences among neonates, children, and adults that may affect medication dosing and which might help in the appropriate labeling of medicines for pediatric use. The USP is reviewing the literature and developing tables for drugs, using evidence-based information.

This overview of pediatric dosing and dosage forms covers issues that peditric health care providers face daily, such as age-related drug pharmacokinetic and pharmacodynamic changes that occur secondarily to physiologic changes in maturing neonates, infants, children, and adolescents that can affect drug absorption from various routes of administration as well as drug distribution, metabolism, and elimination. To be more knowledgeable about pharmacokinetic changes, therapeutic drug monitoring (TDM) must be undertaken for drugs with narrow therapeutic indexes and for those for which pharmacodynamic data (i.e., pharmacologic response that correlates to the drug concentration at the receptor site) correlates with pharmacokinetic information. Also addressed will be drug administration by various routes including intravenous (i.v.), oral (p.o.), intramuscular (i.m.), subcutaneous (s.c.), percutaneous, rectal, otic, nasal, ophthalmic, and inhalation. Another issue discussed is product selection for pediatric patients.

To better understand changes in drug disposition, the pediatric population needs to be categorized into various groups because children vary markedly in their absorption, distribution, metabolism, and elimination of medications. This occurs because neonates, infants, children, adolescents, and adults have different body compositions (i.e., as to their percentages of body water and fat) and have their body organs in different stages of development.

PEDIATRIC PHARMACOKINETICS AND PHARMACODYNAMICS

Effect of Developmental Physiologic Changes on Pharmacokinetics and Pharmacodynamics of Drugs

Rational pediatric pharmacotherapy is primarily based on the knowledge about a particular drug, including its pharmacokinetics and pharmacodynamics, that may be modified by physiologic maturation of the child from birth through adolescence. Physiologic changes that occur can affect drug absorption, distribution, metabolism, and elimination. The most dramatic changes occur during the neonatal period.

Oral Absorption

Drug absorption from the gastrointestinal (GI) tract is dependent on patient factors, physicochemical properties of the orally administered drug, and the drug formulation. Patient factors that affect GI absorption include absorptive surface area, maturation of the mucosal membrane, gastric and duodenal pH, gastric emptying time, GI motility, enzyme activity, bacterial colonization of the GI tract, and dietary intake, including the specific gastric content status at the time when a medication is ingested. Patient factors are influenced by rapid maturational changes that occur throughout early childhood, but which occur primarily during the first few months of life.

Most drugs are absorbed across the GI tract by passive diffusion, but a variety of drug physicochemical factors influence the extent of absorption. These factors include molecular weight, lipid solubility, ionization as well as disintegration and dissolution rates. In addition, drug absorption may be dependent on the dosage form selected (e.g., a liquid, a tablet that may need to be crushed, or a sustained-release product), and the particular brand selected. For timed- release preparations, the release characteristics must also be taken into consideration.

Gastric pH

When examining patient-specific factors such as gastric pH, which affect oral absorption, it should be noted that infants born vaginally who are at least 32-weeks gestation, usually have gastric pHs between 6 and 8 at birth. Gastric pH then falls rapidly within a few hours after delivery to a pH of less than 3. The initial gastric pH is alkaline compared to that of adults and results from the presence of amniotic fluid in the infant's stomach. Thereafter, gastric pH remains acidic until approximately day 10, then a nadir in acid production occurs between days 10 and 30 of life. Then gastric acid production begins to increase, but gastric pH and maximal gastric output may not mirror that of adults on a per kilogram basis until after the neonatal period.

Gastric emptying and gastrointestinal motility

Gastric emptying time in neonates, especially those less than 24 h of age, may be variable. It may not reach adult levels until 6–8 months of age and may be associated with diet. Gastrointestinal transit time may be prolonged and peristaltic activity unpredictable in young infants; both appear affected by the feeding. Lebenthal and colleagues noted that breast-fed infants, older than 45 days of age, had gastric transit times longer than 10h while formula-fed infants had transit times less than 10 h. It should also be noted that young infants have a propensity to reflux their gastric contents because of GI immaturity. All these factors affect the extent to which a drug may be absorbed.

Enzyme activity and microflora in the gastrointestinal tract

Pancreatic enzyme activity may be low at birth, but enzymes such as amylase, lipase, and trypsin develop to adult levels within the first year of life. Premature infants appear to have lower amylase levels than do full-term infants. Low concentrations of pancreatic enzymes may be the reason why newborns have a decreased ability to cleave prodrug esters such as chloramphenicol palmitate. Lipid-soluble drugs may not be well absorbed by neonates because of low lipase concentrations and bile acid pool. More information is needed about the microflora of the GI tract and its effect on drug absorption. In addition, the effects of various diets and antibiotic use can alter the microflora of the GI tract.

Absorptive surface area

The surface area of the small intestine in young infants is proportionately greater than in adults. This physiologic difference may allow for increased drug absorption from the GI tract.

Intramuscular Absorption

When a child is unable to take a medication orally or the drug is unavailable for oral use, there may be a need to administer a drug parenterally by either the i.v. or i.m. route. Of these, the latter may be less desirable because of pain, irritation, and decreased drug delivery as compared to i.v. administration. Drug absorption after i.m. administration depends on various physicochemical and patient factors. Physicochemical factors to be considered include lipid or water solubility, drug concentration, and surface area. When addressing drug solubility, it should be noted that lipophilic drugs readily diffuse through the capillary walls of endothelial cells whereas water-soluble drugs diffuse at fairly rapid rates from interstitial fluid to plasma via pores in capillary membranes. A lipid-soluble drug may be more rapidly absorbed i.m., but a water-soluble drug may be more desirable because the drug must be stable in an aqueous solution until administered. After administration, the drug must then be water soluble at physiologic pH until absorption occurs.

Drug absorption may be dependent on concentration, but available data do not allow us to determine whether an increased or decreased drug concentration results in better absorption. An increase in the osmolality of a pharmaceutical preparation secondary to the addition of another substance such as an excipient may decrease or slow down i.m. adsorption. Absorption occurs more rapidly when diffusion involves a large area of muscle or the drug spreads over a large muscle mass. The massaging of an injection site after i.m. administration increases the rate of absorption.

A physiologic determination of i.m. drug absorption is dependent on the adequacy of blood flow to muscle groups used for drug administration. Absorption rates differ at injection sites because blood flow varies among different muscle groups. For example, the absorption of a drug-administered i.m. in the deltoid muscle is faster than from the vastus lateralis that, in turn, is more rapid than from the gluteus. This occurs because blood flow to the deltoid muscle is 7% higher than to vastus lateralis and 17% higher than to gluteal muscle groups. Physiologic conditions that reduce blood flow to a muscle group may adversely alter the rate and/or extent of a drug- administered i.m. Decreased perfusion or hemostatic decompensation, frequently observed in ill neonates and young infants, may reduce i.m. drug absorption. Drug absorption may be adversely affected in neonates who receive a skeletal muscle-paralyzing agent such as pancuronium because of decreased muscle contraction. A small muscle mass in neonates and young infants may also reduce the ability of a drug to be adequately absorbed.

The injection technique used may alter i.m. absorption. This was noted when needles of different lengths were used. The use of a longer needle (38 vs. 31 mm, $1^1/_2$ vs. $1^1/_4$ in.) for i.m. administration in adult patients resulted in higher diazepam serum concentrations. This probably occurred because the drug administered with the shorter needle was actually administered s.c. rather than i.m.

Some drugs are absorbed more slowly after i.m. than oral administration; examples include diazepam, digoxin, and phenytoin. This probably occurs because these drugs require a mixture of alcohol, propylene glycol, and water for solubility, and they are insoluble in the muscle after i.m. administration. Complications associated with i.m. administration include nerve injury, muscle contracture, and abscess formation. Less common problems include intramuscular hemorrhage, cellulitis, skin pigmentation, tissue necrosis, muscle atrophy, gangrene, and cyst or scar formation. In addition, injury may occur from broken needles and inadvertent injection into a joint or vein.

Subcutaneous Absorption

The s.c. route is used for the administration of drugs such as insulin that require slow absorption. Injection technique and patient factors, such as fluid status and physical build, are important. Exercise, elevation or warming of the injection site, or inadvertently administrating a drug i.m. rather than s.c. can increase absorption and be dangerous in some situations, such as hypoglycemia occurring in a diabetic patient from excessive insulin absorption. Adverse effects that can occur secondarily to s.c. administration include tissue ischemia, sterile and non-sterile abscesses, lipodystrophy, cysts, and granulomatous formation.

Intraosseous Drug Absorption

If an i.v. line cannot be placed, the intraosseous drug administration route can be used for pediatric patients during, for example, cardiopulmonary resuscitation (CPR) because drug delivery by this route is similar to that for i.v. administration. If drug or fluid deliver by this route is sluggish, a saline flush can be used to clear the needle. Intraosseous administration is used to deliver medications such as epinephrine, atropine, sodium bicarbonate, dopamine, diazepam, isoproterenol, phenytoin, phenobarbital, dexamethasone, and various antibiotics.

Percutaneous or Transdermal Absorption

The percutaneous (transdermal or topical) route for systemic drug delivery is used infrequently for pediatric patients. Medications are typically applied to the skin for their local effect. In the future, this route may be used more frequently for systemic effects as more transdermal systems are developed for drug delivery. The *percutaneous absorption* or the transdermal delivery of a drug occurs in the following manner. Initially a topically applied drug is absorbed into the stratum corneum and diffuses through that layer of skin into the epidermis and then into the dermis where drug molecules reach capillaries and enter the circulatory system. Diffusion through the stratum corneum is the rate-determining step unless skin perfusion is decreased. If the latter case, diffusion is controlled by the transfer of drug molecules into capillaries rather than by the diffusion process previously explained.

Percutaneous or transdermal absorption is affected by

1. Patient age
2. Application site
3. State of hydration of the stratum corneum
4. Thickness and intactness of the stratum corneum
5. Physical characteristics of the solute
6. Physical characteristics of the vehicle or solvent

Drug diffusion may be explained by Eq. (1):

$$J = \frac{K_m \times D_m \times C_s}{l} \qquad \ldots(1)$$

where J is flux, K_m is the partition coefficient, D_m is the diffusion constant under specific conditions such as temperature and hydration, C_s is the concentration gradient, and l is the length or thickness of stratum corneum.

Lipid-soluble drugs are better absorbed into the stratum corneum than are water-soluble drugs, but the latter do not easily traverse the stratum corneum. Thus, lipid-soluble drugs are more likely to be stored in the stratum corneum, whereas water-soluble drugs are more likely to diffuse across the stratum corneum to the epidermis and dermis.

Patient age

Drug absorption transdermally is not appreciably different in various age groups of patients except for neonates less than 32-week gestation at birth. Drug absorption is increased in premature neonates, because the stratum corneum is not completely formed at birth. An example of increased drug absorption occurred in two premature neonates who were repeatedly washed with 3% hexachlorophene and developed encephalopathy secondary to drug absorption. The absorption of the corticosteroid betamethasone valerate after topical application in children resulted in hypothalamus- pituitary-adrenal axis suppression. Children may have increased drug absorption from the percutaneous application of drugs not because of higher absorption rate but because of a greater topical application or a larger dose per kilogram. Examples of deaths in children from percutaneous drug absorption include those caused by salicylic acid and phenol absorption. Toxicity has also been noted with the topical application of iodine and alcohol-containing products.

Application site

The ability of a drug to be absorbed transdermally depends on the thickness of the stratum corneum. For example, absorption occurs more readily through abdominal skin than through skin on the plantar surface of the foot. Topical absorption may be enhanced from a particular site by the application of an occlusive dressing.

Status of the stratum corneum

Percutaneous absorption of a drug is enhanced by the hydration of the stratum corneum. Such hydration affects the absorption of hydrophilic drugs more than lipophilic drugs. Drugs will penetrate damaged skin more than intact skin. Skin damaged because of dryness will allow for increased drug penetration through areas where the skin is cracked or broken.

Solute

The penetration of the solute (or drug) depends on its polarity and on the polarity of the delivery vehicle.

Vehicle or solvent

Drug-delivery vehicles typically used for topical application include lotions, ointments, creams, emulsions, and gels. Substances such as emulsifiers may be added to the drug and vehicle to improve the texture of an emulsion, a stabilizer to preserve drug stability, the vehicle, or both, a thickening agent to increase viscosity, or a humectant to draw moisture into the skin. It is particularly important to consider the vehicle and other additives when selecting a topical drug preparation for a neonate, especially when premature, because of the greater possibility of absorption of not only the drug but also other product ingredients. Toxic reactions have occurred in neonates from ingredients considered "inactive."

Transdermal Drug-Delivery Systems

Drugs chosen for delivery via a transdermal drug-delivery system must adequately penetrate the skin in such a way that the system determines the delivery rate that should be fairly constant. In addition, the drug must not irritate or sensitize the skin. It is hoped that in the future more drugs will be developed for transdermal delivery. This could become an alternative route for drug delivery to children who have difficulty with oral administration.

Endotracheal Absorption

The endotracheal (ET) route has been used to administer medications during CPR when other routes, such as the i.v. route, are unavailable. It provides rapid access as well as rapid drug absorption and distribution. Some studies have shown that the time to reach peak absorption is similar to that for the i.v. route, but serum concentrations achieved were 10–33% of that achieved with i.v. administration, resulting in a weaker response. A depot effect has also been demonstrated for drugs such as epinephrine. Work needs to be done to determine the optimal dose by this route, drug-delivery vehicle, and the most effective delivery technique.

Rectal Absorption

The rectal route is used for local and systemic therapy for the following reasons:

1. Nausea or vomiting
2. Rejection of oral education because of its taste, texture, etc
3. Upper GI disease that might affect absorption
4. Medication absorption affected by food or gastric emptying
5. Medication is readily decomposed in gastric fluid but may be stable in rectal fluid
6. First-pass effect of high-clearance drug may be partially avoided

Absorption from the rectum depends on various physiological factors such as surface area, blood supply, pH, fluid volume, and possible metabolism by microorganisms in the rectum. The rectum is perfused by the inferior and middle rectal arteries, whereas the superior, the middle, and the inferior rectal veins drain the rectum. The latter two are directly connected to the systemic circulation; the superior rectal vein drains into the portal system. Drugs absorbed from the lower rectum are carried directly into the systemic circulation, whereas drugs absorbed from the upper rectum are subjected to hepatic first-pass effect. Therefore, a high-clearance drug should be more bioavailable after rectal than oral administration. The volume of fluid in the rectum, the pH of that fluid, and the presence of stool in the rectal vault may affect drug absorption. Because the fluid volume is usually low compared to that in other areas of the GI tract, a drug may not be completely soluble. In addition, a variety of organisms colonize the rectum, and it is debated whether these organisms are involved in drug metabolism. Absorption is also influenced by the dosage form used. For example, drugs are rapidly absorbed rectally from aqueous or alcoholic solutions, whereas absorption from a suppository depends on its base, the presence of a surfactant, particle size of the active ingredient(s), and drug concentration. The following problems may be associated with the rectal route for drug administration.

1. Decreased absorption secondary to defecation of the rectally administered pharmaceutical product
2. Less absorption rectally than orally because the absorbing surface area of the rectum is smaller
3. Dissolution problems for rectally administered medications because of lower fluid volume in the rectum than in the stomach, duodenum, etc
4. Microorganisms in rectum may cause degradation of some medications
5. Patient or parent acceptance.

Distribution

A drug is distributed by moving from a patient's systemic circulation to various compartments, tissues, and cells. Distribution depends on patient factors, drug physiochemical properties, and the route of drug administration. Patient factors that influence drug distribution or the volume of drug distribution (V_d) include body composition, perfusion, protein- and tissue-binding characteristics, and permeability. Many of these characteristics are age dependent. Drug physiochemical properties that may influence distribution include molecular weight, pK_a, and partition coefficient.

Differences in body composition

Age-related changes in body composition can alter the V_d of a drug. At birth, 85% of the weight of a premature infant may be water, compared to approximately 75% as total body water (TBW) in a full-term infant. Neonates have the highest percentage of extracellular water (65% of TBW in premature infants as compared to 35–44% in full-term neonates and 20% in adults). The intracellular water (ICW) is more stable throughout life (i.e., 25% in premature neonates, 33% in full-term neonates, and 40% in adults). An infant's percentage of TBW approaches that of an adult male by 1 year of age (60% TBW); it reaches the same about the time of puberty or 12 years of age. Women have a lower percentage of TBW (50%) than men do because they have a higher concentration of body fat. Thus, neonates, because of their high TBW, have a higher V_d for water-soluble drugs such as aminoglycosides than older children or adults. For example, the V_d for an aminoglycoside such as gentamicin approximates that of extracellular cellular fluid volume, 0.5–1.2 L/ kg for a neonate, but only 0.2–0.3 L/kg for an older child or an adult.

Adipose tissue increases from as little as 0.5% in a premature infant to approximately 16% of body weight for a full-term infant. Boys experiene a spurt in body fat between the ages of 5 and 10 years, and then a gradual decrease in fat content until about 17 years of age; girls usually have a rapid increase in adipose tissue at puberty. Thus, one would expect neonates and young infants to have a decreased V_d for lipid-soluble drugs. This has been noted for diazepam in neonates who have exhibited an apparent V_d of 1.4–1.8 L/kg compared to 2.2–2.6L/kg in adults.

Protein binding

Neonates have lower concentrations of various plasma proteins (e.g., albumin concentrations about 80% of those in adults) for drug binding, but the albumin present may also have a lower affinity for binding drugs than noted for adults who are receiving the same medications. This lower affinity for binding drugs may result in a competition for various albumin-binding sites with substances such as bilirubin. Plasma protein binding noted in adults is usually achieved in children by the age of 1 year.

In neonates drugs such as various penicillins, phenobarbital, phenytoin, and theophylline have lower protein-binding affinity than in adults. This may increase the concentration of free or pharmacological active drug in neonates, and may also change the apparent volume of distribution. Thus, neonates may require different doses on a mg/kg basis compared to that for adults for these drugs to achieve appropriate therapeutic serum concentrations.

In addition to binding to plasma proteins in the neonate, some drugs such as sulfonamides may displace plasma bilirubin from binding sites. This may increase an infant's risk for developing kernicterus. The significance of drugs displacing bilirubin is controversial because bilirubin may have a greater affinity for albumin than drugs have.

Tissue binding

The binding of drugs to various body tissues appears to vary with age; for example, digoxin binding to erythrocytes is higher in neonates than in adults. This may be due to the increased number of binding sties on neonatal erythrocytes.

Drug penetration into the central nervous system

A drug is more likely to cross into the central nervous system (CNS) of a neonate rather than an older child or an adult. This most likely occurs because its CNS is less mature and the blood–brain barrier is less formed. This is an important consideration when antimicrobial therapy is needed for the treatment of bacterial meningitis or anticonvulsant for seizures.

Metabolism

Although drug metabolism can occur in various body organs including the lungs, GI tract, liver, and kidneys as well as in the blood, the liver is the primary organ for metabolism. Most drugs are metabolized from lipid-soluble parent compounds to more polar, less lipophilic metabolites that are more readily eliminated renally.

Hepatic metabolism

Most drug metabolism occurs in the liver by phase I or phase II metabolic processes. Phase I reactions primarily biotransform an active drug to a more water-soluble compound that typically is inactive or has less activity than the parent compound. Oxidation, reduction, hydralysis, and hydroxylation are examples of phase I reactions Oxidation is primarily catalyzed by the cytochrome (CYP) P450 system that has a multitude of isozymes (at least 13 primary enzymes) with a multitude of isozymes of specific gene families. It appears that isozymes CYP450 1A2, 2D6, 2C19, and 3A3/4 are involved in drug metabolism in humans. Oxidizing enzyme systems appear to mature after birth so that by the age of 6 months, activity is similar to or even exceeds adult levels.

Phase II reactions (glucuronidation, sulfation, acetylation, and glutathione conjugation) usually involve the conjugation of active drugs with endogenous molecules to form metabolites that are more water soluble; glucuronidation is the most thoroughly studied reaction. It is postulated that maternal glucocorticoids inhibit the development of glucuronyltransferase, the enzyme involved in glucuronidation in utero. After birth this metabolic system matures rapidly and reaches adult levels by the age of 2 years.

Sulfate conjugation appears to be fully developed immediately prior to or at the time of birth. Infants and young children readily sulfate acetaminophen; in adults the major metabolic route is glucuronidation. Little is known about acetylation in neonates or infants. It is believed that neonates have an extremely low capacity for acetylation at birth, but this pathway matures at approximately 20 days of age.

Theophylline is an example of a drug that is readily metabolized in neonates by *N*-methylation to caffeine (process not relevant clinically in older infants, children, and adults). It is also a compound that has pharmacologic activity versus apnea (like theophylline), but which may have toxicity when it is not readily metabolized by the liver, and its elimination is slowed by immature kidneys.

Neonates require close monitoring if their mothers received enzyme inducers such as phenytoin, phenobarbital, carbamazepine, or rifampin during pregnancy or if they need one of these drugs themselves. Examples of drugs that inhibit the metabolism of other medications include cimetidine, erythromycin, and ketoconazole.

Renal Elimination

The kidneys are the major route for drug elimination, especially for water-soluble compounds or the metabolites of lipid-soluble drugs. Renal drug elimination is dependent on renal blood flow, glomerular filtration, and tubular secretion and reabsorption. These functions appear to mature at different rates in the neonate and infant. Full-term infants achieve renal blood flow similar to that of adults by the age of 5–12 months; glomerular filtration approaches adult values by the age of 3–5 months. Premature neonates exhibit lower rates for glomerular filtration at birth than do full-term neonates, and more time is required of them postnatally to develop filtration ability. This is probably due to their lack of as many functional nephrons at birth. Tubular function is less mature in the neonate at birth than is glomerular filtration, and it matures at a slower rate. Tubular function begins to approach adult values by 7 months of age. Renal function is equal to that of adults by 1 year of age.

Aminoglycosides (e.g., gentamicin, tobramycin, amikacin) and digoxin are drugs whose eliminations are affected by renal maturation. The renal elimination of aminoglycosides in neonates and young infants parallels the maturation of glomerular function and correlates with creatinine clearance. The renal elimination of digoxin parallels kidney maturation. Dosage adjustment for this drug is necessary as renal function matures in neonates and young infants. In addition, older infants and children require higher mg/kg doses of digoxin than do adults to achieve the same serum concentrations. This may be due to decreased digoxin absorption or increased renal elimination.

Therapeutic Drug Monitoring

Therapeutic drug monitoring should encompass the entire drug-use process including drug selection, product selection, administration route, patient age, appropriate dosing on a mg/kg or mg/m^2 basis, and monitoring serum concentrations when appropriate and observing the patient for optimal drug effect(s) and possible adverse drug events.

Important Differences in Pediatric Serum Drug Concentrations

For many drugs, especially for those with narrow therapeutic indexes, serum concentration ranges have been determined that correlate to minimum and maximum therapeutic effects as well as to the development of toxicity. Therapeutic serum concentration ranges for various drugs have been developed for adults, and these data have been applied to pediatric patients including neonates. Such data may be appropriate to monitor drug therapy in children, but possibly not in children of all ages or possibly not in children at all. For example, Painter et al. noted that neonates need higher serum phenobarbital concentrations than do older children and adults to terminate seizures. Gilman et al. observed that higher phenobarbital loading doses were needed to achieve serum concentrations in neonates that would reduce the occurrence of seizures. Thus, there may be a need for different serum concentration ranges for various drugs needed by different age groups of patients for a similar pharmacodynamic or therapeutic outcome.

Free serum concentrations, rather than total concentrations, of some drugs such as phenytoin may need to be monitored in some patients, including neonates, who have low serum albumin. Gilman has advocated the possibility of using individualized dosing and serum concentration range for pediatric patients because children, especially neonates, have rapidly maturing functions of various organs and changes in albumin for drug binding.

Serum concentration monitoring of various drugs administered to pediatric patients may appropriately give information about the drug but not its metabolites. This may be a problem when children metabolize specific drugs differently than adults with resulting differences in metabolite concentrations or the presence of different metabolites. This has been noted when premature infants have been administered theophylline for central apnea. A major metabolite of theophylline in neonates is caffeine, although only small concentrations of this metabolite are noted in older children and adults. Caffeine is effective in treating apnea, and thus may add to the effectiveness of theophylline. This may help explain why lower theophylline serum concentrations may be needed for apnea rather than asthma. In addition, the presence of the 4-en metabolite of valproic acid noted in the serum of infants and young children, but not adults, receiving this medication for seizures may be responsible for the hepatoxicity of this drug in young pediatric patients.

Serum Drug Concentrations

Because of the cost associated with therapeutic drug monitoring, serum drug concentrations must be drawn appropriately to provide useful information. Drugs typically followed pharmacokinetically are those with narrow therapeutic indexes for which there is an association between pharmacokinetic and pharmacodynamic data or toxicity. For many drugs, especially for those administered orally, the determination of trough concentrations (serum concentrations obtained prior to administration) may be most appropriate.

This eliminates differences in absorption rates that could influence peak concentrations (e.g., orally administered phenobarbital, phenytoin, carbamazepine, or valproic acid). Trough concentrations may be important for drugs such as digoxin that take time to distribute to tissue receptors in such a way that serum concentrations reflect pharmacodynamic effects. Peak concentrations are best used for determining toxicity and therapeutic effects of drugs with short half-lives.

Technical Factors

Sample size and timing of blood drawing forserum concentration determination

Because of the small blood volume and the small size of veins, it is technically difficult to draw blood from neonates, infants, and young children for therapeutic drug monitoring, and it is therefore important to determine the best drawing schedule. For example, when are peak and trough data needed compared to trough data only? For anticonvulsants administered orally or i.v., trough concentrations are needed, whereas for amino-glycosides it may be important to obtain both peaks and troughs.

Dosing Regimens

Drugs for pediatric patients should be dosed on a mg/kg or a mg/m^2 basis using information available for the patient's age group. In addition, the patient s renal and hepatic functions must be considered. The route for administration must be determined based on the severity of the illness, the availability of the medication for a particular route of administration, and whether the patient is able to take a medication orally.

The Bibliography succeeding the References at the end of this chapter contains a list of handbooks and other references that are useful sources of dosing information for neonatal and/or pediatric pediatrics. In addition, drug information centers in pediatric hospitals or university settings are another excellent resource for pediatric drug information.

Excipients or Additives in Medications

Pharmaceutical products may contain, in addition to the active or therapeutic agent(s), a variety of other ingredients that are termed inactive or inert that are categorized as excipients or additives (flavorings, sweeteners, preservatives, stabilizers, diluents, lubricants, etc.). The words inert or inactive are misnomers for some excipients because some have been shown to cause adverse effects. Neonates and young children are at risk for such adverse effects, because they may not be able to metabolize or eliminate an ingredient in a pharmaceutical product in the same manner as an adult. In addition, patients of various ages have experienced allergic reactions to excipients such as tartrazine dyes.

Benzyl alcohol is a preservative that may be present in multidose vials of bacteriostatic sodium chloride and bacteriostatic water for injection and pharmaceuticals available in multidose vials for parenteral use. An association between the presence of benzyl alcohol in solutions used for flushing intravascular catheters and to reconstitute medications and a gasping syndrome and deaths in neonates was first reported in the early 1980s. The neonates also displayed clinical findings such as an elevated anion gap, metabolic acidosis, CNS depression, seizures, respiratory failure, renal and hepatic failures, cardiovascular collapse, and death. Those at highest risk were premature infants who weighted less than 1250 g at birth. In a study by Benda et al., premature neonates who survived benzyl alcohol administration were compared to neonates born after the use of benzyl alcohol-containing flush solutions was discontinued. They noted that survivors had a higher incidence of cerebral palsy (50%) compared to infants who did not receive benzyl alcohol flushes (2.4%) ($P < 0.001$). In addition, the incidence of cerebral palsy and developmental delay was 53.9 versus 11.9% in the two populations ($P < 0.001$). The cause is probably associated with benzyl alcohol use and the inability of neonates, especially those who are premature, to adequately metabolize benzyl alcohol. The American Academy of Pediatrics, the Centers for Disease Control, and the FDA recommend that the administration of products containing benzyl alcohol be avoided in infants. Preservative-free i.v. flush solutions are recommended.

Initially, it was believed that benzyl alcohol was only toxic in neonates who received doses greater than 99 mg/kg, but it has been suggested that lower doses may be toxic, resulting in kernicterus and intraventricular hemorrhages. Therefore, pharmaceutical preparations and fluids containing benzyl alcohol should be avoided in premature neonates.

Benzoic acid and sodium benzoate are added in low concentrations to various pharmaceutical preparations as bacteriostatic and fungistatic agents. Hypersensitivity reactions to benzoates have occurred when administered to allergic patients, such as those with asthma, those who do not tolerate aspirin, and those with a history of urticaria. Hyperbilirubinemia and systemic effects attributed to benzyl alcohol may occur in premature neonates because benzyl alcohol is metabolized to benzoic acid.

Propylene glycol is found as a solvent in some i.v. multiple vitamin preparations and a variety of pharmaceutical preparations for parenteral administration including phenytoin, digoxin, and diazepam. MacDonald et al. noted that neonates who received MVI-12 (propylene glycol dose of approximately 3 g/day) versus those who received MVI concentrate (propylene glycol dose of approximately 300mg/day) had a significant increase in seizures. In addition, infants in the first group suffered from hyperbilirubinemia and renal failure.

Serum hyperosmolality has been reported in infants who received vitamin preparations, and in burn patients due to the topical absorption of propylene glycol-containing products. In addition, burn patients have experienced metabolic acidosis with a high anion gap, decreased ionized calcium concentrations, acute renal failure, and death from topical propylene glycol absorption. Problems associated with the oral ingestion of propylene glycol-containing products by children include CNS depression, seizures, and cardiac dysrhythmias. Hypotension, cardiac dysrhythmias, respiratory depression, and seizures have occurred after the rapid administration of phenytoin that may be associated with the propylene glycol.

The American Academy of Pediatrics Committee on Drugs recommends that medications intended for pediatric use be ethanol free. If, because of stability or solubility problems with the active ingredients(s), liquid medications need ethanol as an ingredient, but they should not contain more than 5% v/v ethanol. The Academy also recommends that the ingestion of a single dose of an ethanol-containing product by a pediatric patient should not result in blood ethanol concentrations greater than 25 mg/100 mL, the volume of a packaged liquid medication should be of a minimal amount so that its entire ingestion would not result in a lethal dose and safety closures should be on all medicinals containing greater than 5% v/v ethanol. In addition, the Academy suggests that children under 6 years of age who need an ethanol-containing OTC preparation be under medical supervision and that doses of any ethanol-containing product be spaced at intervals to avoid ethanol accumulation.

The Academy of Pediatrics made their recommendations concerning ethanol exposure from medications based on potential acute and chronic ethanol-related problems. Acutely, the coadministration of ethanol may alter drug adsorption or metabolism, and may result in drug interactions (e.g., increased sedation when taken with sedatives). Disulfiram-like reactions have occurred after the ingestion of an alcohol-containing medication or when an ethanol-containing product is used in conjunction with medications such as metronidazole, sulfonamides, chloramphenicol, or cefamandole. The CNS effects (muscle incoordination, a longer reaction time, behavioral changes) are the most commonly reported acute adverse reactions associated with ethanol ingestion. Such reactions have occurred with blood ethanol concentrations in the range of 1–100 mg/100 ml. Lethal ethanol doses in children occur at approximately 3 gm/kg although deaths due to ethanol-induced hypoglycemia have occurred at lower doses or because of interactions with other medications. Chronic ethanol exposure may induce hepatic enzymes, and may thus alter the clearance of drugs such as phenytoin, phenobarbital, and warfarin. Examples of other additives that have been problematic in pediatric patients include lactose, tartrazine dyes and sulfites.

It is therefore important for health care professionals, and especially those who are responsible for selecting and administering medications to premature neonates, to examine pharmaceutical preparations for the presence of inactive ingredients as well as for the active drug. The provision of medications should be based on choosing the safest preparations possible. Various brands of medications should be compared to ensure that products without hazardous excipients. In the hospital setting, pharmacy and therapeutics committees and the pharmacy department play important roles in this process because they compare pharmaceutical preparations for formulary selection. In the outpatient setting, physicians and pharmacists must responsibly select the most appropriate brand of a particular medication. Kumar, Rawlings, and Beaman recommend that labeling for pharmaceutical products should include the names and the amounts of excipients as well as active ingredients to help health care professionals select appropriate drug products for neonates.

Intravenous Administration

Without being properly instructed about methods used for administering i.v. medications to pediatric patients, health care personnel may give a medication incorrectly, resulting in an inappropriate or unexpected therapeutic response. Therefore, it is important that health care personnel (nurses, physicians, pharmacists) understand how medications are administered by this route. The i.v. route is most frequently chosen for medication delivery when a patient's clinical condition requires that a medication be administered by the most expeditious and complete method possible. In addition, some drugs are only available for i.v. administration. Although this route is the most reliable for drug delivery to the systemic circulation, problems can occur that reduce and/or delay medication delivery because of the product selected, dosage volume needed, or frequency of administration, but problems can also be associated with the i.v. delivery system used. The latter occur most frequently when a small medication volume is administered at a slow rate as is often needed for a neonate or young infant.

Disposable IV Equipment, Effects on Drug Delivery

Infusion rates and location of injection sites

The first article to explore problems that can occur with i.v. drug delivery to pediatric patients was published in 1979 by Gould and Roberts. They demonstrated in their study using an in vitro system for drug administration that infusion rates as well as the location of the injection sites in the i.v. infusion system influence the infusion profile of i.v. administered medications. It was reported that at a slow infusion rate of 3 ml/h, a drug takes longer to be infused and that the time for infusion time depends on the site of administration (i.e., the further the drug injection from a patient, the longer to administer 95% of the medication. Thus, it took approximately 400 min to infuse gentamicin at an infusion rate of 3 ml/h via a Y-site in the administration system. However, the same drug administered at a butterfly injection site at the same fluid flow rate reduced the length of time to administer 95% of the drug to less than 20 min. Gould and Roberts also stated that the time needed for drug administration in their i.v. system was longer than what had been expected.

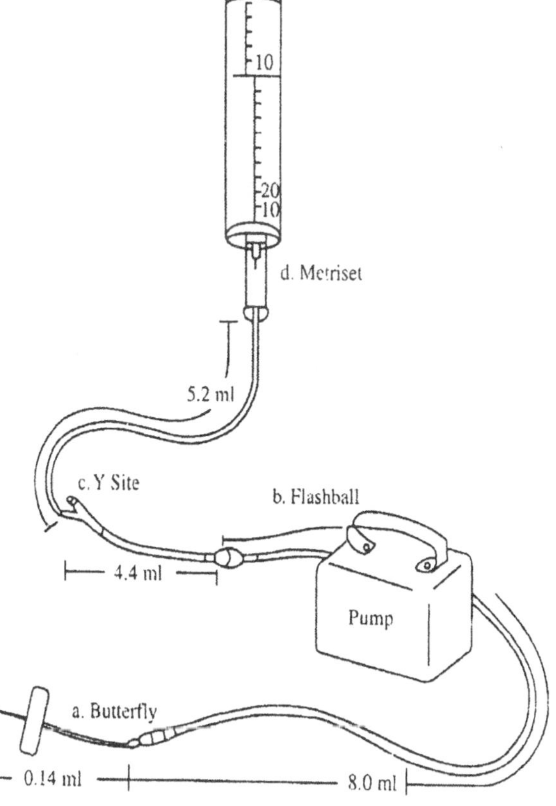

Fig. 14.1. Intravenous administration system.

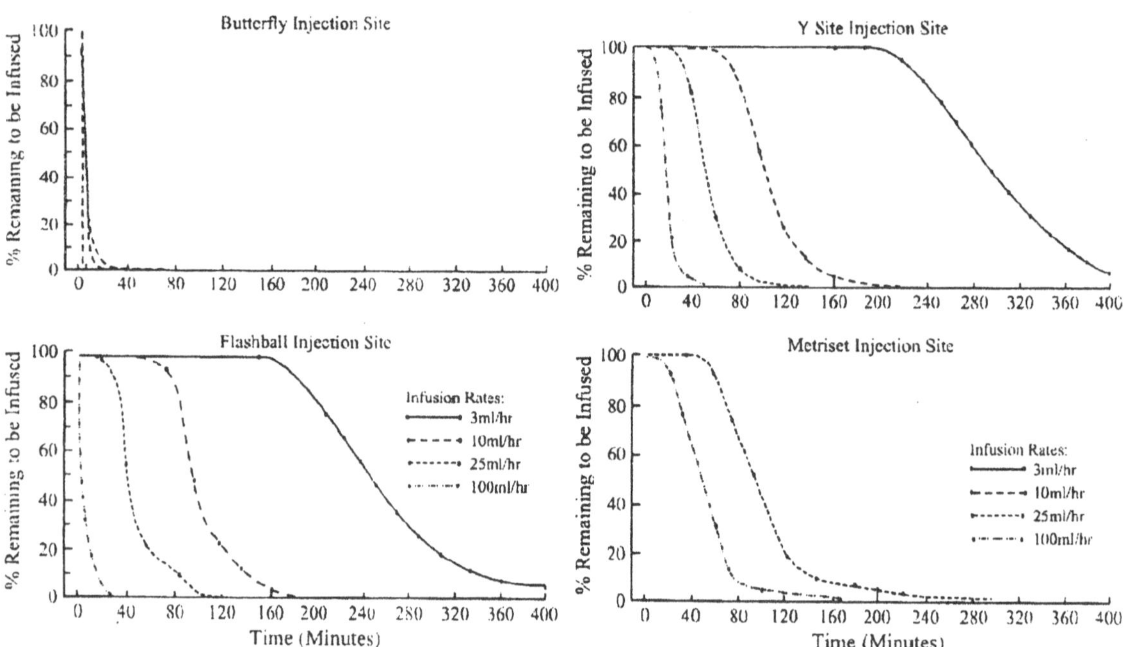

Fig. 14.2. Influence of i.v. flow rate on the infusion profile of gentamicin.

Type of injection site

Leff and Roberts demonstrated that the amount of drug received by a pediatric patient and the drug-delivery rate are influenced by the type of injection site (Y-site, T-type, T-connector, stopcock, etc.) and the volume (dead space) contained in the particular site. For the delivery of small dosage volumes (less than 1 ml) i.v. tubing should have microinjection sites that prevent a drug from being sequestered in the injection site. In addition, the amount of i.v. fluid needed to adequately flush microinjection sites to clear the medication would be less than needed to flush injection sites found on tubing used to administer drugs to adults.

Fluid flow dynamics

Another characteristic of i.v. tubing that affects drug delivery is fluid flow dynamics. It appears that flow in i.v. tubing is best characterized by laminar flow, and the radius of the tubing. Poiseuille's law describes flow in i.v. tubing as

$$q_v = \frac{Pr^4}{4nL} \quad \ldots(2)$$

where q_v is the volumetric flow rate, P is the pressure change in the i.v. tubing, r is the radius of the i.v. tubing, n is the viscosity of the fluid, and L is the length of the i.v. tubing.

Thus, for i.v. delivery to pediatric patients, micro- bore tubing with an intraluminal diameter of <0.06 in. should be used rather than macrobore tubing. The use of microbore tubing allows the use of longer tubing lengths without significantly increasing delivery time.

Filters

A filter, especially one with a large reservoir volume, may prolong and/or reduce drug delivery. This occurs if the drug and its diluent are of different densities and there is a layering out of the drug in the filter. Therefore, a filter with a smaller reservoir volume should be selected.

Drug and Fluid Considerations for Intravenous Drug Administration

Characteristics of the drug and the fluid such as drug volume, osmolality, pH, and density may affect i.v. drug delivery. The frequency and duration of drug administration is also important as is the need for the infusion system to handle multiple drugs. This may lead to drug incompatibilities and problems in medication scheduling.

Osmolality and pH

Osmolality and pH must be considered when preparing a drug solution for i.v. administration to pediatric patients. Problems such as tissue irritation, pain on injection, phlebitis, electrolyte shifts, and even intraventricular hemorrhages in neonates have been associated with the administration of drug solutions with high osmolalities. Drug solutions should have osmolalities similar to serum osmolality, if possible. To control the osmolality, a drug can be diluted with a vehicle selected for i.v. infusion via a syringe infusion system or the i.v. flow rate can be adjusted to achieve a particular drug-vehicle osmolality.

Density

If the density of a drug is significantly different from that of the diluent, the drug may layer out on the filter or in the i.v. tubing. The latter occurs more frequently if macrobore tubing, a low flow rate, the i.v. system, or if the tubing is in a particular position. A density problem can be avoided by using microbore tubing which promotes mixing; this is especially important when i.v. flow rates are low, as are needed for neonates or young infants.

Frequency and Duration of Drug Administration; Multiple Drugs

To ensure that frequent doses are administered at appropriate intervals or that multiple drugs are administered to avoid drug incompatibilities, a syringe infusion pump can be used to administer drug volumes over a specific length of time. This helps avoid a situation where part of a drug dose is left in the tubing when the i.v. set is changed, as has been reported for manual administration techniques. More than one syringe pump can be used to simultaneously administer compatible drugs in a parallel system into a micro-Y-site or stopcock.

Types of Intravenous Administration

Drugs may require i.v. administration as continuous infusions or at intervals (q4h, q6h, q12h, etc.). Manual methods require the administration of the drug into the i.v. system at an injection site (Y-site, T-connector, stopcock, etc.), added to the i.v. solution in a mixing chamber, or added to an i.v. bag to be administered via gravity. A syringe pump or another mechanical device may be used for drug administration.

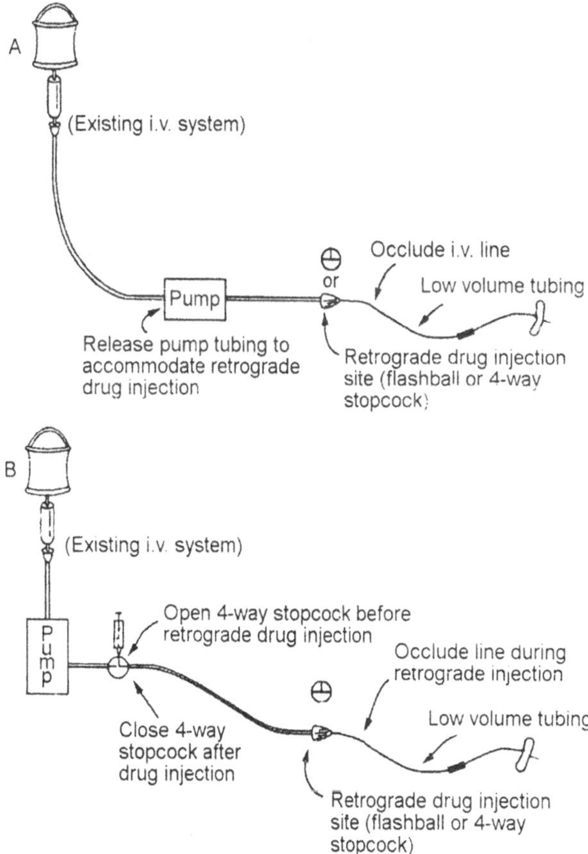

Fig. 14.3. Examples of retrograde system setups.

Manual administration

Manual administration is not as accurate as using a syringe pump for drug administration. It has been used for small volumes of medication (<3 ml), a low flow rate (<20 ml/h), or if the antegrade (forward toward the patient) injection of a drug bolus is safe. If a medication is to be administered antegrade, it should be administered slowly into a microinjection site toward the patient; microbore tubing should be placed between the injection site and the patient to reduce the time to get the drug to the patient. Leff and Roberts recommended that the volume of the drug to be injected by the antegrade technique should be a smaller volume than the tubing fluid volume between the injection site and the patient. If the medication volume is too large to be safely given by antegrade administration, but the i.v. fluid flow rate is low (<20 ml/h), the drug may be administered by a retrograde technique.

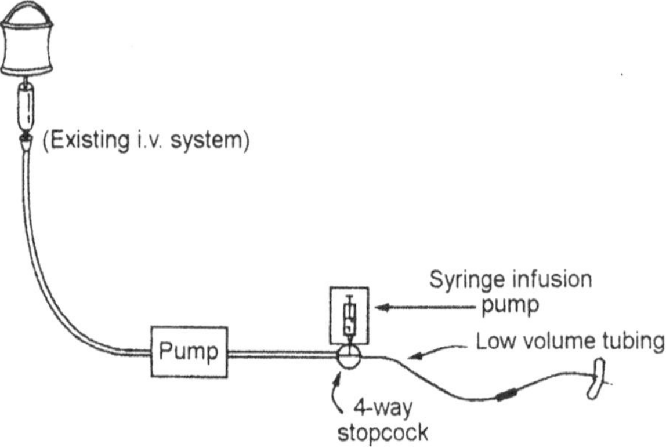

Fig. 14.4. Syringe pump setup with drug administered separately of the primary i.v. fluid flow rate.

Mechanical system for drug administration

If a mechanical system is chosen for drug administration, the appropriate infusion device must be selected based on its operating mechanism, flow accuracy, flow continuity, and ability to detect occlusions. Other important factors include an alarm system, ease of operation, ability to be cleaned easily, and safety from children inadvertently trying to change pump settings. A syringe pump is best for delivering small dosage volumes and when intermittent intervals are needed for medications. It is the mechanical device most often selected for medication administration because it can be used for intermittent administration of small and large doses, or for the continuous infusion of medications at low rates. A drug can be administered separately from the primary i.v. fluid flow rate, with the drug and the fluid mixing for a short distance therefore in microbore tubing before reaching the patient. In addition to being able to more accurately deliver medications than by manual methods, syringe pump systems have the advantage of being able to separate the administration of incompatible drugs, reduce difficulties associated with the administration of multiple doses, and shorten the time required to administer medications.

Additional Comments about IV Drug Administration

Reed and Gal recommended the following steps to decrease problems associated with i.v. drug administration to pediatric patients:

1. Standardize and document total time for drug administration.
2. Document the volume of any solution used to flush an i.v. dose.
3. Standardize infusion techniques for drugs administration, especially for those with a narrow therapeutic index.
4. Use the largest gauge cannula that can be used.
5. Standardize dilution and infusion volumes for drugs given by intermittent i.v. injection, and avoid attaching lines for drug infusion to a central hub with solutions infused at widely disparate rates, and
6. Use low-volume i.v. tubing and use the most distal sites for drug administration.

In addition, one must remember that for infants the amount of fluid required for drug administration may take away from the amount of fluid available for nutrition. Thus, with medication administration, the fluid volume must be as restrictive as possible so that the bulk of the daily fluid intake can be saved for nutrition. Health care providers must closely monitor daily fluid intake from all sources to prevent fluid overload and must also watch the osmolality of medications with diluents.

Administration of Oral Medications

The oral route is typically the preferred route for medication administration to pediatric patients. Other routes may be used, if the patient cannot take a medication orally because of vomiting, being unable to swallow, or the medication is unavailable for oral use. In addition, for specific problems it may be better to deliver the medication directly to the area being treated, for example, inhalation, ophthalmic administration, or otic administration.

Dosage Forms

Oral liquids

Liquid medications are the most commonly administered oral medications to pediatric patients because of the ease of swallowing by infants and young children who cannot swallow solid dosage forms. However, availability of some medications as liquid formulations may be limited. If not available in liquid form, a solid dosage form may need to be modified by the pharmacist, other health care provider, or by the parent. If a solid dosage form is modified, for example a suspension is prepared, will the drug be stable and for how long, and will it be absorbed differently than the original dosage form? These are just a few questions that must be answered about the extemporaneous preparation of a drug product for a pediatric patient.

Alcohol-free products should be selected for pediatric patients whenever possible. Furthermore, the inactive ingredients or excipients contained in an oral preparation should be identified. this is especially important if the patient is known to have had an adverse reaction to a particular excipient or there is another reason to avoid a particular additive in a medication. The Committee on Drugs of the American Academy of Pediatrics recommended that pharmaceutical products contain a qualitative listing of inactive ingredients in order that products containing these substance could be avoided in patients who had problems with specific adjuvants. Kumar, Rawlings, and Beaman contains lists of inactive ingredients (sweeteners, flavorings, dyes, and preservatives) found in many liquid medications such as analgesics, antipyretics, antihistamine decongestants, cough and cold remedies, antidiarrheal agents, and theophylline preparations. The authors of the previous article and Golightly et al. have reviewed adverse effects associated with many inactive ingredients.

Liquid medications, taken orally, can cause diarrhea and other GI symptoms, or they may aggravate GI distress that a patient is already experiencing. These GI effects can be associated with the high osmolality of some oral liquids. Osmolalities have been determined for various oral liquids. For preparations containing propylene glycol, or various sugars (e.g., sucrose, mannitol, glucose), osmolalities were noted to be high. It is important to compare various brands of liquid medications because they may contain different excipients and may have different osmolalities.

Sustained-Release Preparations

Most medications have shorter half-lives in children than in adults, and therefore children may need sustained-release products to maintain serum concentrations in the therapeutic range. For example, a sustained-release theophylline product may be needed for a child with asthma. It may need to be administered every 8 h to the child as compared to every 12 h for a healthy, non-smoking adult to maintain therapeutic serum concentrations. When choosing a sustained- release theophylline preparation for a child, it must be remembered that because of differences in release properties, theophylline sustained-release products are not interchangeable. A product selected for the pediatric asthma patient should be reliably absorbed with a minimal serum concentration variation and not a preparation that has exhibited a difference in bioavailability when administered with or without food.

Extemporaneous liquid preparations

Because many medications are not available as liquid preparations, there are times when powder papers or suspensions must be prepared.

Product selection

Products for oral administration should be in a dosage form most readily taken by the child. If the child is old enough to participate in the decision-making process, he or she may state a preference for a liquid, chewable tablet, tablet, or capsule, if the needed drug is available in a variety of dosage forms and appropriate dosage. If a liquid medication is needed, a product should be chosen based on texture, taste, and ease of administration. Other factors that must be considered are the absence of alcohol and dyes, and an osmolality that is close to physiologic (280–290 mOsm/kg). Are there excipients or adjuvants in the product, and if so, what are they and what is their concentration? Is there bioavailability information or pharmacokinetic information for the oral medication in pediatric patients, and if so, in what age groups? Is there information about the extemporaneous product that is to be prepared?

Rebecca Chater, a North Carolina pharmacist, recommends that pediatric patients be involved in medication counseling in order to improve their understanding of why a medication is needed. In the counseling process, the word medication should be used and not drug because of the connotation associated with the latter in today's society. Wheeler recommends that, when possible, a product be selected that requires the fewest number of doses administered per day, for example, every 12 h dosing rather than every 8 h, so the medication does not need to be taken to school or day care for administration. If a medication must be given outside of the home, she recommends that two small labeled bottles be dispensed or one large bottle with a small empty bottle labeled to be used for medication administration at day care or school. Health care providers including nurses, pharmacists, and physicians should demonstrate to parents and older children how medications should be administered and offer appropriate dosing devices (oral syringe, dropper, cylindrical medication spoon, or a small-volume doser with attachable nipple) to enable parents to accurately measure liquid products. A household teaspoon or tablespoon should not be used for medication administration because they are inaccurate. Kraus and Stohlmeyer explain the use of a new oral liquid medication delivery system that can be used for infants and young children who still use a bottle for feeding.

Administration techniques

The following information is presented to help health care providers counsel parents and older children on how medication should be administered by various routes.

Oral liquids

An oral liquid medication needed for an infant or young child should be shaken well, if required, accurately using an appropriate device. If a dropper or an oral syringe is used, the liquid should be administered toward the inner cheek. Administration in the front of the mouth may allow the child to spit out the medication, whereas administration toward the back of the mouth may result in gagging or choking. The oral syringe should be of an appropriate size to allow for administration into the inner cheek.

Oral solid dosage forms

A medication available only as a solid dosage form, may be prepared as an extemporaneous liquid (e.g., suspension) or it may be modified for oral use, for example, by crushing. As mentioned previously, a sustained-release product should not be crushed or chewed. For a solid, non-sustained-release medication, the product can be crushed and mixed with a small amount of food just prior to administration. Examples of foods that may be used for mixing include applesauce, yogurt, or instant pudding, but the medication should not be added to an entire dish of food or to infant formula, because the infant or child may not eat/drink the entire portion and thus not receive the total amount of medication.

Other Routes

Intramuscular Administration

Absorption of i.m. administered medications depends on the injection site because perfusion of individual muscle groups differs. For example, drug absorption from the deltoid muscle is faster than that from the vastus lateralis that is more rapid than from the gluteus. In addition, lower perfusion or hemostatic decompensation, frequently observed in ill neonates and young infants, may reduce i.m. absorption. It may also be decreased in neonates who receive a skeletal muscle-paralyzing agent such as pancuronium because of decreased muscle contraction. In addition, the smaller muscle mass of neonates and young infants provides a small absorptive area. The injection technique and the length of the needle used may affect drug absorption, and thus serum concentrations. For example, using a longer needle ($1^1/_2$ vs. $1^1/_4$ in. or 3.8 vs. 3.1 cm.) for i.m. administration resulted in higher diazepam serum concentrations in adults. Therefore, it is important to select the appropriate site for drug administration as well as the appropriate length and needle bore. Sites that can be used for i.m. administration include anterior thigh and vastus lateralis, gluteal area and deltoid.

The midanterior thigh (rectus femoris) and the middle third of the vastus lateralis are used for i.m. administration to young infants as well as to older children. These sites are better developed and larger than other muscle groups that are used for drug administration to older children or adults. With the patient lying supine, the "needle should be inserted in the upper lateral quadrant of the thigh, directed inferiorly at an angle of 45° with the long axis of the leg and posteriorly at a 45° angle" to the surface on which the patient is lying. The person administering the injection should compress the tissues of the injection site to help stabilize the extremity. A 1-in. (2.5-cm) needle has been recommended for pediatric patients by Bergeson, Singer, and Kaplan while Newton, Newton, and Fudin recommend a 23–26 gauge $1^1/_2$ in. (3.8 cm) needle. The volume of drug that can be administered in this manner is 0.1–1 ml in infants and 0.1–5 ml in older children and adults.

The gluteal musculature develops as the infant or child increases his or her mobility; it becomes a more suitable injection site in children who are walking. Damage to the sciatic nerve is the major problem associated with this injection site, and it occurs more commonly in infants because of their lack of gluteal muscle mass. Injury to the gluteal nerve, resulting in muscle atrophy, has occurred even when the injection technique was appropriately performed. Other nerves including the pudendal, posterior femoral cutaneous, and the inferior cluneal nerves have been damaged because of poor injection technique. All techniques involve the determination of the upper outer quadrant. After the location of the upper outer quadrant is determined, the needle should be inserted at a 90° angle to the surface on which the patient is lying, not to the patient's skin. This site can be used for older children. A 1-in. (2.5 cm) needle has been recommended. The volume of drug that can be administered in this manner is 0.1–5 ml for older children and adults.

The ventrogluteal (gluteus medius and minimus) site may be less hazardous for i.m. administration than the dorsogluteal (gluteus maximus) site. The person administering a drug i.m. ventrogluteally should first note the anatomical landmarks (anterior superior iliac spine, tubercle of the iliac crest, and upper border of the greater trochanter). The needle is inserted into a triangular area bounded by these landmarks while the patient is in the supine position. The location for this injection can be determined

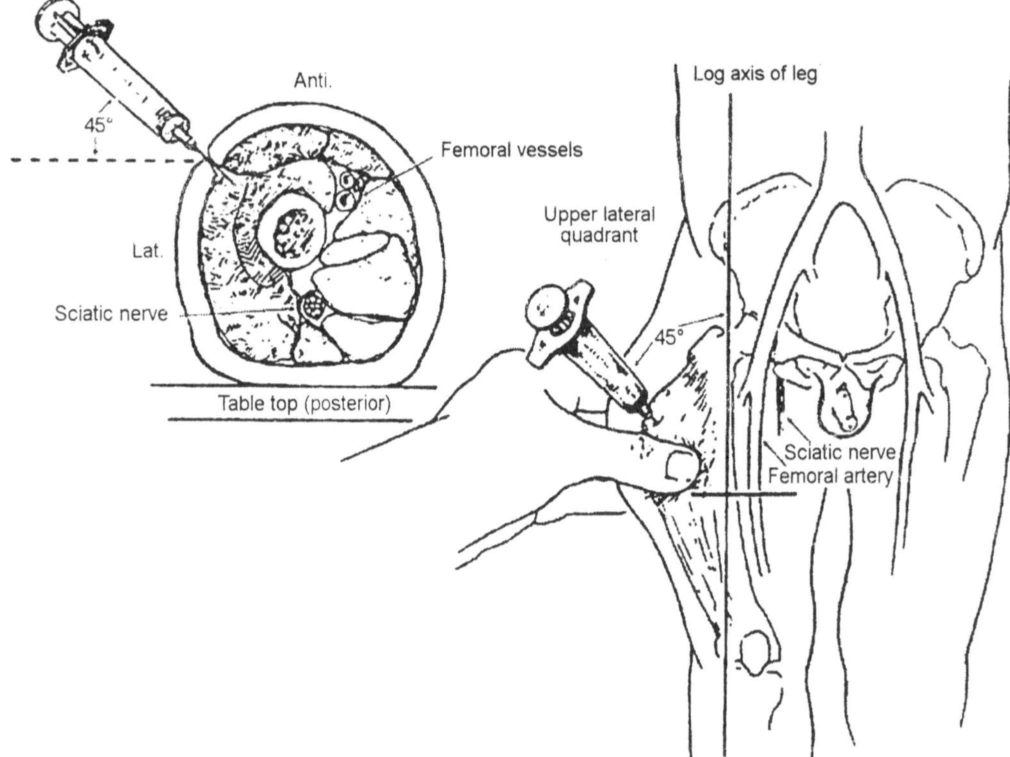

Fig. 14.5. A technique for anterior lateral-thigh intramuscular injection.

"by placing the palm over the greater trochanter, the index finger over the anterior superior iliac spine, and spreading the index and middle fingers as far as possible."

The deltoid muscle can be used for i.m. injections in older children, but it is not an option for young infants and children because of their limited muscle mass. Although there are few complications associated with this administration route, nerve injury can occur. The area for deltoid administration should be fully visible so that the anatomical landmarks can be visualized. Then the needle for deltoid injection should enter the muscle halfway between the acromium process and the deltoid tuberosity to avoid hitting the underlying nerves. The drug volume that can be administered by this route to older children and adults is 0.1–2 ml. The recommended needle length for older children is 1-in. (2.5 cm).

Subcutaneous Administration

The s.c. route is used for drug administration, such as insulin, that requires slow absorption. It is not commonly employed for medication administration for pediatric patients but is used for specific drugs. Typically a 1/2- or 1-in. (1.25- or 2.5 cm) needle is used with the volume of drug that can be administered by this route ranging from 0.1–1 ml (drug volume administered depends on patient size).

Percutaneous Administration

The skin should be thoroughly cleaned prior to applying a topical ointment, cream, etc. A thin layer of ointment or cream should be applied to the prescribed area to reduce the possibility of a toxic reaction. The area of the skin where the medication is applied should not be covered or occluded unless instructed to do so by the physician because this procedure may increase drug absorption. Specific information should be given on how to cover the area.

Rectal Administration

Before the administration of a rectal suppository, the child's r-ctal area should be thoroughly cleaned. The infant or child should be placed on his or her side or stomach. The wrapper should be removed from the suppository and its pointed end should be inserted into the rectum above the anal sphincter. (If only half a suppository is prescribed, the suppository should be cut lengthwise before administration.) A finger cot or finger wrapped in plastic can be used for administering the suppository. Because an infant or small child cannot adequately retain a suppository in the rectum, the buttocks can be held together firmly for a few minutes after rectal administration to hold the suppository in place.

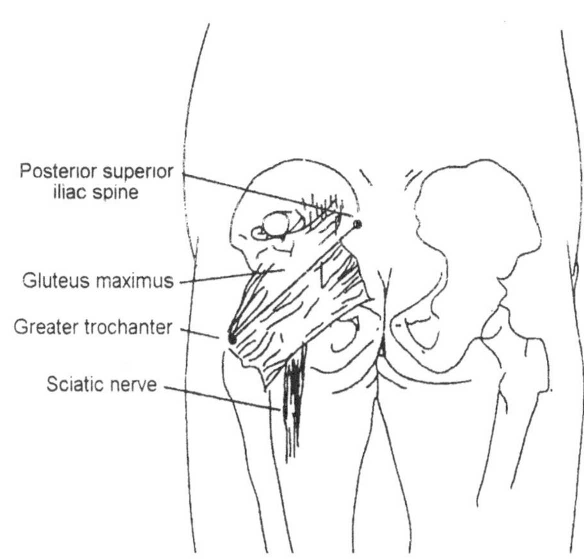

Fig. 14.6. A technique for gluteal-area intramuscular injection.

Otic preparations should be at room temperature prior to administration. If the otic product is a suspension, it should be gently shaken for approximately 10 sec. before administration. The child should be lying on his or her side, and the earlobe should be gently pulled down and back to straighten the outer ear canal (for adults the earlobe is pulled up and back). Then the prescribed number of drops should be instilled into the ear without placing the dropper in the ear canal. The patient should be kept in a position with the ear tilted for approximately 2 min to help keep the drops in the ear. This procedure may be repeated for the treatment of the other ear, if needed. The tip of the dropper should wiped with a clean tissue after use.

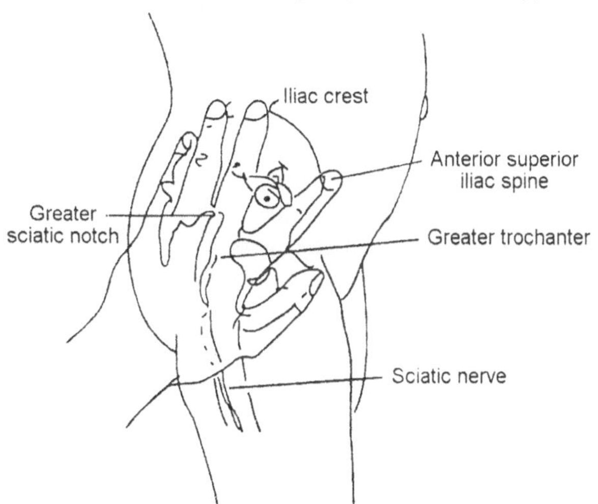

Fig. 14.7. von Hochstetter technique for ventrogluteal intra-muscular injection.

Nasal Administration

For adults, the first step in administering nose drops or a nasal spray is blowing the nose to clear the nasal passages of mucus and other secretions, but infants and young children are unable to do this. Therefore, the nasal passages may need be cleared with a bulb syringe prior to medication administration. A child should lie down on his or her back, or a young infant or child should be placed in a lying position, and the head should be tilted slightly backwards. An appropriate amount of medication should then be placed in each nostril. Thereafter, the infant or child should remain quiet for a few minutes to allow the medication to be absorbed. The dropper should be rinsed with hot water before it is returned to the medication container.

Ophthalmic Administration

An ophthalmic medication should be at room temperature prior to administration. If the eye drops are in a suspension, the container should be gently shaken before administration. A child old enough to follow directions should tilt his or her head slightly backward and to the side so that the eye drops will not drain into the tear ducts near the nose. The eyelids should be separated and the patient should be asked to look up. The appropriate amount of medication is instilled into the lower eyelid, using the medication dropper, which should be accomplished without touching the eyelids. The patient should look downward for a few seconds after drug administration. The eye(s) should then be closed for several minutes in order to spread the medication across the eyeball and be absorbed if the effect is to be systemic. In addition, it has been recommended to gently put pressure on the inside corner of the eye for at least a minute to retard drainage of the medication. If a squeeze bottle is used, the appropriate amount of medication should be gently squeezed into the eye(s). For each of these methods, the dropper or the tip of the squeeze bottle should be kept away from the eye or skin to avoid contamination of the administration device. The dropper should not rinsed after use because this could lead to contamination of the dropper and the medication. The package insert should be reviewed for specific information.

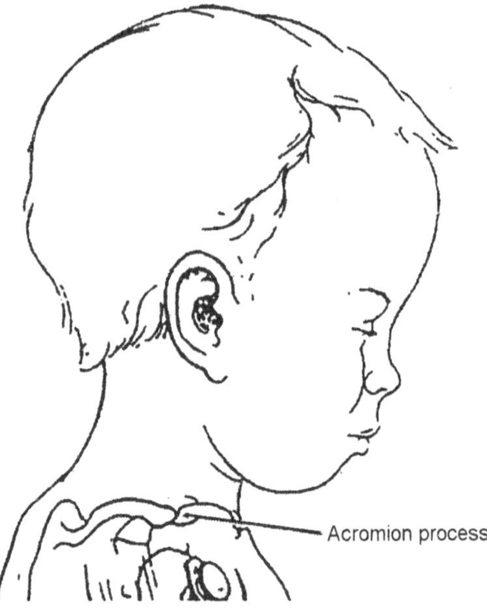

Fig. 14.8. A technique for deltoid intramuscular injection.

Another method for administering eyedrops to children recommends that the drops be applied to the inner canthus of the eye while the patient keeps his/ her eyes closed until told to open them after medication administration. Approximately 66% of the medication administered in this fashion was absorbed. In addition, this method may increase compliance and make children more cooperative. For the administration of an ophthalmic ointment to a child who can cooperate, the child should tilt his or her head backwards and look up. After the hands have been washed, the person to administer the medication should gently pull down the lower eyelid(s) for drug administration. A thin layer of ointment should then be placed in the lower eyelid(s). Afterwards, the eyelid(s) should be closed for 1 to 2 min to allow for the spreading of the medication and absorption. During this process, the tip of the ophthalmic applicator should not touch the eye. After administration is completed, the tip of the applicator tube should be cleaned with a clean tissue and be tightly capped. The package insert should also be reviewed for specific information.

Inhalers

For the use of an inhaled medication (e.g., β_2-agonists, corticosteroids, antivirals, cromolyn, etc.), it is crucial for the child and parents to understand the mechanism of the metered dose inhaler (MDI) or nebulizer, if used. The package insert should also be reviewed for information about the specific drug product. A decision may also need to be made as to whether a spacer may be needed for use with the medication canister.

15

Good Manufacturing Practices

The Current Good Manufacturing Practice (cGMP) regulations for finished pharmaceuticals that have been promulgated by the U.S. Food and Drug Administration (FDA) have been a subject of active discussion since they were first published with the passage of the Kefauver–Harris Drug Amendments in 1962. GMPs were intended to establish minimum manufacturing and control practices for the pharmaceutical industry and focus on what needed to be done rather than how it should be done. Failure to comply with the current Good Manufacturing Practice regulations as set forth in the "Code of Federal Regulations," 21 CFR Parts 210 and 211, constitutes adulteration of a drug that is entered into interstate commerce and is therefore subject to regulatory action. These requirements apply to human and animal drugs. The regulations in Part 210 are introductory in nature; Part 211 contains the more detailed and descriptive regulations.

In the late 1970s, the FDA organized a task force to study the GMPs. Revised GMPs were published in September 1978, and became official in March 1979. At that time, the FDA also considered establishing more specific GMP regulations for products such as small-volume parenterals, medicinal gases and drug substances, to supplement the existing umbrella regulations.

Today, separate GMPs are in effect for biologics and foods but have not yet been promulgated for small-volume parenterals, medicinal gases or drug substances. In attempting to create regulations for specific products, the FDA concluded that it would be better to first issue guidances and guidelines rather than to revise regulations. Thus, what is put forth in 21 CFR Part 211 is supplemented with a number of guidances, guidelines and Compliance Policy Guides. There remain some differences, however, between guidances and guidelines from the Center for Biologics Evaluation and Research (CBER), the Center for Drug Evaluation and Research (CDER), and the Compliance Policy Guides, sometimes leaving a firm's cGMP status subject to the interpretation of a field investigator.

Based on the amount of time needed to promulgate a revision of the regulations, it is understandable that it is preferable to work with guidances, guidelines, and compliance policy guides. Current GMPs are supposed to be, as their title indicates, a description of the current manufacturing and control practices that are acceptable for a pharmaceutical company selling products in the United States. Although these cGMPs are not enforced in some foreign countries, an FDA inspection in a foreign country, based on current GMPs, can be the key to importing and marketing a product in the United States.

The FDA is required to inspect a firm every 2 years for compliance to cGMPs. With the advent of programs such as the new drug preapproval inspection program implemented in 1990, inspections may be more frequent and have expanded into areas not previously investigated regularly by the FDA, such as clinical manufacturing. An unsatisfactory inspection can delay approval of new products and lead to further regulatory action by the FDA, such as seizure and injunction, for existing products. The penalties can apply to the individual or both the firm and individuals.

The GMPs as set forth in 21 CFR Part 211 also have been applied to drug substances and clinical products. Guidelines and guidances have been issued to describe the FDA interpretation of 21 CFR Part 211 pertaining to drug substances and the production of investigational drugs and reinforce the agency's understanding that cGMPs are applicable. The FDA has reinforced the connection between registration of drugs and the manufacture of active pharmaceutical ingredients by the issuance of guides to industry. Recently, the FDA has issued for comment a draft guidance for "Good Manufacturing Practice for the Manufacturing, Processing, and Holding of an Active Pharmaceutical Ingredient." Finalization of these draft cGMP principles is being written into a guideline that is being coordinated through the International Conference on Harmonization of Technical Requirements for the Registration of Pharmaceuticals for Human Use (ICH) toward publication of a guidance for active pharmaceutical ingredients that will be standardized and followed by manufacturers in the United States, Europe, and Japan. As a sidenote, active pharmaceutical ingredients have also been called drug substances and bulk pharmaceutical chemicals. The "Status of Current Good Manufacturing Practice Regulations for Finished Pharmaceuticals" is as follows:

(a) The regulations set forth in this part and in parts 211 through 226 of this chapter contain the minimum current good manufacturing practice for methods to be used in, and the facilities or controls to be used for, the manufacture, processing, packing, or holding of a drug to assure that such drug meets the requirements of the act as to safety, and has the identity and strength and meets the quality and purity characteristics that it purports or is represented to possess.

(b) The failure to comply with any regulation set forth in this part and in parts 211 through 226 of this chapter in the manufacture, processing, packing, or holding of a drug shall render such drug to be adulterated under section 501(a)(2)(B) of the act and such drug, as well as the person who is responsible for the failure to comply, shall be subject to regulatory action.

The "Applicability of Current Good Manufacturing Practice Regulations for Finished Pharmaceuticals" is as follows:

(a) The regulations in this part and in parts 211 through 226 of this chapter as they may pertain to a drug and in parts 600 through 680 of this chapter as they may pertain to a biological product for human use, shall be considered to supplement, not supersede, each other, unless the regulations explicitly provide otherwise. In the event that it is impossible to comply with all applicable regulations in these parts, the regulations specifically applicable to the drug in question shall supersede the more general.

(b) If a person engages in only some operations subject to the regulations in this part and in parts 211 through 226 and parts 600 through 680 of this chapter, and not in others, that person need only comply with those regulations applicable to the operations in which he or she is engaged.

This article reviews Part 211, Current Good Manufacturing Practice for Finished Pharmaceuticals. Title 21, Parts 600 through 680 for biological products, supplement but do not supersede the regulations in this part, unless the regulations explicitly provide otherwise. The focus of Good Manufacturing Practice for all products is on a quality control unit that has the responsibility and authority to approve or reject all components, drug product containers, closures, in- process materials, finished product, and production and control documentation. "Quality Control Unit" refers to any person or organizational element designated by the firm to be responsible for the duties relating to quality control. Specific subparts of Part 211 are summarized and described later. This article is not intended to reproduce the complete GMPs, but certain parts are excerpted for emphasis.

Organization and Personnel

Responsibilities of Quality Control Unit

(a) There shall be a quality control unit that shall have the responsibility and authority to approve or reject all components, drug product containers, closures, in-process materials, packaging material, labeling, and drug products, and the authority to review production records to assure that no errors have occurred or, if errors have occurred, that they have been fully investigated. The quality control unit shall be responsible for approving or rejecting drug products manufactured, processed, packed, or held under contract by another company.

(b) Adequate laboratory facilities for the testing and approval (or rejection) of components, drug product containers, closures, packaging materials, in-process materials, and drug products shall be available to the quality control unit.

(c) The quality control unit shall have the responsibility for approving or rejecting all procedures or specifications impacting on the identity, strength, quality, and purity of the drug product.

(d) The responsibilities and procedures applicable to the quality control unit shall be in writing; such written procedures shall be followed.

The intent of this subpart is to ensure that there is a group within the organization that can review and judge the acceptability of procedures used to produce pharmaceutical products on an independent basis, as well as judging the products themselves, before they are entered into interstate commerce. The FDA has emphasized separation of the quality control unit from production (organizationally). In addition, the FDA considers the organizational level to which the quality control unit reports very important. From a legal perspective, the chief executive officer (CEO) or president of a firm is considered the most responsible official and thereby becomes the most liable. Therefore, he is subject to criminal prosecution should the organization be found to violate the Food, Drug and Cosmetic (FDC) Act. One of the most serious infractions is fraud, that is, the intent to mislead the FDA. Hence, it is incumbent on the CEO to have well-qualified personnel in the organization and an organizational structure that reinforces quality.

Personnel Qualifications

This section emphasizes the training of personnel both in cGMP and in their specific responsibilities with regard to manufacturing, processing, packing or holding of a drug product and functions to provide assurance that the drug product has the safety, identity, strength, quality, and purity that it purports or is represented to possess. This section also requires that there be a sufficient number of qualified personnel.

(a) Each person engaged in the manufacture, processing, packing, or holding of a drug product shall have education, training, and experience, or any combination thereof, to enable that person to perform the assigned functions. Training shall be in the particular operations that the employee performs and in current good manufacturing practice (including the current good manufacturing practice regulations in this chapter and written procedures required by these regulations) as they relate to the employee's functions. Training in current good manufacturing practice shall be conducted by qualified individuals on a continuing basis and with sufficient frequency to assure that employees remain familiar with cGMP requirements applicable to them.

(b) Each person responsible for supervising the manufacture, processing, packing, or holding of a drug product shall have the education, training, and experience, or any combination thereof, to perform assigned functions in such a manner as to provide assurance that the drug product has the safety, identity, strength, quality, and purity that it purports or is represented to possess.

(c) There shall be an adequate number of qualified personnel to perform and supervise the manufacture, processing, packing, or holding of each drug product.

This section makes it clear that the quality control unit is not the only group responsible for the quality of products and conformance with GMP. Because the quality of a product must be "built in," control (at the manufacturing level) of raw materials and process control are important.

Buildings and Facilities

This section requires that the buildings and facilities are adequate, provide specifically defined areas for certain operations and are designed to prevent mix-ups. Included are design and construction features; lighting; ventilation, air filtration, air heating and cooling; plumbing; sewage and refuse disposal; washing and toilet facilities; sanitation; and maintenance. Lighting, ventilation, air filtration, and air heating and cooling must be adequate. Again, the word adequate is used frequently. This is where an individual investigator's and firm's interpretations can differ. This section also requires written procedures associated with sanitation and that the facilities should be maintained in a good state of repair. Although it may seem obvious that maintenance should be performed regularly, it can happen that preventative maintenance programs compete with production requirements for attention; however, an in-depth preventative maintenance program should be in place.

Equipment

This section addresses equipment design, size, and location, as well as construction, cleaning and maintenance. Similar to the requirements for buildings and facilities, it is necessary to provide appropriate equipment for the manufacture of a product and ensure that the equipment material of construction is not reactive, additive, or absorptive. In the 1978 version of the GMPs, requirements for equipment cleaning and use logs, as well as written procedures for equipment cleaning and maintenance were added. These requirements aid in the investigation and solution of problems by identifying batches that may also be implicated in a particular problem.

Control of Components and Drug Product Containers and Closures

This section relates to the receipt, identification, storage, handling, sampling, testing, and approval or rejection of components and drug product containers and closures, and the requirements for written procedures for each. It also covers the use of approved materials, retesting of approved material, and prevention of use of rejected materials. Although the requirements of this section indicate that each lot be appropriately identified as to its status and that materials in different statuses be stored separately, the implementation of computerized warehouses has made it possible to eliminate status labels and physical separation of quarantined and approved materials. Rejected materials are usually handled separately. These practices are not to imply that a computerized system can be used without appropriate assurance of controls. The current GMP requirement that materials must be tested or examined for all specifications and released prior to use is in conflict with the philosophy of vendor certification, which is based on a consistent, reliable record of good quality. Only vendors with well-controlled processes and a good record of acceptable batches qualify for such a program. Thus, a material could be put into use based on the quality record of the supplier (vendor), even if testing is only for identification. This section also requires the use of oldest approved stock first, retesting of approved stock "as appropriate," and controls for drug product containers and closures. It prohibits use of rejected components and drug product containers and closures.

Production and Process Controls

This section focuses again on the need for written procedures and formal authorization by the quality control unit for any deviation from written procedures. Areas covered are addition of components;

calculation of yield; equipment identification; sampling and testing of in-process materials and drug products; time limitations on production; control of microbiological contamination; and reprocessing.

Many drug companies are using electronic means of verifying component names or item codes, receiving and control numbers, weights, or measures, and even the verification of component addition to a batch. There is a range of acceptability on the part of the FDA of electronic means of verification and batch documentation; however, the validation of such systems must be performed to accept electronic means of identification and verification.

The process controls required in this section should be based on process capabilities rather than conforming with a checklist based on the regulations. This would mean that tests not typically used for a particular dosage form may be appropriate, whereas other more commonly used tests may be without any value. This not only depends on the validation of the process but also equipment and process qualification. In addition, the need for microbiological controls can be greatly reduced by knowing whether a product supports microbial growth and whether the environment in the production area is maintained at a sufficiently low bioburden. Clearly, certain products require close attention to the production environment because of the ingredients and the end use.

Many firms use the so-called clean-zone concept, in which the restrictions on personnel entering a production area and the required protective clothing are based on the nature of a product—whether the product is prone to the growth of microbes or whether it is required to be sterile. Even for products not required to be sterile or that are not supportive of microbial growth, this concept controls the production environment through reduction of bioburden.

Reprocessing frequently receives considerable attention from the FDA. Over the years, reprocessing appears to have decreased, not only because of FDA pressures, but also because more products and processes are being validated and better controls are being exercised during production. At times, however, there is the need to reprocess, but it requires authorization of the quality control unit.

For a product covered by a New Drug Application (NDA) or Abbreviated New Drug Application (ANDA), provision for reprocessing must be included in the approved registration document. Although it is not always possible in the filing of an NDA or ANDA to foresee all reasons why a product may need to be reprocessed, a procedure for reprocessing can be evaluated and included in the registration document. If not included in the approved registration document, the regulations require submission of a supplemental application and prior approval in order to market a reprocessed batch.

To some people, batch or lot yield may seem to be more of a business concern rather than a regulatory or technical matter. However, GMPs require that yield tolerances be established and that yields outside of the tolerances be investigated. The need for an investigation is to determine that yields outside of normal limits can be an indication of problems during production that would not be evident with routine testing. A minor deviation may be relatively insignificant and could simply mean that the yield tolerances need to be reevaluated, a procedure that should be followed periodically.

It may seem that the identification of equipment in the processing record is also a superfluous burden. If several pieces of equipment have been shown to be used interchangeably, one might question the reason for this additional documentation; however, when a problem arises, it is necessary to know exactly which equipment was used. It may be possible to trace this back by reviewing equipment cleaning and use logs, but the investigation is simplified by having this information in the batch record. Recording variable batch information concerning the equipment, such as tablet compressing speeds, is also necessary.

Packaging and Labeling Controls

This subpart covers one of the aspects of pharmaceutical production that has received much attention because of recalls, including an increase in recalls related to labeling errors or product mix-ups associated with the packaging and labeling operation. Specific requirements identified in this section recently include the following.

Materials Examination and Usage Criteria

1. Use of gang-printed labeling for different drug products, or different strengths or net contents of the same drug product, is prohibited unless the labeling from gang-printed sheets is adequately differentiated by size, shape, or color.
2. If cut labeling is used, packaging, and labeling operations shall include one of the following special control procedures:
   (a) Dedication of labeling and packaging lines to each different strength of each different drug product;
   (b) Use of appropriate electronic or electromechanical equipment to conduct a 100% examination for correct labeling during or after completion of finishing operations; or
   (c) Use of visual inspection to conduct a 100% examination for correct labeling during or after completion of finishing operations for hand- applied labeling. Such examination shall. be performed by one person and independently verified by a second person.
4. Printing devices on, or associated with, manufacturing lines used to imprint labeling upon the drug product unit label or case shall be monitored to assure that all imprinting conforms to the print specified in the batch production record.

Labeling Issuance

Procedures shall be utilized to reconcile the quantities of labeling issued, used and returned, and shall require evaluation of discrepancies found between the quantity of drug product finished and the quantity of labeling issued when such discrepancies are outside narrow preset limits based on historical operating data.

Packaging and Labeling Operations

Identification and handling of filled drug product containers that are set aside and held in unlabeled condition for future labeling operations to preclude mislabeling of individual containers, lots, or portions of lots. Identification need not be applied to each individual container but shall be sufficient to determine name, strength, quantity of contents, and lot or control number of each container.

These requirements reflect an increased use of electronic means to ensure correct labeling and tight controls on the practice of filling containers that will be labeled at a later date. A time-consuming operation required in the current GMPs is associated with the reconciliation of labels. The recalls and associated investigations demonstrate that unless 100% accountability can be achieved in the reconciliation process, there will not be an effective means of ensuring correct labeling. Section 211.132 was revised on February 2, 1989, to describe tamper-resistant packaging and labeling requirements for over-the-counter (OTC) human drug products. Compliance Policy Guide 7132a. 17 was issued in 1992 to describe the standardized tamper-resistant packaging requirements. This section also covers information concerning requests for packaging and labeling exemptions. It allows changes in packaging and labeling to comply with the requirements for OTC products subject to approved NDAs to be implemented prior to FDA approval as provided for in Section 314.70(c). Manufacturing changes to provide for sealed capsules require prior FDA approval under Section 314.70(b). Section 211.132 states that none of the requirements for "*special packaging*" (child-resistant packaging), as defined in Section 310.3[1] and required under the Poison Prevention Packaging Act of 1970, are affected. Subpart G also covers drug product inspection and expiration dating. The expiration date that is required in Section 211.137 relates to stability studies performed on the drug product described in 21 CFR 211.166. It requires that expiration dates be related to storage conditions stated on the product labeling.

Furthermore, the programs established are to use stability-indicating methods, under controlled conditions, in the marketed container-closure system and on an adequate number of batches to determine the appropriate expiration date. The FDA has issued guidelines on stability testing which outline in more detail the requirement to establish a stability program to determine and support the expiration date of a product. A new draft guidance for stability testing was published by the FDA in 1998, and discussions with comments to finalize this guidance are still continuing.

Holding and Distribution

This section covers warehousing and distribution and the procedures required for the quarantine of drug products before release by the quality control unit, storage of drug products under appropriate conditions, procedures to ensure use of the oldest approved stock first, and a system for documenting the distribution of each lot of drug product. This is another area where computerized systems are being used extensively. During inspections, the FDA review includes evaluation of the validation of any computerized systems and controls.

Laboratory Controls

This entire section refers to the requirements covering the testing of drug products and their components prior to release for distribution. It also covers stability testing and special testing, including testing for penicillin, if a reasonable possibility exists that a non- penicillin drug product has been exposed to cross- contamination with penicillin and laboratory animals. Additional information can be found in the Good Laboratory Practices, 21 CFR 58. Reserve samples arc required to be maintained for active ingredients and drug products. These specific requirements are elucidated in 211.170. The section on reserve samples also requires that a visual inspection of reserve samples of drug products be conducted at least once a year for evidence of deterioration. Fundamental to the testing requirements is the need for validated methods with established and documented accuracy, sensitivity, specificity, and reproducibility. It is also necessary to have meaningful sampling and testing plans that meet statistical quality control criteria. Judgments made with regard to sampling procedures should be based on the quality of the process control or the reliability of the vendor who supplies a raw material, drug substance, or packaging component.

Records and Reports

This section details the records and reports required to be maintained for pharmaceutical drug products, their components, and the equipment used in the processing of a drug product. Through these records, the entire history of a batch can be traced. The records cover equipment cleaning and use logs; component, container, closure, and labeling records; master production and control records and production record review; laboratory records; distribution records; and complaint files. Because this amount of recordkeeping can be voluminous, Section 211.180(d) allows for microfilm, microfiche, or other accurate reproductions of the original records for storage. Many firms are using the electronic generation of batch and analytical records. It is important to be able to retrieve all of the above records easily during an FDA inspection. Electronic methods must be supplemented with proper procedures to ensure that the records do not deteriorate over a period of time and can be retrieved when the computer systems used to generate the records have been revised or replaced.

This section also requires a master production and control record for each product, from which the batch production and control records are generated. These records must include complete instructions concerning the manufacture of a batch and precautions to be followed. Prior to the commercial distribution of a drug product into interstate commerce, all executed production and control records must be reviewed. If there is a discrepancy or a failure of any batch or any of its components to meet specifications, there must be an investigation and a written report of the findings. The investigation are to extend to other batches of the same or other drug products that may have been associated with the out of specification batch or discrepancy. Another part of this section covers complaint files, which are reviewed regularly during FDA inspections. In fact, a complaint file review may be the sole reason for an inspection if the FDA receives a complaint directly from a pharmacist, which may be a cause for concern. Sometimes the FDA will visit a firm to follow up on a complaint, even though the firm may not have been informed by the complainant. In the event that a complaint is received by a firm, it should be evaluated and a response sent to the complainant. It may be necessary also to conduct an investigation and prompt further action regarding the product or batch in the marketplace.

Returned and Salvaged Drug Products

This section requires that extensive records be maintained on returned drug products including ultimate disposition. Again, if the reason that a drug product is returned implicates other batches, an investigation is to be conducted in accordance with 211.192. Drug product salvaging is not allowed for drug products that have been subjected to improper storage conditions. If there is a question as to whether drug products have been subjected to such conditions, they may be salvaged only if there is evidence from laboratory tests that all applicable standards of identity, strength, quality, and purity have been met. In addition, evidence is required from the inspection of the premises that the drug products and associated packaging were not subjected to improper storage conditions as a result of a disaster or accident. Understandably, the value of the material to be salvaged is taken into consideration when such rigorous requirements exist for salvaging. Compliance with cGMP requires that responsible employees in a firm be knowledgeable about the practices that other firms follow in order to comply. FDA investigators visit many firms and find a broad picture of current manufacturing and control practices. Thus, Current Good Manufacturing Practices are "state of the art," constantly changing. To be in regulatory compliance, a firm must review their procedures and systems regularly and revise them as necessary.

16

PROTEIN ENGINEERING

During the past decade, the incorporation of noncoded amino acids into proteins has emerged as a novel and promising approach in protein science. In its infancy, the approach of protein engineering was essentially restricted to the possibility to chemically modify, in a rather unspecific fashion, particular amino acid side chains in proteins. More recently, the advent of recombinant DNA technology allowed the site-specific alteration of a given polypeptide chain at a glance, thus, greatly expanding the tools available for studying the molecular mechanisms of protein folding, stability, and function. Nevertheless, a quantitative description of the physical and chemical basis that makes a polypeptide chain efficiently fold into a stable and functionally active conformation is still elusive. This mainly originates from the fact that nature combined, in a yet unknown manner, different properties (i.e., hydrophobicity, conformational propensity, polarizability, and hydrogen bonding capability) into the 20 standard protein amino acids, thus making it difficult, if not impossible, to univocally relate the change in protein stability or function to the variation of physico-chemical properties caused by amino acid exchange(s). In this view, incorporation of noncoded amino acids with tailored side chains, allowing investigators to finely tune the structure at a protein site, would facilitate to dissect the effects of a given mutation in terms of one or a few physicochemical properties, thus, greatly expanding the scope of physical-organic chemistry in the study of proteins.

Incorporation of noncoded amino acids has been widely exploited in the study of bioactive peptides. However, the results of these studies provide only a qualitative picture of the mechanism of the ligand-receptor interaction, and thus, they are of limited predictive power, as also documented by the explosion in the last few years of serendipity-based approaches in peptide design and drug discovery. These difficulties stem primarily from the fact that introduction of single or multiple amino acid exchanges into a short peptide is expected not only to alter the interaction energy at the binding site(s) of the receptor, but also to affect (in a yet unpredictable way) fundamental properties of the free ligand, including electrostatic potential, hydration energy, and conformational entropy. Contrary to short peptides (5–20 amino acids), longer polypeptide chains (>50 amino acids) are generally characterized by a well-defined and stable three-dimensional (3D) structure, thus serving as macromolecular scaffolds, by keeping the global properties of the molecule rather constant and allowing the changes in binding free energy to be related in a more predictable way to the local variations of the physico-chemical properties at the mutation site(s). Hence, the incorporation of noncoded amino acids into proteins represents a further, (almost) obligatory extension of the studies aimed at elucidating the relationships existing among the structure, stability, and function in proteins (i.e., protein engineering). In this view, several different strategies have been pursued to incorporate non-coded amino acids, including peptide synthesis native chemical ligation, enzyme-catalyzed semisynthesis, biosynthetic incorporation *via* auxotrophic bacterial strain expression, and nonsense suppression methodologies in cell-free or whole-cell expression systems. Both native chemical ligation and enzymatic semi-synthesis require careful tailoring of the experimental procedures, whereas biosynthetic incorporation methods are not site-specific and are restricted to those cases when the structure of the noncoded amino acid (e.g., p-fluorephenylalanine, selenomethionine, and 7-zatryptophan) is similar to that of the natural counterpart to be replaced. On the other hand, despite significant advancements during the last decade, genetic methods are still limited by exceedingly low amounts of the resulting mutant protein, usually micrograms, that impair a thorough structural and functional characterization. However, stepwise solid-phase chemical synthesis remains the easiest and fastest approach to site-specifically incorporate in high yields any noncoded amino acid into even long (50–80 amino acids) polypeptide chains approaching the size of real proteins.

Relevant applications from our laboratory, regarding protein engineering with noncoded amino acids as a tool in the study of protein folding and function, will be presented. In particular, we will discuss the use of noncoded amino acids in structure-activity relationship (SAR) studies of hirudin binding to thrombin, as well as the incorporation of noncoded analogs of tryptophan and tyrosine (i.e., 7-azatryptophan and 3-nitrotyrosine) as spectroscopic probes for studying the hirudin–thrombin interaction.

Hirudin-Thrombin Interaction

Thrombin is a serine protease of the chymotrypsin family that plays a key role at the interface among coagulation, infammation, and cell growth, and it exerts either procoagulant or anticoagulant functions in hemostasis. The procoagulant role entails conversion of fibrinogen into fibrin and platelets activation, whereas the anticoagulant role regards the activation of protein C. The most effective modulator of thrombin function in solution is Na^+, which triggers the transition of the enzyme from an anticoagulant (*slow*) form to a procoagulant (*fast*) form. The Na^+-bound (*fast*) form displays procoagulant properties, because it cleaves more specifically fibrinogen and the protease-activated receptor (PAR), whereas the Na^+-free (*slow*) form is anticoagulant because it retains the normal activity toward protein C but cannot promote acceptable hydrolysis of procoagulant substrates. The importance of Na^+ on thrombin function is outlined by the fact that under physiological conditions the two forms are almost equally populated and that natural thrombin variants with compromised Na^+ binding result in bleeding phenotypes. In this view, molecules capable of affecting the equilibrium between these two forms can have great potential therapeutic impact on the treatment of coagulative disorders.

Among natural anticoagulants, hirudin is the most potent and specific inhibitor of thrombin, with a dissociation constant in the 20–200-fM range. Due to its important pharmacological implications, the hirudin–thrombin pair has been the object of thorough structural and biochemical investigations. With respect to this, structural studies conducted on hirudin in the free and thrombin-bound state indicate that this inhibitor is composed of a compact N-terminal region, encompassing residues 1–47 and cross-linked by three disulfide bridges, and a flexible negatively charged C-terminal tail that binds to the fibrinogen-recognition site (exosite I) on thrombin. The N-terminal domain covers the active site of thrombin and through its first three amino acids extensively penetrates into the specificity pockets of the enzyme.

Notably, the N-terminal tripeptide makes about half of the total contacts observed for the binding of the core domain 1–47 to thrombin and accounts for ~30% of the total free energy of binding. By limited proteolysis of full-length hirudin, we could produce the peptide fragment corresponding to the N-terminal domain 1–47 of hirudin HM2. Although far less active (at least 2×10^5-fold) than intact hirudin, this fragment (like the parent hirudin molecule) binds ~30-fold more tightly to the *fast* form of thrombin than to the *slow* form, which suggests that the structural determinants for this behavior are stored in the N-terminal domain. Hence, mutational studies on hirudin fragment 1–47 can be useful not only to investigate the physico-chemical determinants responsible for the extraordinary affinity and specificity of hirudin for thrombin, but also to probe the structural properties of the enzyme in the *slow* or *fast* forms.

SELECTION OF AMINO ACID REPLACEMENTS

Val1

Nuclear magnetic resonance (NMR) studies indicate that Val1 is almost fully exposed to solvent and highly flexible in the free hirudin. Conversely, in the thrombin-bound state, Val1 is completely buried into the active site of the enzyme and fixed into a single side-chain conformation. In particular, the α-NH_2 group of Val1 forms a hydrogen bond with the Oγ of the catalytic Ser195, whereas its side chain makes numerous hydrophobic contacts with Tyr60A and Trp60D, shaping the S2 of the enzyme. This loop, absent in other homologous trypsin-like proteases, defines the S2 specificity site on thrombin and narrows the access to the active site such that only small-sized apolar residues are allowed.

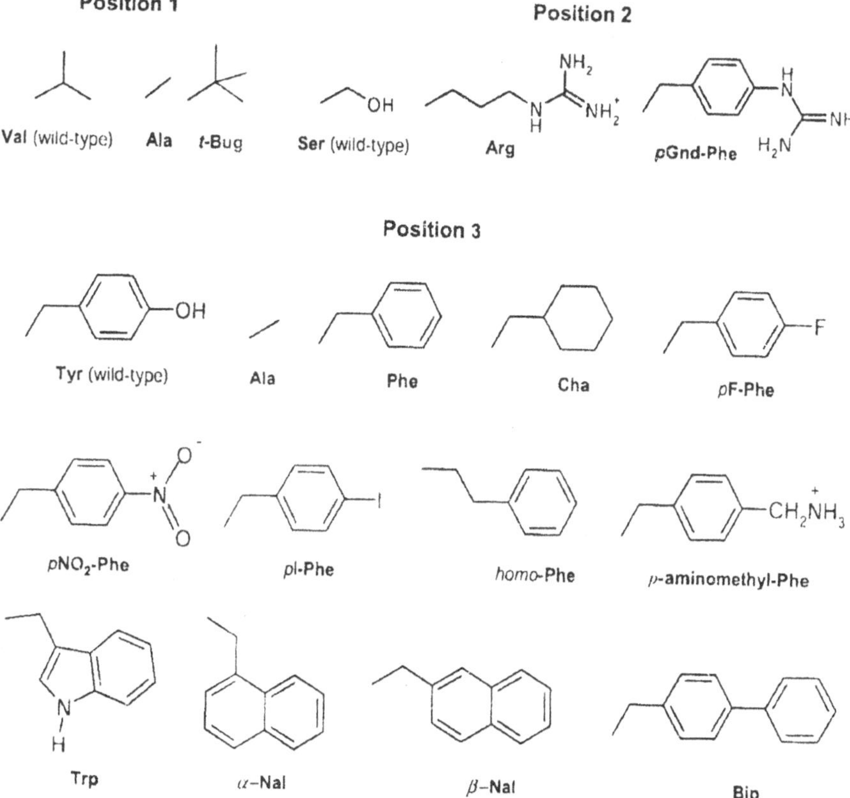

Fig. 16.1. Amino acid replacements introduced into the hirudin fragment 1-47.

Considering the structural properties of hirudin in the free and bound state and the steric requirements at the S2 site of thrombin, we shaved the Val1 side chain with Ala or replaced it with *tert*-butylglycine (*t*Bug). In fact, both Val and *t*Bug have comparable side-chain volume and strong β-forming propensities, with minimum energy points at φ/ψ = −90°, 100° for Val and φ/ψ = −130°, 140° for *t*Bug. On the other hand, the addition of a methyl group to the Cβ of valine is expected to restrict the backbone conformations available to *t*Bug to about one third of those allowed to Val.

Ser2

Analysis of the 3D structure of hirudin thrombin complex reveals that position 2 of hirudin is located at the entrance to, but does not enter, the primary specificity (S1) site. Hence, the occupancy of the S1 site is not strictly required for binding. To evaluate the effects of perturbation of Asp189, located at the bottom of the S1 site, on the affinity of hirduin fragment 1–47 to thrombin, we have replaced Ser2 with Arg and its more rigid analog, *p*-guanidophenylalanine (*p*Gnd-Phe).

Tyr3

Contrary to the high conformational flexibility observed for the first two residues of hirudin, Tyr3 has a well-defined conformation in both the free and the bound state. In the hirudin–thrombin complex, the side chain of Tyr3 projects into the apolar binding site of thrombin (the S3 site), which is formed by a large hydrophobic cavity comprising residues Trp215, Leu99, and Ile174. The importance of position 3 is confirmed by the fact that Tyr3 is highly conserved through the hirudin family. To probe the S3 site of thrombin, we introduced at position 3 of hirudin 1–47 relatively large structural and chemical diversity by systematically replacing Tyr3 with natural and non-natural amino acids having different side-chain volume, hydrophobicity, electronic, and conformational properties.

Structure-Activity Relationships

Chemical synthesis of peptide analogs of the N-terminal domain 1–47 of hirudin was carried out by a combination of manual and automated solid-phase synthesis using the synthetic strategy previously described. The crude peptides with the Cys-residues in the reduced state were allowed to fold (2 mg/mL) under air-oxidizing conditions in bicarbonate buffer, pH 8.3, in the presence of 100-μM β-mercaptoethanol. As an example, the reversed phase (RP)–high-performance liquid chromatography (HPLC) analyses of the crude synthetic analog Tyr3*homo*-Phe in the reduced and disulfide-oxidized state are reported. The chemical identity of the disulfide folded peptides was established by N-terminal sequence ana lysis and electrospray ionization (ESI)–time-of-flight (TOF) mass spectrometry, and for some synthetic peptides, the exact topology of disulfide bonds was established by enzymatic fingerprint analysis. All peptides were purified by preparative RP–HPLC, lyophilized, and used for subsequent conformational and functional characterization. The results of conformational characterization, conducted by far- and near-Ultraviolet (UV) circular dichroism (CD) indicated that amino acid exchanges do not appreciably affect the conformation of hirudin fragment 1–47, allowing us to interpret the differences in affinity to thrombin exclusively on the basis of the variation of the physico-chemical properties at the mutation site. The inhibitory potency of the synthetic analogs toward the pro-coagulant (*fast*) and anticoagulant (*slow*) form of thrombin was determined by measuring at 405 nm the release of *p*-nitroaniline from the synthetic substrate D-Phe-Pro-Arg-*p*-NA, under temperature (25°C) and salt conditions in which the enzyme predominantly (>90%) exists in the *fast* (0.2-M NaCl) or in the *slow* (0.2-M choline chloride ChCl) form.

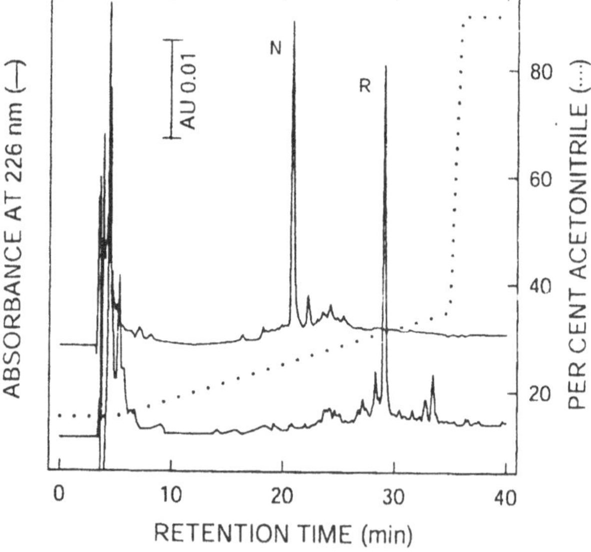

Fig. 16.2. RP-HPLC analysis of the crude synthetic analog Tyr3homo-Phe in the reduced and disulfide oxidized state.

Val1 → X

Shaving of Val1 with Ala (Val1Ala) reduces affinity for the *fast* and *slow* form of thrombin by 15-and 3-fold, respectively. On the other hand, replacement of Val1 with *tert*-butylglycine (*t*Bug) enhances the affinity of fragment 1–47 for the fast form of thrombin by about 3-fold, with a gain in the free energy of binding (ΔG_b) of 0.65 kcal/mol. This result is unprecedented, considering that almost all mutations at this position reported so far dramatically decrease binding.

Model building studies indicate that *t*Bug fits snugly into the S2 subsite of the enzyme without steric hindrance and buries approximately the same amount of apolar surface as Val1 upon binding to thrombin. Likely, the enhanced binding of V1tBug is due to the higher symmetry of the *tert*-butyl group of *t*Bug over the isopropyl side chain of Val. In the case of *t*Bug, three energetically equivalent side-chain rotamers of *t*Bug can bind thrombin into the functionally active conformation, leading to a reduction of the entropy change of binding compared with Val ($\Delta S_{b,\mathrm{Val}\to t\mathrm{Bug}}$), which binds thrombin in only one totamer (i.e., the *trans* rotamer). An estimate of $\Delta S_{b,\mathrm{Val}\to t\mathrm{Bug}}$ can be obtained from the equation $\Delta S_{b,\mathrm{Val}\to t\mathrm{Bug}} = R \cdot \ln(\gamma_{b,t\mathrm{Bug}}/\gamma_{b,\mathrm{Val}}) = R \cdot \ln(3/1)$, where $\gamma_{b,t\mathrm{Bug}}$ and $\gamma_{b,\mathrm{Val}}$ are the number of functionally active conformations allowed to *t*Bug and Val in the hirudin–thrombin complex, respectively. Thus, a relative stabilization of $\Delta G_{\mathrm{Val}\to t\mathrm{Bug}} = -T \cdot \Delta S_{\mathrm{Val}\to t\mathrm{Bug}} = -0.65$ kcal/mol at 298K is expected for the Val1*t*Bug analog over the natural species, in excellent agreement with the experimental value ($\Delta G_{\mathrm{Val}\to t\mathrm{Bug}} = -0.63$ kcal/mol) reported. Our results suggest that proper introduction of symmetric groups into amino acid side chains can significantly improve binding by increasing the entropy of the ligand in the bound state, thus reducing the overall change in ΔS_b. With this respect, amino acid substitutions like valine → *tert*-butylglycine or leucine → *tert*-butylalanine represent safe mutations, enabling us to improve binding with minimal steric requirements.

Ser2 → X

Replacement of Ser2 with Arg or its more rigid analog *p*Gnd-Phe induces a strong enhancement of the affinity of fragment 1–47 for thrombin, which is partly anticipated by modeling studies showing that the Arg side chain can be electrostatically coupled to Asp189, positioned at the bottom of the S1 site. Notably, perturbation of Asp189 enhances the affinity of hirudin preferentially for the *slow* form of the thrombin.

Tyr3 → X: Effect of Side-Chain Volume and Hydrophobicity

The effects of coarse variations in the side-chain volume at position 3 on the binding to the *fast* or *slow* form were investigated by replacing Tyr3 with a smaller amino acid, like Ala, and with much larger residues, like Trp, α- and β-naphthylalanine (αNal and βNal), and biphenylalanine (Bip). Thrombin dinding data indicate that shaving of Tyr3 at Cβ reduces affinity almost exclusively for the *fast* form of thrombin, whereas enlargement of the side-chain volume at position 3 enhances binding in all cases, but preferentially to the procoagulant *fast* form of the enzyme. The lower affinity of Tyr3Ala can be reasonably explained either by the lower hydrophobicity of Ala or by the loss of numerous van der Waals contacts with the S3 site of the enzyme. Modeling of the Tyr3Ala–thrombin complex reveals that shaving of the Tyr3 side chain creates a cavity of about 150 Å^3 at the inhibitor–enzyme interface within the S3 region, which allows penetration of water at the binding interface, with a resulting destabilization of the hirudin–thrombin complex. Increasing the side-chain volume at position 3 also increases the hydrophobic effect, due to the burial of larger apolar surface upon binding. Strikingly, replacement of Ala with Bip enhances the affinity of hirudin 1–47 for thrombin by more than 1.3×10^4 times. Clearly, thrombin binding data indicate that hydrophobicity is a major driving force for interaction. However, in the following we show that, beyond hydrophobicity, both side-chain orientation and electronic effects also play an important role in binding.

Tyr3 → X: Orientation Effects

Trp is less hydrophobic than αNal. Nevertheless, the corresponding 1–47 analogs Tyr3Trp and Tyr3αNal display very similar inhibitory activity. Conversely, although αNal and βNal have the same hydrophobicity value, Tyr3βNal is sixfold more potent than Tyr3αNal. Model building studies and accessible surface area (ASA) calculations provide reasonable explanation for these results. In fact, both Trp and αNal have similar side-chain orientation and bury approximately the same amount of apolar surface area upon complex formation. In addition, the side-chain of the residue in position 3 points toward the S2 site of thrombin in both Tyr3Trp and Tyr3αNal. Conversely, the βNal isomer in the analog Tyr3βNal buries a larger amount of apolar surface area upon binding, and it favorably interacts with in the S3 site. Further support to the importance of orientation effects to the binding of hirudin to thrombin comes from the low affinity of the analog of hirudin 1–47 in which Tyr3 was replaced by *homo*-Phe. Although *homo*-Phe is much more hydrophobic than Tyr and Phe, the analog Tyr3*homo*Phe is less potent than the wild-type species and Tyr3Phe analogs by 4- and 40-fold, respectively. Due to steric clashes, the side chain of *homo*-Phe cannot favorably interact with the apolar S3 site, but more likely it points toward Tyr60A and Trp60D in the S2 site, leaving an uncompensated cavity at the S3 site.

An important aspect emerging from our work is that the intrinsic aversion of nonpolar groups for water is the dominant driving force for ligand binding only when the removal of these groups from the aqueous solvent leads to favorable specific interactions with the receptor binding-site(s), which suggest that ligand–receptor association is strongly influenced by both hydrophobic and shape-dependent packing effects.

Tyr3 → X: Electronic Effects

Aromatic–aromatic interactions have been identified as important factors for protein stability and binding. Indeed, edge-to-face interaction between two aromatic side chains allows the δ^+ hydrogen atoms of the edge of one aromatic ring to approach the δ^- π-electron cloud of the other ring, favorably contributing to protein stability and binding by 0.6–1.3 kcal/mol. Analysis of the 3D structure of the hirudin–thrombin complex reveals that the δ^+ hydrogens on the edge of the Tyr3 ring can favorably interact in a T-shaped conformation with the δ^- π-electron cloud of the aromatic ring of Trp215 at the S3 site on thrombin. To probe the importance of aromatic–aromatic interactions in the hirudin–thrombin system, we replaced Tyr3 with Phe and its saturated analog, cyclohexylalanine (Cha). Compared with Tyr or Phe, Cha is similar in size but significantly more hydrophobic. Hence, if hydrophobicity were the dominant driving force for binding, Tyr3Cha would be expected to be a more potent inhibitor than the wild-type and Tyr3Phe derivatives. Conversely, the Tyr3 → Phe exchange improves affinity for thrombin by 10-fold, whereas saturation of the aromatic ring of Phe (by Phe → Cha substitution) reduces binding by a similar amount. These findings clearly indicate that the enhanced affinity of Tyr3Phe and wild-type species over Tyr3Cha is primarily due to the stabilizing interaction with Trp215, which is possible only for the aromatic side chain of Phe or Tyr and not for its saturated analog, Cha, thus demonstrating that, beyond hydrophobicity, electronic effects, and specifically aromatic–aromatic interactions, can markedly modulate binding.

With the aim to strengthen aromatic–aromatic interactions, we systematically replaced Tyr3 with noncoded amino acids retaining the aromatic nucleus of Tyr, as well as similar size and hydrophobicity, but possessing electron-withdrawing substituents on the aromatic ring (i.e., *p*-fluoro-, *p*-iodo-, *p*-nitro-Phe, *p*-aminomethyl-Phe). The presence of electron-attracting groups in the *para*-position of Phe3 was expected to enhance binding by making the hydrogens of the aromatic nucleus at position 3 more electron-deficient, thus reinforcing the aromatic electrostatic interaction with the π-electron cloud of Trp215. Contrary to expectations, electron-withdrawing substituents failed to improve thrombin binding.

Conversely, their presence resulted in a significant reduction in the affinity by 4 (i.e., Tyr3*p*F-Phe) to 46-fold (i.e., Tyr3*p*NO_2-Phe) in respect to that of Tyr3Phe. Rather surprisingly, the presence of *p*-aminomethyl-Phe (*p*AM-Phe), carrying a net positive charge at position 3 (pK_a 9.36), reduced affinity for the *fast* form of thrombin by only threefold and did not affect the binding strength to the *slow* form. Notably, the charged amino-group of *p*AM-Phe is shielded from water and buried into the apolar S3 site. Both theoretical and experimental work estimated an energy cost of 9–10 kcal/mol to bury a charge in the protein interior. In our case, the difference of hydrophobicity between *p*-aminomethyl-Phe and Tyr or Phe would yield an unfavourable increase of ΔG_b to thrombin by 3.8 and 4.8 kcal/mol, respectively. Therefore, the low energetic penalty of 0.72 and 0.03 kcal/ mol experimentally derived for the binding of Tyr3*p*AM-Phe to the *fast* or *slow* form of the enzyme would lead us to reconsider the apolar properties of the S3 site or, more reasonably, to invoke specific interactions of the charged amino group within the S3 site (see below) that would compensate for its unfavorable desolvation properties.

Given the apolar character of the S3 site, traditionally referred to as the "aryl binding site" of thrombin, we first attempted to relate the affinity of the synthetic analogs of hirudin fragment 1–47 for the fast form of thrombin to the hydrophobicity value of the amino acid side chain at position 3. The contribution of hydrophobicity to the free energy change of binding (ΔG_b) was estimated using the approach of Eisenberg and McLachlan, which assumes that desolvation free energy change of binding, $\Delta G_{desolv} = G_{desolv}(\text{complex}) - [G_{desolv}(\text{thrombin}) + G_{desolv}(\text{hirudin})] = -\Sigma_i \Delta\sigma_i \times \Delta ASA_i$, is related to the amount of polar and apolar surface area of both ligand and receptor that becomes buried upon complex formation. ΔASA_i is the change in the ASA for the atom-type *i* upon binding of hirudin to thrombin, and $\Delta\sigma_i$ (i.e., the atomic solvation parameter) is the solvation free energy change per unit area of atom type *i* that becomes buried upon binding. Desolvation free energy change of binding for a mutated hirudin analog (M) was calculated relatively to that of the wild-type fragment 1–47 (WT) as $\Delta\Delta G_{desolv} = \Delta G_{desolv}(M) - \Delta G_{desolv}(WT)$. Data clearly indicate that the experimental free energy change of ΔG_b is linearly related to the

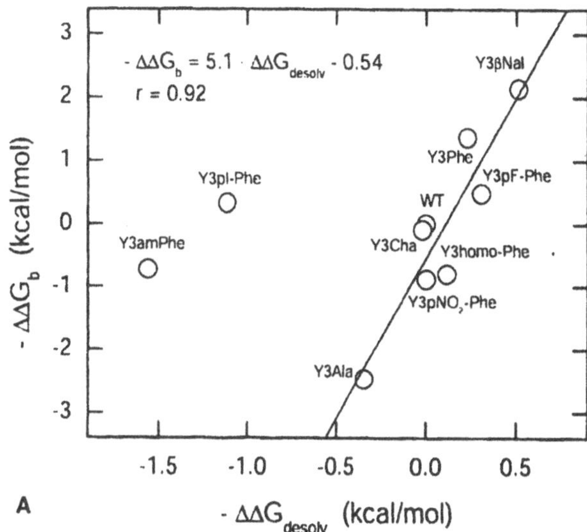

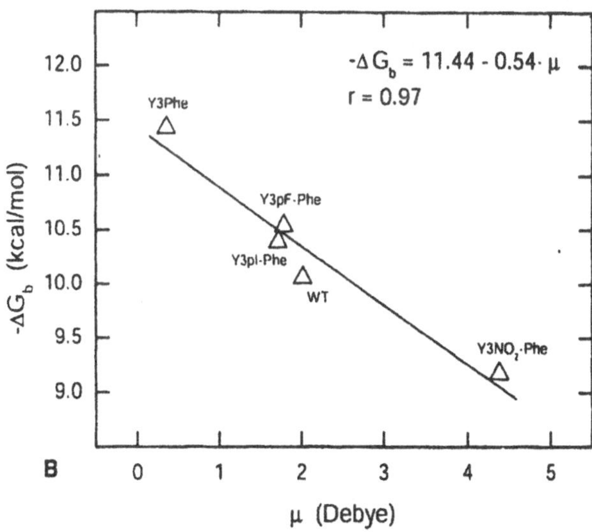

Fig. 16.3. A–Plot of the experimental free energy change of binding to the fast form of thrombin ($-\Delta\Delta G_b$) for the synthetic analogs of fragment 1-47 mutated at position 3 as a function of free energy change of desolvation ($\Delta\Delta G_{desolv}$) upon hirudin-thrombin interaction. B–Plot of ΔG_b versus the electric dipole moment μ of the amino acid side chain at position 3.

variation of desolvation free energy (ΔG_{desolv}), which is calculated on theoretical grounds. Only two data points strongly deviate from the regression line, namely Tyr3*p*I-Phe and Tyr3*p*AM-Phe. In particular, these analogs were found to bind thrombin much more tightly than predicted by desolvation free energy calculations.

Structural analysis of the corresponding complexes with thrombin reveals that both the iodine atom of *p*I-Phe and the charged nitrogen of *p*AM-Phe can productively interact with the aromatic nucleus of Trp215 at the S3 site, thus compensating (or overwhelming) their unfavorable desolvation free energy of binding. In the case of the Tyr3*p*I-Phe analog, the favorable interaction of iodine with Trp215 is predominantly driven by dispersive forces related to the high polarizability of iodine. In this regard, I_2 forms stable complexes with benzene. On the other hand, the surprisingly high affinity of the Tyr3*p*AM-Phe analog can be rationalized by taking into account a specific charge–π interaction between the protonated amino group of *p*-aminomethyl-Phe and the it-electrons of Trp215. Since the seminal work of Burley and Petsko on "*weakly polar interactions*," a great deal of experimental evidences have been accumulated over the years, leading to the conclusion that "nonconventional" hydrogen bonds of the type X–H... π and cation–π interactions can play a key role in protein structure and stability, as well as in ligand recognition. With respect to this, theoretical calculations indicate that, among many other possible combinations of cations and aromatics, the interaction of $NH4^+$ (or K^+) with indole provides the most favorable interaction energy. These predictions have been confirmed by a comprehensive structural analysis of X–H... π hydrogen bonding in proteins, in which the indolyl nucleus of Trp was found by far to be the most frequent π-acceptor of hydrogen and Lys-Trp to be the most represented donor–acceptor pair.

To better understand the physical nature of these forces driving the hirudin– thrombin interaction, we plotted the experimental ΔG_b of hirudin analogs *versus* the electric dipole moment, μ, of the *para*-X substituted (X = -H, -F, -I, -OH and -NO_2) amino acid side chain at position 3. The data indicate that the affinity of hirudin fragment 1–47 for thrombin is inversely related to the value of μ, which suggests that hirudin–thrombin interaction is destabilized by the presence of a partial negative charge at the *para*-position of the phenyl ring, as in the case of *p*NO2-Phe, where the two oxygen atoms are strongly electron-dense. A reasonable explanation for these results may be found in the specific electrostatic interactions with the electronic π-system of Trp215, which for *p*-aminomethyl-Phe are attractive, whereas for *p*NO2-Phe are repulsive. Taken together, our results indicate that the relative change in the affinity of hirudin 1–47 analogs can be accounted for by the apolar character of the ligand quite well, but on the other hand, they also emphasize the importance of "*hidden interactions*," mainly of electrostatic nature, in strengthening hirudin-thrombin binding. If a reasonable estimate of the hydrophobic effect can be obtained by calculating the free energy change due to desolvation of apolar surfaces that become buried upon ligand–receptor association, electrostatic effects are much more difficult to evaluate and predict, because they are mediated by weakly polar interactions, whose strength is strongly dependent on the electron density and polarizability, as well as on the orientation and distance of the interacting groups, such that even subtle perturbations in the ligand or receptor structure may dramatically alter binding. In this perspective, the possibility to introduce at a given protein site noncoded amino acids with larger structural and chemical diversity will improve our understanding of the mechanisms dictating molecular recognitions in proteins.

Cumulative Amino Acid Substitutions in Hirudin Yield a Highly Potent Thrombin Inhibitor

Hirudin offers numerous advantages over the existing anticoagulants heparins and cumarins, and its use in clinical practice has been recently introduced. However, hirudin administration necessitates careful dose-titration, and bleeding effects are not rare. These problems stem primarily from the intrinsic instability of the highly flexible C-terminal tail of full-length hirudin to degradation by endogenous proteases, generating truncated N-terminal fragments that, however, are dramatically less potent as thrombin inhibitors than the intact molecule.

To minimize the hirudin sequence binding to thrombin and to improve its therapeutic profile, several N-terminal fragments of hirudin have been prepared as potential anticoagulants. Their use would provide a more predictable effect *in vivo* compared with intact hirudin, due to their stability to denaturants and proteolytic attack and lower immunogenicity. Moreover, N-terminal core fragments targeting solely the active site of thrombin are expected to have a safer therapeutic profile, in keeping with the notion that active-site reversible inhibitors of thrombin display a better antithrombotic/hemorrhagic balance than bivalent inhibitors. However, a major limitation of these fragments resides in their poor affinity for thrombin (K_d = 30–400 nM), compared with hirudin (K_d = 0.2–1.0 pM).

To possibly obtain a mini-hirudin retaining the highly potent antithrombin activity of full length hirudin, but lacking the susceptibility to proteolysis, we selected the best-performing amino acid exchanges tested in our previous work (i.e., Val1*t*Bug, Ser2Arg, and Tyr3βNal) and combined them in the same analog, denoted as BugArgNal [65], which was synthesized in high yields by standard Fmoc chemistry. The introduction of only three mutations at the N-terminal end of hirudin fragment 1–47 yields a molecule that inhibits the *fast* or *slow* form by 2670- and 6820-fold more effectively than the natural counterpart and that binds exclusively at the active site of thrombin with an affinity ($K_{d,fast}$ = 15 pM, $K_{d,slow}$ = 220 pM) comparable with that of full-length hirudin ($K_{d,fast}$ = 0.2 pM, $K_{d,slow}$ = 5.5 pM). Strikingly, BugArgNal induced a change in the coagulative parameters (i.e., thrombin time, prothrombin time, and activated partial thromboplastin time) comparable with that evoked by intact hirudin (unpublished data). BugArgNal is also highly stable to low pH and resistant to the action of numerous proteases, including trypsin, chymotrypsin, thermolysin, and pepsin, and like full-lemgth hirudin, it displays almost absolute selectivity for thrombin over other closely related, physiologically important serine proteases, including plasmin, factor Xa, and tissue plasminogen activator, up to the highest concentration of inhibitor tested (10 μM). Only a slight inhibition was observed for factor Xa, with an estimated K_d value higher than 8 μM.

The issue of protease selectivity is crucial in the design of novel thrombin inhibitors, because inhibition of other physiologically relevant serine-proteases (e.g., tissue plasminogen activator and plasmin) can impair their clinical use. The results reported in this study demonstrate that the presence of an Arg-residue at the N-terminal end of hirudin fragment 1–47 strongly improves binding, while retaining the extraordinary selectivity of the natural product.

This is in contrast with the results obtained for low-molecular-weight inhibitors, where it is paradigmatic that the introduction of a positive charge at P1-position improves binding, but strongly reduces selectivity, because the positive charge of the inhibitor interacts in the S1 site of thrombin with Asp189, which is highly conserved among the endogenous enzymes prevalent in the vascular system. Likely, in the case of BugArgNal, many weak favorable contacts operate at the inhibitor–thrombin interface to cooperatively encode protease specificity.

The effects of the amino acid replacements are additive in both the *fast* and the *slow* forms of thrombin, indicating that S1, S2, and S3 sites behave independently; that is, perturbation of a given site of the enzyme does not affect the binding properties of the other two sites. This result is of particular relevance, because it would allow the properties of a multiple mutant to be inferred directly from those of the singly mutated species and to engineer incremental increases in binding strength and selectivity for either allosteric form of thrombin. For instance, substitution of Val1 with *t*Bug, Ser2 with Arg, and Tyr3 with Bip would yield a synthetic analog about 15,750 more potent than the wild-type species, with a predicted K_d value of about 2.5 pM.

Structural Mapping of Thrombin Recognition Sites in the Na^+-Bound and Na^+-Free Form

The effect of Na^+ binding on thrombin function is allosteric in nature, and several crystal structures of the enzyme with and without Na^+ bound have been recently reported. The structures of the pseudo-wild-type thrombin mutant (Arg77aAla), reported by Di Cera et al., in the presence or absence of Na^+, display only small changes in the side-chain orientation of Ser195 in the active site, Asp189 in the S1 site, Glu192 and Asp222 on the protein surface, and some rearrangement of the water molecules filling the S1 site. Conversely, the structures of the *fast* and *slow* form reported by Huntington et al. show significant differences at the level of the S2 and S3 sites, which in the *slow* form protrude onto the protein surface and limit the access to the catalytic pocket. In particular, the apolar cavity of the S3 site is restricted by protrusion of Trp215, which is possibly caused by reorientation of the underlying Phe227 and 168–182 disulfide bond. Partial unfolding of the Na^+ site is observed, with a collapse of the 148-loop onto the groove leading to the catalytic pocket. Furthermore, all putative structures of the *fast* and slow forms reported so far display numerous contacts between thrombin monomers in the crystal lattice, and therefore, the packing effects can also influence the thrombin structure in the crystal.

Hence, we decided to use the N-terminal hirudin domain 1–47 as a molecular probe of the solution conformation of thrombin recognition sites in the *fast* and *slow* form. The guiding idea is that structural information on thrombin sites in the two allosteric forms can be gained from the physico-chemical properties of the mutated residue at position 1–3 of hirudin and from the effects of the perturbations introduced on the value of coupling free energy ΔG_c, which is the difference in standard free energy of binding of the inhibitor to the *fast* and *slow* form of thrombin, $\Delta G_c = \Delta G^F - \Delta G^S$. Thrombin binding data can be summarized as follows: First, Ala-shaving at either position 1 or position 3 reduces affinity almost exclusively for the fast form; second, side-chain enlargement at position 3 with bulky and hydrophobic amino acids (i.e., βNal and Bip) strongly enhances affinity for both forms, but preferentially for the fast form; third, electrostatic perturbation of the primary specificity site S1, by Ser2 → Arg or Ser2 → *p*Gnd-Phe exchange, enhances affinity preferentially for the slow form. These data were analyzed within the theoretical framework of site-specific thermodynamics and used to extract structural information on the specificity sites of thrombin in the two allosteric forms:

$$\begin{array}{ccccc} & & \Delta G^S & & \\ & S & \Leftrightarrow & SI & \\ \Delta G^0 & \Downarrow & & \Downarrow & \Delta G^1 \\ & F & \Leftrightarrow & FI & \\ & & \Delta G^F & & \end{array}$$

The *slow* (*S*) and *fast* (*F*) forms bind the inhibitor (*I*) with a standard free energy change ΔG^S and ΔG^F, whereas ΔG^0 and ΔG^1 represent the free energy changes for switching from the *slow* to the *fast* form in the absence or presence of the inhibitor. The coupling free energy (ΔG_c) for the cycle is given by the equation $\Delta G_c = \Delta G^F - \Delta G^S = \Delta G^1 - \Delta G^0$, where ΔG^F and ÄG^S can be determined experimentally. The preferential loss (or gain) in affinity of a mutated inhibitor for one of the two allosteric forms of the enzyme is a measure of the energetic contribution of the interactions being lost (or gained) upon mutation and provide strong, albeit indirect, means for identifying those regions on thrombin that have different structural features in the *slow* or *fast* form. On the other hand, mutations that affect both forms to the same extent reveal that the perturbations introduced in the inhibitor are important for binding to thrombin and that the site is not involved in the *slow*→*fast* transition or, otherwise, that the entity of the perturbation introduced is too small to elicit a different behavior at that site in the two allosteric forms. In addition, because Na^+ binds the hirudin–thrombin complex with ~20-fold higher affinity than the free enzyme ($\Delta G^\circ \neq \Delta G^1$), then from the linkage principles mentioned above, it follows that the inhibitor must bind with different affinity to the *slow* and *fast* forms ($\Delta G^f \neq \Delta G^s$), ruling out other possibilities.

In the case of Tyr3 → Ala and Val1 → Ala exchanges, elimination of the interactions of Tyr and Val side chains beyond the Cβ strongly reduces affinity for the *fast* form, by 65- and 15-fold, respectively, whereas it is practically ineffective on the *slow* form, which suggests that the presence of Tyr and Val is crucial to enhance binding exclusively to the procoagulant *fast* form. On the other hand, the presence of the larger side chain of βNal at position 3 enhances affinity for the *fast* form by about 40-fold and by only 15-fold for the *slow* form. Taken together these results suggest that the S3 site of thrombin in the procoagulant (*fast*) form is in a more open and accessible conformation in respect to the less forgiving structure it acquires in the anticoagulant *slow* form. Also consistent with our model are the effects of the replacement of Ser2 with Arg or *p*Gnd-Phe, whose long, charged side chain is expected to facilitate penetration of the inhibitor into thrombin recognition sites, to a greater extent in the case of the more closed *slow* form than in the case of the *fast* form of the enzyme, which is already accessible for binding. From the effects of amino acid substitutions on the affinity of fragment 1–47 for the enzyme allosteric forms, we conclude that the specificity sites of thrombin in the Na^+-bound form are in a more open and permissible conformation, compared with the more closed structure they assume in the Na^+-free form.

The structural picture of thrombin allosteric forms proposed above is consistent with detailed molecular dynamics (MD) simulations carried out for 18 ns in full explicit water, showing two well-defined conformational minima on the energy landscape. After about 5 ns, a concerted conformational transition, involving the S2/S3 sites, the 148-loop, and the fibrinogen binding site, leading the thrombin molecule from a more compact and closed form, which we propose can be related to the anticoagulant (*slow*) form in the Na^+-free state, to a more open and accessible conformation, which we propose can be related to the procoagulant (*fast*) form in the Na^+-bound state. Moreover, the results of MD analysis outline the high degree of correlation existing between the motions of all these regions of thrombin, all occurring after about 5 ns, and suggest that a structural network is present, capable of communicating the conformational changes, induced by Na^+ binding, between different structural domains of the enzyme.

Our model also provides reasonable explanation for the fact that those substrates that are related to the procoagulant activities of thrombin (e.g., fibrinogen, PAR-1, and factor XIII) orient a bulky side chain deep into the S3 site of the enzyme and, as expected, are cleaved by the *fast* form of thrombin 20–40-fold more efficiently than by the *slow* form. In particular, fibrinogen interacts at the S3 site of the enzyme through the bulky Phe8 having a side-chain volume of 127 $Å^3$, PAR-1 through Leu38 (Leu = 100 $Å^3$) [1nrs.pdb; 79], and factor XIII through two Val-residues (Val29 and Val34; Val = 79 $Å^3$) [1de7.pdb; 80]. On the other hand, protein C, which is related to the anticoagulant function of thrombin, does not seem to extensively interact with the S3 site of the enzyme, and as expected, it is cleaved with similar specificity by either the *slow* or the *fast* form (ΔG_c = 0.2 kcal/mol).

Incorporation of Noncoded Amino Acids as Spectroscopic Probes in the Study of Protein Folding and Binding

A major application of protein engineering with noncoded amino acids regards the introduction into proteins of biophysical probes possessing physico-chemical properties (e.g., side-chain volume, hydrophobicity) similar to those of the corresponding natural amino acids, but spectral features distinct from those of the natural counterparts and highly sensitive to the chemical environment in which the probe is located. Hence, by the use of the so-called "spectrally enhanced proteins", it should be possible to effectively monitor the local structure and dynamics of the mutated protein during key events, such as protein folding and denaturation or ligand binding, without significantly perturbing the kinetics and equilibrium properties of the process under investigation. With respect to this, in a recent study, Cohen et al. could site-specifically introduce 6-dimethylamino-2-acyl-naphthylalanine (Aladan) into the B1 domain of staphylococcal protein G to obtain estimates of the local dielectric constant of the protein at different sites.

More specifically, the development of new spectroscopic tools for studying protein–protein interactions is central to many disciplines, including structural biology, biotechnology, and drug discovery [84]. Traditionally, the change in tryptophan (Trp) fluorescence has been exploited to study ligand–protein interactions. However, the fluorescence signal of many proteins is insensitive to ligand binding, because fluorescence changes are mostly restricted to those cases where Trp-residues are embedded in the ligand–protein interface or when the ligand binding induces conformational changes in the protein, remote from the binding region and involving one or more Trp-residues. Furthermore, the presence of multiple tryptophans in proteins may lead to compensating effects that often complicate interpretation of the fluorescence data.

To overcome these problems, several extrinsic spectroscopic probes, characterized by well-defined spectral properties, have been covalently bound to protein functional groups (i.e., Cys and Lys), to act as energy donors or acceptors in fluorescence resonance energy transfer (FRET) studies. This approach, however, is limited by possible labeling heterogeneity, nonquantitative modification, structural alteration of the proteins resulting from the labeling *per se*, and perturbation of the binding process, due to the large size of the fluorescent labels used. In the following, we show the utility of two noncoded analogs of tyrosine and tryptophan, namely 3-nitrotyrosine (NT) and 7-azatryptophan (AW), in the study of hirudin folding and binding to thrombin.

7-Azatryptophan

Among the noncoded tryptophan analogs studied so far (i.e., 5-hydroxy- and 5-metoxy-Trp, benzo [b]thiophenylalanine and the spectrally silent fluorotryptophans), 7-azatryptophan (AW), an isostere of tryptophan (W), displays interesting absorption and fluorescence properties. Unlike tryptophan, free AW displays single exponential fluorescence decay and the presence of a nitrogen-atom at position 7 in the indolyl-nucleus results in a red shift of 10 nm in the absorption and 46 nm in the emission of AW compared with Trp. Furthermore, the fluorescence λ_{max} and quantum yield of 7-azaindole (7AI) are strongly influenced by the polarity of the chemical environment. In particular, on going from cyclohexane to water the emission fluorescence of 7AI is shifted from 325 to 400 nm and the quantum yield is decreased by 10-fold. The quantum yield of AW increases from 0.01 in aqueous solution, pH 7, to 0.25 in acetonitrile. Hence, it should be possible to selectively excite the fluorescence of AW at the red edge of its absorption (between 310 and 320 nm), where Tyr does not absorb and the contribution

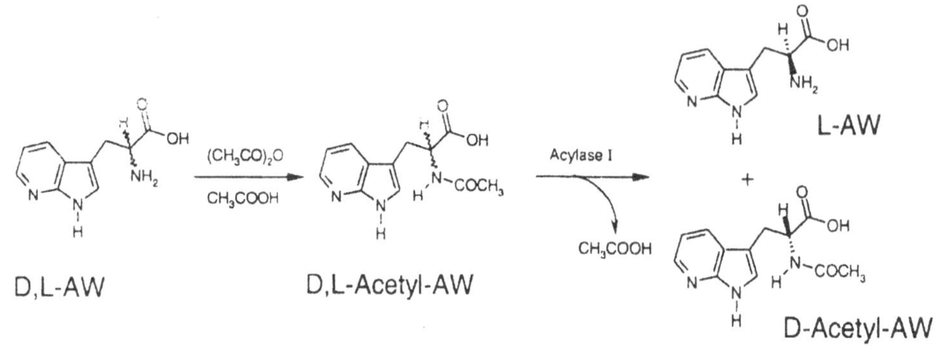

Fig. 16.4.

of Trp is negligible and, thus, investigate protein folding and binding processes through variation of the AW fluorescence signal.

Recently, we exploited the unique spectroscopic properties of AW to probe the disulfide-coupled folding of the hirudin N-terminal domain 1–47 and the binding to its the target enzyme, thrombin [90]. Before chemical synthesis, the resolution of the commercially available enantiomeric mixture of AW was carried out by treating the racemic mixture with acetic anhydride and subsequent enantioselective deacylation with immobilized *Aspergillus oryzae* acylase-I to yield L-AW. Purified L-AW was then reacted with 9-fluorenylmethoxycarbonyl chloride (Fmoc-Cl), to quantitatively obtain the Fmoc-derivative, which was subsequently used in the solid-phase synthesis of the analog of hirudin 1–47 in which Tyr3 was replaced by AW.

The replacement of tryptophan with the isosteric 7-azatryptophan leads to a significant reduction (~10-fold) in the affinity of fragment 1–47 for the *fast* form of thrombin, indicating that exchange of even a single atom (C → N) can substantially affect binding to the enzyme. These results can be explained by the lower hydrophobicity of 7-azatryptophan compared with that of tryptophan, as given by the values of octanol→water partition coefficient (logP) of indole ($logP_{indole}$ = 2.33) and 7-azaindole ($logP_{azaindole}$ = 1.72), determined experimentally.

The results of spectroscopic characterization indicate that the λ_{max} values in the absorption and fluorescence spectra of Y3AW are red-shifted by ~10 and 40 nm, respectively, compared with those of Y3W. The fluorescence spectra of Y3AW with the six Cys-residues in the fully reduced or correctly folded state are compared with those of the corresponding Y3W analog. The emission spectrum of the reduced, unfolded Y3AW reveals the presence of two distinct, well-resolved bands at 305 and 397 nm, assigned to the contribution of Tyr13 and AW at position 3, respectively. In the folded state the Tyr-band disappears, whereas the fluorescence of AW is blue-shifted to 390 nm and enhanced by about 20%. Our results can be rationalized by considering that in the reduced state, hirudin fragment 1–47 is in a random coil conformation, with the donor (Tyr13) and acceptor (AW3) amino acids far apart in space. In the native state, the chain folding brings Tyr13 in close proximity to AW3 and allows the energy absorbed by Tyr to be efficiently transferred to AW. In the case of Y3W, a single band at 350 nm is observed in the native state, whereas in the reduced state the contribution of Tyr13 appears as a very weak shoulder at 303 nm, overwhelmed by the stronger emission of Trp3 at 355 nm. This actually makes it difficult (if not impossible) to follow the folding process of hirudin by Tyr → Trp energy transfer measurements.

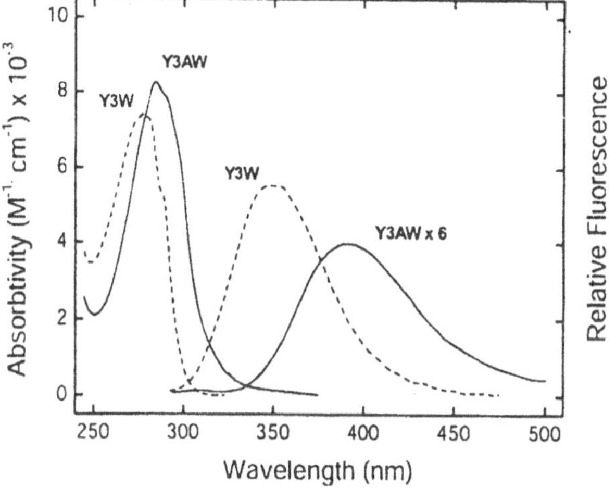

Fig. 16.5. UV absorption and emission fluorescence spectra of Y3AW (—) and Y3W (--) analogs of hirudin fragment 1-47.

The strong dependence of the fluorescence properties of AW on solvent polarity was exploited to investigate the binding of Y3AW analog to thrombin. To minimize the contribution of the nine Trp-residues present in the thrombin sequence, we excited AW at the red edge of its absorption range (320 nm), where the contribution of Trp is expected to be negligible. The spectra clearly indicate that the fluorescence of AW is strongly quenched upon binding to thrombin. Given the known solvent-dependent emission of AW and the apolar character of the S2/S3 binding sites of thrombin, this result is surprising.

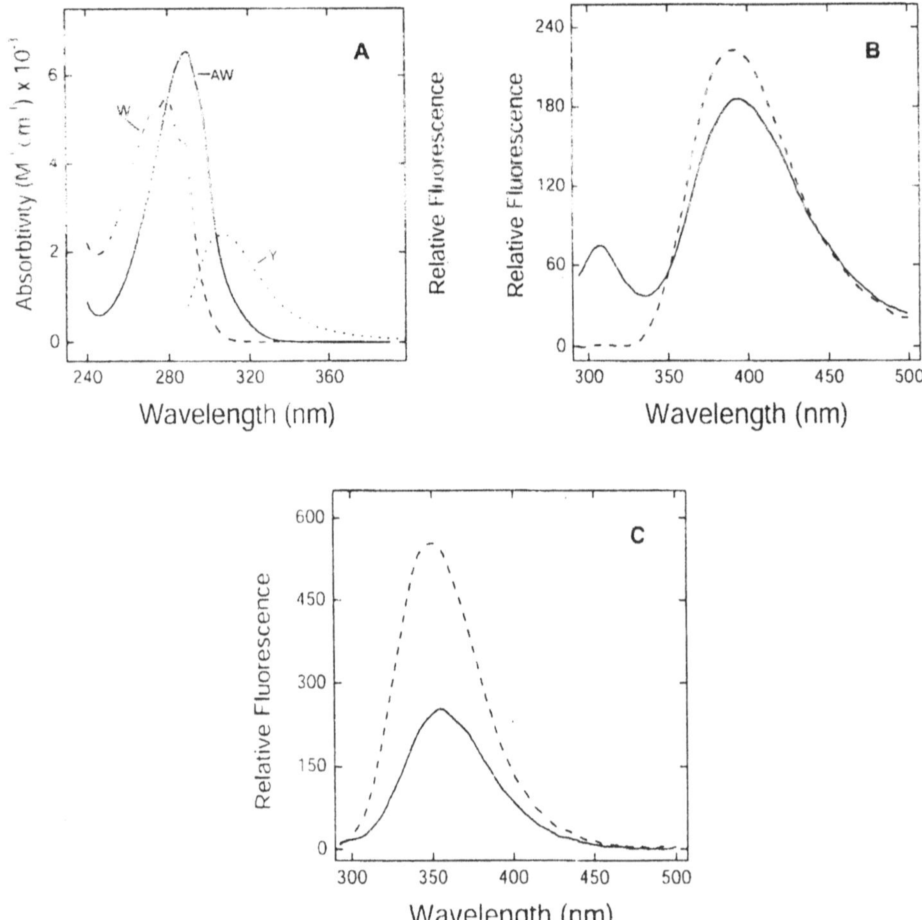

Fig. 16.6. Disulfide oxidative folding of Y3AW analog monitored by fluorescence spectroscopy.

In fact, we would have expected that binding of Y3AW to thrombin is accompanied by a blue-shifted emission of AW and a substantial increase in its fluorescence intensity. The fluorescence spectra of the model compound 7-azaindole (7AI) in different solvents well document the extraordinary dependence of the fluorescence signal of 7AI on the solvent polarity, shifting from 325 nm in cyclohexane to 345 nm in diethylether and 362 nm in acetonitrile. In particular, in water-restricted environments (e.g., water-saturated diethyl ether), the fluorescence signal is dramatically reduced, due to the formation of a 1:1 7AI-H_2O cyclic adduct that promotes formation in the excited state of a "tautomer" species that is poorly fluorescent.

In the light of these considerations, the strong quenching effect on the fluorescence of 7AW, observed upon binding of Y3AW to thrombin, can be explained on the basis of the model structure of Y3AW bound to thrombin. The ^{1}NH group of AW interacts with water molecule w432, whereas N^7 may be linked to Tyr60a through a water bridge involving the structural water molecule w606. Hence, the rigid, structural water molecules at the hirudin–thrombin interface can have a crucial role in quenching the fluorescence of 7AW, because they promote the nonradiative decay of AW in the excited state more effectively than the labile water molecules solvating the 7AW in the free Y3AW analog. In conclusion, our data demonstrate that the incorporation of 7-azatryptophan into proteins can be of broad applicability in structure-activity relationship studies, where a Trp-isostere is required, or as a spectroscopic probe in the study of protein folding and binding.

3-Nitrotyrosine

3-Nitrotyrosine (NT) is produced *in vivo* by reaction of protein tyrosines with peroxynitrite. The NT side chain is only 30 Å^3 larger than the unmodified Tyr, and the presence of the electron-withdrawing nitro-group makes the phenolic hydrogen of free NT about 10^3-fold more acidic (pK_a 6.8). At pH < pK_a, where the neutral form is predominant, NT is more hydrophobic than Tyr, whereas at higher pH, where NT exists in the ionized form, it is much more polar. NT can form an internal hydrogen bond, and its absorption properties are strongly of free NT displays a major band at 422 nm, characteristic of the ionized form, whereas at acidic pH a prominent band appears at 355 nm, assigned to the contribution of the neutral form. NT is essentially nonfluorescent and absorbs radiation in the wavelength range where both Tyr and Trp emit fluorescence, with a Trp-to-NT Förster's distance (i.e., the donor-acceptor distance at which the FRET efficiency is 50%) as large as 26 Å. For these reasons, NT has great potential as an energy acceptor in FRET studies, and indeed, direct chemical nitration of Tyr was used to investigate the structural and folding properties of calmodulin and apomyoglobin. However, very little is known about the possibility of exploiting the unique spectral properties of NT to study molecular recognition.

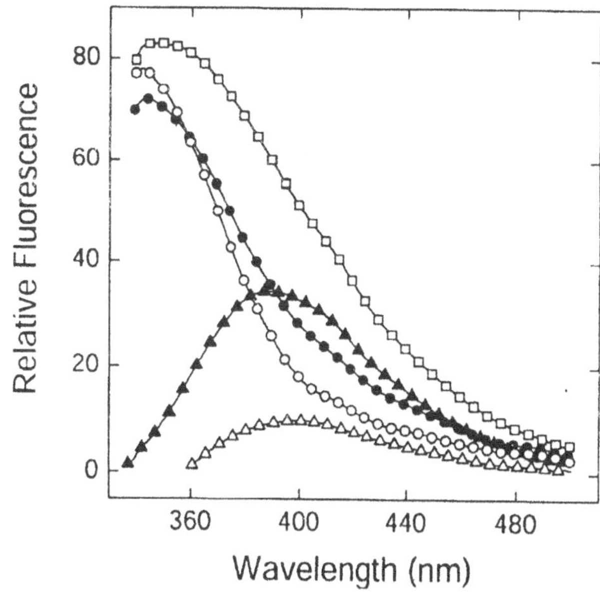

Fig. 16.7. Hirudin-thrombin interaction probed by fluorescence spectroscopy.

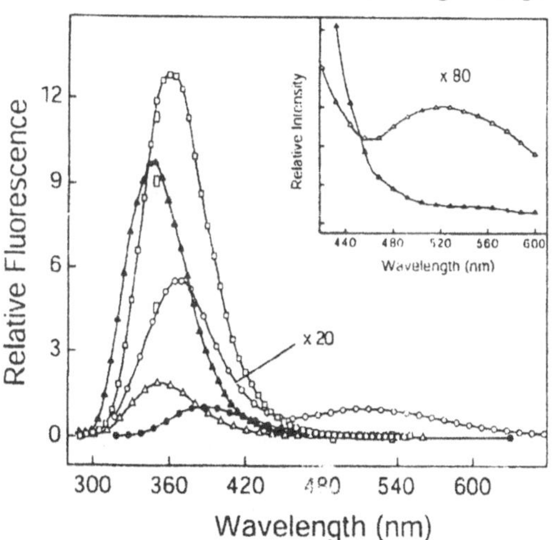

Fig. 16.8. Fluorescence emission spectra of 7-azaindole (7AI) in different solvents.

Hence, we chose the hirudin-thrombin system as a suitable model for evaluating the potentialities of NT as a spectroscopic probe in the study of protein–protein interactions. To this aim, we synthesized two analogs of the N-terminal domain (residues 1–47) of hirudin: Y3NT, in which Tyr3 was replaced by NT, and S2R/Y3NT, containing the cumulative substitutions Ser2→Arg and Tyr3→NT. In the presence of saturating concentrations of Y3NT or S2R/Y3NT, the fluorescence of thrombin is strongly quenched and approaches a similar value, under either *fast* (0.2-M NaCl) and *slow* (0.2-M ChCl) conditions. We have demonstrated that quenching of fluorescence is mainly caused by FRET, occurring between (some of) the Trp-residues of thrombin (i.e., the donors) and the single 3-nitrotyrosine of the inhibitors (i.e., the acceptor).

FRET is a nonradiative decay process occurring between a donor and an acceptor, which interact *via* electromagnetic dipoles transferring the excitation energy of the donor to the acceptor. For a one-donor–one-acceptor system, the efficiency of energy transfer depends on the extent of spectral overlap

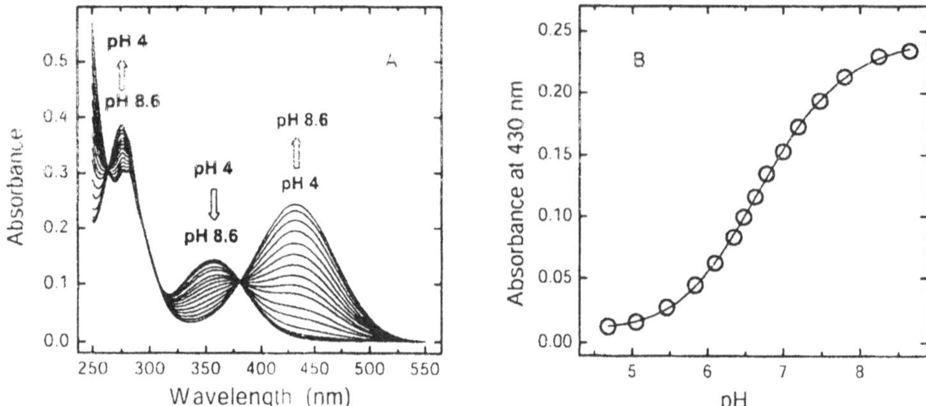

Fig. 16.9. Spectrophotometric titration of Y3NT by UV/Vis absorption spectroscopy.

of the emission spectrum of the donor with the absorption spectrum of the acceptor, on the donor quantum yield, on the inverse sixth power of the distance separating the donor and acceptor, and on their orientation. In the case of hirudin–thrombin interaction, there is an extensive overlap of the emission spectrum of the enzyme (i.e., the donor) with the absorption spectrum of the inhibitor (i.e., the acceptor). In addition, Trp-to-NT energy transfer is also favored by the relatively short distances separating Trp-residues and NT in the enzyme–inhibitor complex. To estimate the possible contribution of spectroscopic effects other than FRET (e.g, unspecific binding, dynamic or static quenching, inner filter effect), the fluorescence of thrombin was measured in the presence of increasing concentrations of free NT. The data indicate that NT slightly (~14%) reduces the fluorescence of the enzyme, in keeping with the notion that nitro-compounds (e.g., nitromethane and nitrobenzene) quench the emission of polycyclic aromatic hydrocarbons mainly by a dynamic mechanism. Moreover, we found that for concentrations of NT-containing analogs lower than 20 μM, inner filter effect can be neglected. These considerations allow us to conclude that quenching of thrombin fluorescence by Y3NT (or S2R/Y3NT) is mainly caused by Trp-to-NT energy transfer.

The quenching data reported above were used to obtain quantitative estimates (i.e., K_d values) of the binding of hirudin analogs to thrombin allosteric forms. For both analogs, the excellent fit of the experimental data to the curve describing one-site binding mechanism is a stringent, albeit indirect, proof of 1:1 binding stoichiometry. The replacement of Tyr3 with NT resulted in a drop in the affinity of Y3NT for thrombin, which was restored in the doubly substituted analog S2R/Y3NT by replacing Ser2 with Arg. The structural model of Y3NT bound to thrombin, based on the crystallographic structure of the hirudin–thrombin complex, reveals that the $-NO_2$ group of NT might be easily accommodated into the S2 specificity site of the enzyme without requiring steric distortion. Likely, the lower affinity of Y3NT reflects the lower hydrophobicity of NT at pH 8.0, where it exists by ~95% in the ionized form. With respect to this, the logP value of 2-nitrophenol, taken as a suitable model of the NT side chain, is -1.47 at pH 8.0, whereas that of phenol, taken as a model of Tyr, is +1.50. Besides hydrophobicity, the presence of the nitro-group introduces a net (i.e., at pH 8.0) negative charge at position 3 of hirudin, which can oppose binding through unfavorable electrostatic interaction with the strong negative potential of the thrombin active site, in agreement with our previous structure-activity relationship studies. The reliability of these data was verified by comparing the K_d values of Y3NT and S2R/Y3NT, obtained by FRET measurements, with those determined by classic enzyme inhibition experiments, in which the rate of thrombin-mediated substrate hydrolysis was measured as a function of inhibitor concentration. Strikingly, the K_d values for the binding of Y3NT and S2R/Y3NT to thrombin

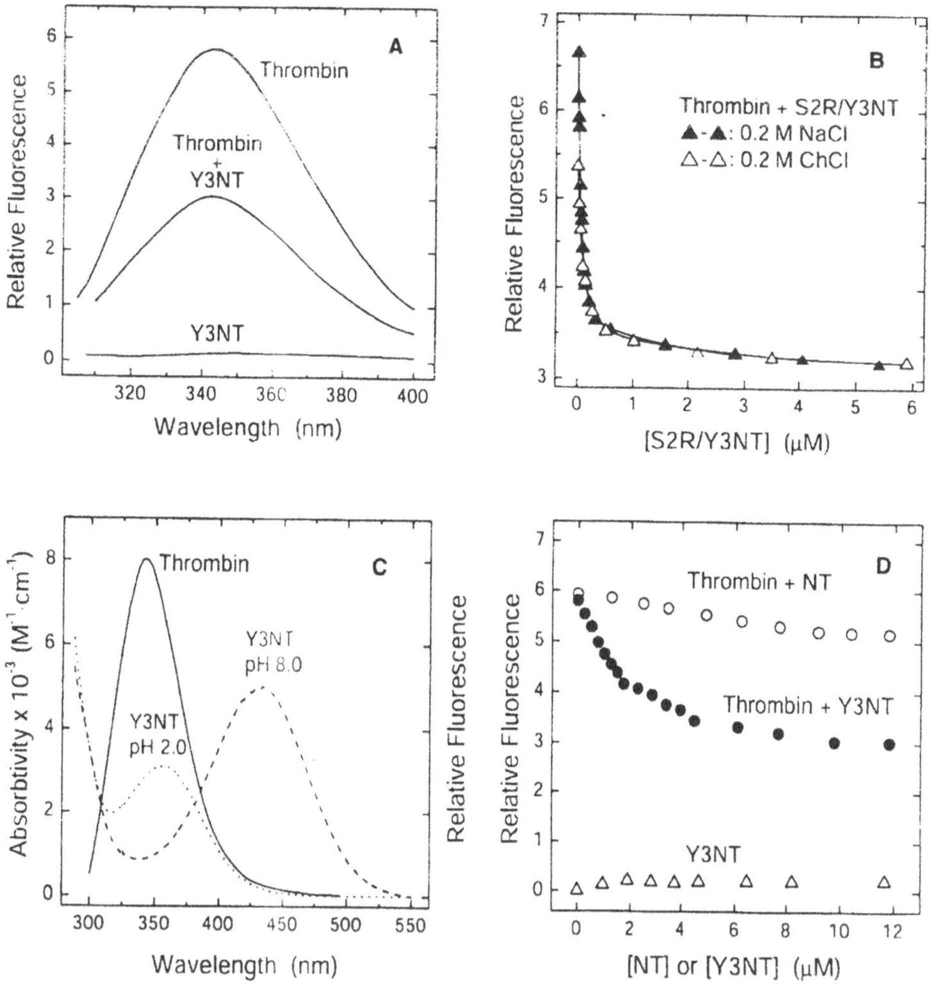

Fig. 16.10. Binding of Y3NT and S2R/Y3NT to thrombin, monitored by Trp-to-NT fluorescence energy transfer.

fast form were determined as 1.4 ± 0.1 μM and 41 ± 2 nM, respectively, in agreement (8–10%) with those obtained by FRET.

Under *fast* conditions, the 430-nm band of S2R/Y3NT, assigned to the contribution of the ionized form of NT at pH 8.0, is reduced by 54%, whereas an additional band of similar intensity appears at about 362 nm, characteristic of NT in the neutral form. Of note, the binding of Y3NT to thrombin *fast* form yields very similar results. These observations can be explained on the basis of the modeled structure of Y3NT bound to thrombin and assuming that NT interacts with the enzyme in the neutral form.

There are three structural water molecules at the enzyme–inhibitor interface (i.e., w432, w606, and w672), characterized by low thermal factors and high occupancy values, can variably interact with NT. In particular, w606, which in the structure of the wild-type hirudin–thrombin complex connects Tyr3′ of the inhibitor to Tyr60a of the enzyme, is suitably positioned as a hydrogen bond donor to stabilize the six-membered ring system of NT. As a result, the contribution of the protonated NT in the bound form appears as a distinct band at about 362 nm in the absorption spectrum of the thrombin–S2R/Y3NT complex. The residual intensity of the 430-nm band is contributed by the ionized form of

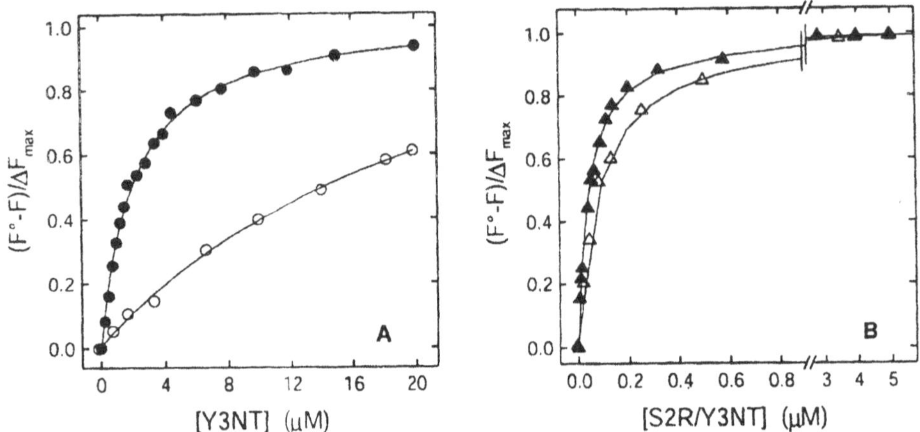

Fig. 16.11. Determination of the dissociation constant (K_d) of the complexes formed by the synthetic analogs Y3NT and S2R/Y3NT with thrombin, under fast (filled symbols) and slow (empty symbols) conditions.

NT in the free inhibitor that exists in equilibrium with the thrombin-bound form. Hence, we conclude that the phenate moiety of NT in the free state becomes protonated to phenol upon binding to thrombin and that a water molecule at the hirudin–thrombin interface, likely w606, functions as a hydrogen donor. Notably, w432 and w606 are conserved in the structure of thrombin bound to hirugen (i.e., the 53-64 peptide of hirudin), where the specificity sites of the enzyme are unoccupied, thus suggesting that these water molecules represent constant spots in the solvation shell of thrombin and, perhaps, key elements for molecular recognition, in keeping with the key role that protein–water interactions play in ligand binding.

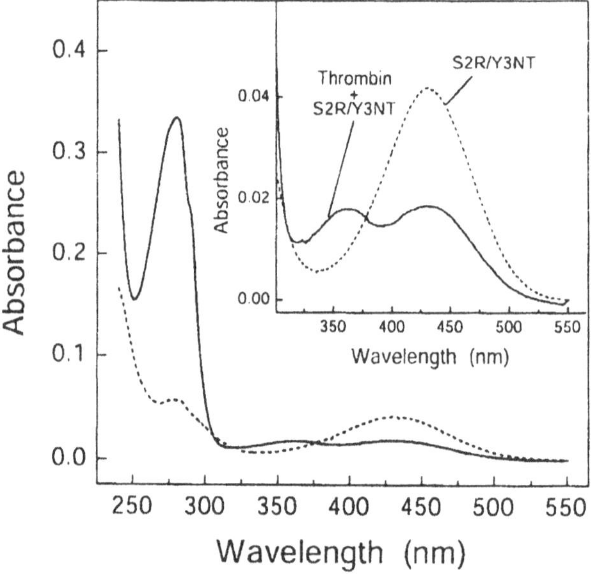

Fig. 16.12. Binding of the synthetic analog S2R/Y3NT to thrombin, monitored by UV/Vis absorption spectroscopy.

Our results demonstrate that NT is a suitable spectroscopic probe for investigating ligand-protein interactions and suggest that its incorporation into proteins may have vast applications for identifying ligand-protein interaction. It is widely accepted that even the knowledge of the structure of the ligand-receptor complex provides only partial information for predicting ligand binding energetics. In this view, we have demonstrated here that it is possible to transfer the quantitative structure-activity relationship (QSAR) approach, traditionally applied to low-molecular-weight bioactive compounds, to the study of recognition in macromolecular systems, such as the hirudin–thrombin complex. Recent advances in chemical and genetic methodologies will, hopefully, allow the researchers to extend this approach to other protein systems of relevant pharmacological application. Moreover, we have shown that incorporation of noncoded amino acids, possessing peculiar spectroscopic properties, can have great potentialities in biotechnology and pharmacological screening.

17

UNEXPECTED BENEFITS

Recombinant human erythropoietin (rHuEPO) is a purified glycoprotein produced by recombinant DNA technology. It is indistinguishable from human urinary erythropoietin in its biologic and immunologic activity. It is commercially available and has absolute indications for the treatment of the anemia associated with chronic renal failure, prematurity, and platinum-based chemotherapy. Other uses have included the anemia associated with multiple myeloma, cancer, myelodysplasia, HIV infection, and other forms of chemotherapy. It has been used to potentiate preoperative autologous blood donation. Less common uses have been in the treatment of the anemia of chronic disease, for perisurgical augmentation and after allogenic bone marrow transplantation.

Endogenous erythropoietin (EPO) is produced primarily by the peritubular capillary endothelium of the kidney in response to tissue hypoxia or anemia. EPO is a hormone that plays a crucial role in the regulation of hematopoiesis and induces the proliferation, maturation, and differentiation of erythroid (red blood cell) precursors. In renal failure, the nonfunctioning kidneys fail to produce adequate amounts of endogenous EPO to support erythropoiesis with resultant anemia. Before the introduction of exogenous erythropoietin in the 1980s, patients in renal failure required repeated blood transfusions.

After 1998 there was a significant increase in the number of cases of pure red cell aplasia (PRCA) associated with subcutaneous injections of rHuEPO in the renal dialysis population. PRCA is a relatively rare condition. It presents as a sudden onset of severe isolated anemia characterized by near-complete absence of erythroid precursors in the bone marrow. Most of the initial reports in the literature before 1998 involved isolated cases, of which 50% had no known cause. After 1998, the PRCA was shown to be related to neutralizing antibodies to erythropoietin that cross-reacted with endogenous EPO. Most of these reported antibody-mediated cases were for patients using Eprex. In total between January 1, 1989 and June 30, 2004, the company reported a total of 206 cases, of which 155 occurred in the peak years of 2001–2003. The mean time from initial exposure to onset of PRCA was 9.1 months.

The rise in cases of PRCA corresponded with the introduction of polysorbate 80 stabilized Eprex in prefilled syringes with uncoated rubber stoppers, which was administered subcutaneously. Previously human serum albumin (HSA) was used to stabilize the product, but this practice was discontinued in several countries due to fears of disease transmission by HSA. Epidemiologic and immunologic data reported by Boven et al. demonstrated that the rise in PRCA was most likely related to leachates from the uncoated stoppers in the presence of the polysorbate 80 stabilizer. These leachates may have potentiated the immunogenicity of the product when administered subcutaneously.

No cases for intravenous administration were reported. Since the introduction of coated stoppers in the prefilled syringes in April 2003 and a concomitant switch to intravenous administration in many dialysis units, the number of reported cases fell from 71 in 2003 to 2 reported cases in the first 4 months of 2004. Even at its peak, the incidence rate for PRCA was relatively low at 4.61/10,000 patient years of exposure to the product.

Erythropoietin as a Potential Growth Factor in Wound Healing

In addition to its ability to stimulate erythropoiesis, EPO enhances cell phagocytosis and reduces macrophage activation, therefore modulating the inflammatory process. These anti-inflammatory effects of EPO may be able to reverse the chronic inflammatory condition that is believed to underlie chronic skin ulcers. By interfering with the chronic inflammatory process EPO may help reduce inflammatory cytokines and degradative enzymes that interfere with many wound healing processes and limit new tissue growth. Recent literature suggests that many chronic wounds persist because of inflammatory processes that alter the wound environment. Analysis of wound fluid taken from healing and chronic wounds revealed that chronic wounds have elevated levels of inflammatory mediators and degradative enzymes that interfere with the healing process.

Healing wounds are characterized by high mitogenic potential, rapid cellular migration, balanced inflammatory cytokines, low proteases, and good cellular response to growth factors. Chronic wounds, however, are characterized by poor mitogenic potential and cell migration, high proteases and inflammatory cytokines, and senescent cells unresponsive to growth factors. EPO's effects on the wound healing process not only include restoring the normal wound environment, but it also has recently been found to interact with vascular endothelial growth factor (VEGF). Together EPO and VEGF stimulate endothelial cell mitosis and motility important in new vessel growth and wound healing. Galeano et al. demonstrated in an artificial wound model in genetically diabetic mice that erythropoietin injections increased VEGF mRNA expression, wound protein content, wound healing, and wound breaking strength.

The additional benefits of EPO are its neurotrophic and neuroprotective functions that may ameliorate neurological damage after spinal cord and brain injury. A specific EPO/EPO receptor system has been found in the central nervous system and in the cerebrospinal fluid, which is independent of the heatopoietic system.

Chronic skin ulcers experienced by patients who have low concentrations of circulating hemoglobin ($\leq$100 g/L) may be difficult to heal because of impairment in tissue oxygenation. There are various types of anemias with differing underlying causes, including nutrient deficiencies, such as iron deficiency anemia, and anemia as the result of chronic disease or chronic inflammatory processes. Iron deficiency anemia results from inadequate intake, absorption, or utilization of iron and/or acute or chronic blood loss. It is characterized by low hemoglobin and other hematological changes combined with microcytic, hypochromic red blood cells. There are low levels of stored iron as indicated by low serum ferritin values. Anemia of chronic disease (ACD) is characterized by low hemoglobin concentrations and other hematological changes with normocytic, normochromic red blood cells. In anemia of chronic disease, red blood cell production is impaired and there may be a shortened red blood cell life span. ACD is also characterized by a normal or elevated serum ferritin level.

ACD is generally not an irondeficiency anemia, and it is refractory to an iron-enhanced diet, iron replacement therapy, either oral or intravenous, and transfusion. In fact, iron supplementation and transfusion are generally contraindicated in ACD because of the risk of iatrogenic hemochromatosis. ACD occurs in individuals with a chronic inflammatory process such as arthritis, critical illness, or chronic skin ulcers. It is thought to be the result of impaired responsiveness of erythroid progenitor cells due to a persistent elevated level of circulating inflammatory cytokines that are known to occur in patients with chronic inflammatory conditions. Ferrucci et al. demonstrated in a study of inflammatory serum markers in a sample of the residents of Chianti Italy that the anemia of inflammation evolved from a pre-anemic state in which normal hemoglobin was maintained in persons with high levels of inflammatory markers by increasing levels of erythropoietin to a clinical anemia in which erythropoietin levels were suppressed possibly through the inhibitory effect of inflammation on erythropoietin production.

However, despite the numerous documented effects of EPO on cellular and physiological events known to be important in the healing process and the management of ACD, few clinical studies are investigating the use of EPO to promote the healing of chronic wounds. In 1992 Turba et al. reported the successful treatment of ACD related to stage IV pressure ulcers. In another hematological disorder, treatment with EPO resulted in the rapid and complete healing of chronic leg ulcer, further improvement in hematological parameters, and relief from chronic pain.

Clinical Experience with Recombinant Human Erythropoietin and Patients with Pressure Ulcers

Spinal cord-injured patients are at high risk of developing pressure ulcers, many of which often become associated with anemia of chronic disease. These ulcers are challenging to heal. Pressure redistribution, nutritional support, management of incontinence, and good local wound care are key components for healing these ulcers. Despite best-practice care, patients with anemia of chronic disease remain difficult to heal.

In an attempt to reverse the anemia of chronic disease, several patients in the Spinal Cord Injury rehabilitation unit at Parkwood Hospital, St. Joseph's Health Care, London, Canada, were treated with subcutaneous erythropoietin. A retrospective chart audit was conducted to review the effectiveness of 6 weeks of subcutaneous erythropoietin 75 IU/kg subcutaneously 3 times weekly in resolving refractory anemia of chronic disease and healing stage IV pressure ulcers. The mean age of the patients was 59, and all had a stage IV pressure ulcer.

All patients received pressure off-loading, nutritional assessment and supplementation, and best-practice local wound care. Comorbid conditions such as diabetes were medically managed. All patients received rHuEPO 75 IU/kg subcutaneously three times weekly for 6 weeks. Iron supple-mentation with oral ferrous gluconate as indicated by ferritin levels was administered.

Mean initial hemoglobin was 88 g/L. After 6 weeks of rHuEPO injections, the mean hemoglobin for the four patients rose to 110 g/L. The mean number of ulcers decreased from 3 to 2.3, and the mean surface area of the largest ulcer decreased from 42.3 cm^2 to 38.4 cm^2. Ulcer depth was decreased by half. The extent of undermining improved in all ulcers. Some patients showed an increased ability to fight intercurrent infections. All patients felt more energetic and were better able to participate in their rehabilitation activities. No adverse effects were observed.

The results were promising enough to suggest that a prospective study is warranted. Such a study would carefully collect all hematologic factors as well as use validated tools for determining ulcer size and appearance. In addition, collecting wound fluid before, during, and after treatment to determine the effect on chronic inflammatory mediators would be useful. Research into effects at the molecular level may be useful.

Future Research

The introduction of human recombinant erythropoietin significantly improved the quality of life for patients on real dialysis by managing the concomitant anemia, which results from end stage renal failure. It has also been successfully employed in several other conditions in which erythropoiesis is suppressed either through disease processes or as a result of treatments.

The emergence of pure red cell aplasia as a complication of treatment with subcutaneous injection in the late 1990s was probably the result of the use of prefilled syringes with uncoated rubber stoppers in which the product was stabilized with polysorbate 80. Leachates from the stoppers most likely potentiated the immunogenicity of the product leading to the production of neutralizing antibodies. Since the reformulation of the product, the incidence of PRCA has been steadily dropping.

Human recombinant erythropoietin shows promise in resolving the refractory anemia of chronic disease associated with stage IV pressure ulcers, and further study is suggested. The results may also suggest that rHuEPO acts as a growth factor either alone or in conjunction with intrinsic factors in the wound. Studies of its role at the molecular level are indicated. Further studies of the neurotrophic and neuroprotective properties observed in rat models hold promise in the area of spinal cord injury research.

INDEX